State Food Crimes

Some states deny their own citizens one of the most fundamental human rights, the right to food. Rhoda E. Howard-Hassmann, a leading scholar of human rights, discusses state food crimes, demonstrating how governments have introduced policies that cause malnutrition or starvation among their citizens and others for whom they are responsible. This book introduces the right to food and discusses historical cases (communist famines in Ukraine, China, and Cambodia, and neglect of starvation by democratic states in Ireland, Germany, and Canada). It then moves to detailed discussion of four contemporary cases: starvation in North Korea and malnutrition in Zimbabwe, Venezuela, and the West Bank and Gaza. These cases are then used to analyze international human rights law, sanctions and food aid, and civil and political rights as they pertain to the right to food. The book concludes by considering the need for a new international treaty on the right to food.

RHODA E. HOWARD-HASSMANN held the position of Canada Research Chair in International Human Rights at Wilfrid Laurier University from 2003 to 2016. Since 1993 she has been a Fellow of the Royal Society of Canada, which awarded her the John William Dawson Medal for Interdisciplinary Research in 2013. She was named a Distinguished Scholar of Human Rights by the Human Rights Sections of the International Studies Association and the American Political Science Association in 2013 and 2006, respectively. Earlier books include *Can Globalization Promote Human Rights?* (2010), *Reparations to Africa* (2008), *Compassionate Canadians: Civic Leaders Discuss Human Rights* (2003), and *Human Rights and the Search for Community* (1995).

State Food Crimes

Rhoda E. Howard-Hassmann
Wilfrid Laurier University, Canada

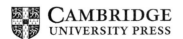
CAMBRIDGE
UNIVERSITY PRESS

CAMBRIDGE
UNIVERSITY PRESS

University Printing House, Cambridge CB2 8BS, United Kingdom

Cambridge University Press is part of the University of Cambridge.

It furthers the University's mission by disseminating knowledge in the pursuit of education, learning, and research at the highest international levels of excellence.

www.cambridge.org
Information on this title: www.cambridge.org/9781107133525

© Rhoda E. Howard-Hassmann 2016

First published 2016

Printed in the United Kingdom by Clays, St Ives plc

A catalogue record for this publication is available from the British Library

ISBN 978-1-107-13352-5 Hardback
ISBN 978-1-107-58996-4 Paperback

In memoriam

PETER BAEHR

1935–2010

beloved colleague, friend, and "older brother"

who survived the hunger winter of 1944–45

and much more

Contents

Part III Implications for the International Human Right to Food

Contents

Acknowledgments

Many colleagues and friends read parts of this manuscript and provided valuable comments for its improvement. Judith Adam, Michal Baer, Alan Dowty, Neve Gordon, Louis Greenspan, Alan and Sara Mendelson, and Raz Segal commented on earlier versions of chapter 7 on the West Bank and Gaza: Alexander Catta, Javier Corrales, Kathryn Hochstetler, Ken Jackson, Francisco López-Bermudez, and Antulio Rosales offered comments on earlier versions of chapter 6 on Venezuela; and Abel Chicanda, Oliver Masakure, Edward Shizha, and Alan Whiteside offered comments on earlier versions of chapter 5 on Zimbabwe. Mark Gibney kindly read a draft of chapter 8. Special thanks to Yehonatan Alsheh, Post-Doctoral Fellow at the Balsillie School of International Affairs from late 2013 to mid-2015, for many conversations and excellent intellectual advice about the West Bank and Gaza as well as about the book as a whole. Others who offered comments were Ann Elizabeth Mayer, John Siebert, Alyssa Cundy, and Laura Ludwin, as well as colleagues too numerous to name who listened to my various presentations of parts of this project over the last five years. I am grateful to all of them for their time and their valuable advice. My apologies to anyone I might have inadvertently omitted from this list.

I am also most grateful to the research assistants who helped me with this project; namely, Elizabeth Baisley, Andrew Basso, David Clement, Matthew Overall, Jinelle Piereder, Rina Patel, Antulio Rosales, Leah Samson, and Kwang-Sheng Wen. Thanks as always to the Canada Research Chairs Program, which since 2003 has been funding my research and providing the release time from teaching necessary for writing, and to Wilfrid Laurier University for nominating me for my chair. Wendy Webb, Administrative Assistant to the Chair until 2012, and Mayura Stratopoulos, Administrative Assistant from 2012 to 2015, were also extremely helpful, efficient, and devoted to this project.

I thank the editors and reviewers of the following journals in which articles on which I have drawn for this book were published: "The Right to Food under Hugo Chavez," *Human Rights Quarterly*, vol. 37, no. 4,

2015; "North Korea: A Case for a New International Treaty on the Right to Food," *Asia-Pacific Journal on Human Rights and the Law*, vol. 15, nos. 1&2, 2015, pp. 31–50; "State-Induced Famine and Penal Starvation in North Korea," *Genocide Studies and Prevention*, vol. 7, nos. 2/3, 2012, pp. 147–65; "Faminogenesis: State Policies that Undermine the Right to Food (A Lecture in Memory of Peter Baehr)," *Netherlands Quarterly of Human Rights*, vol. 29, no. 4, 2011, pp. 560–77; and "Mugabe's Zimbabwe 2000–2009: Massive Human Rights Violations and the Failure to Protect," *Human Rights Quarterly*, vol. 32, no. 4, 2010, pp. 898–920. I am also grateful to the two reviewers of this manuscript for their very helpful comments on two drafts.

Special thanks to Susan Dicklitch for suggesting the title to this book and to David Marcus, whose brilliant 2003 article started me thinking about state food crimes.

As usual my husband, Peter McCabe, suffered graciously through this entire project. I am, as always, deeply in his intellectual and personal debt.

Part I

Introduction and Background

1   State Food Crimes

This book discusses state food crimes; that is, crimes by states that deny their own citizens and others for whom they are directly responsible one of their most fundamental human rights, the right to food. The worst type of deprivation of food is famine. Not only are famines not pure natural disasters, they are often consequences of national policy decisions that benefit political elites at the expense of the populations whose well-being is entrusted to them. As de Waal argues, "The occurrence of famine is an indictment of the ethics of the country in which it has occurred" (de Waal 1991, 77). Through the use of four late twentieth and early twenty-first century case studies described in Part II, this book demonstrates that some states – or political elites in those states – deliberately deprive their citizens of food while others neglect to ensure that their citizens, or others for whom they are responsible, have adequate nutrition. The four cases are North Korea in the 1990s and twenty-first century; Zimbabwe since 2000; Venezuela since 1999; and the West Bank and Gaza (WBG) in the 1990s and twenty-first century. The factual descriptions of food policies in these countries end as of April 2015.

I draw these four cases from different areas of the world and different political systems. North Korea, an Asian country, was a pseudo-Communist dynastic regime. Zimbabwe in the 2000s became an authoritarian regime ruled by a small clique of family and allies surrounding President Robert Mugabe. Venezuela was ruled from 1999 to 2013 by an increasingly authoritarian populist, Hugo Chávez, succeeded by Nicolás Maduro, who intensified Chávez's policies. Israel, internally a democracy, was an occupying power in the West Bank and exercised effective control over Gaza.

Many countries in which famine exists are at war. I have deliberately chosen three cases – North Korea, Zimbabwe, and Venezuela – in which war is not a complicating variable. In the case of WBG, the Gaza War of 2009 is one reason why Palestinians suffered malnutrition, but the main reason for malnutrition in the West Bank was colonialism. I have also chosen states with functioning (however corrupt or malevolent)

3

governments, rather than failed states: thus, for example, I have chosen Zimbabwe over Somalia.

I chose these cases to illustrate different degrees of abuse of the right to food and different political and economic mechanisms that resulted in its abuse. I do not suggest that the cases are comparable in the severity of abuse of this right. North Korea is by far the worst case, followed by Zimbabwe. In Venezuela, food shortages caused by government policy had not, by 2015, resulted in massive malnutrition, as in Zimbabwe, or starvation, as in North Korea. In WBG, conflict and colonialism had contributed to widespread malnutrition, but not starvation. Thus, the state food crimes I discuss are of different levels of severity and caused by different economic and political policies.

I refer to state "crimes" in both the legal and moral senses. Legally, state food crimes fall under various aspects of international law, the most explicit of which is as a crime against humanity. Under the Rome Statute of the International Criminal Court (ICC), the crime of extermination includes deprivation of access to food (International Criminal Court 1998, Article 7,2, b). Deprivation of food is also a war crime under the Geneva Conventions, discussed in Chapter 8. Not all of what I consider to be state food crime is so under international law, however; thus, one of my aims is to persuade readers that there should be a broader interpretation of state food crimes than currently exists. (A similar, but not identical, argument was made by Jappah and Smith in 2012 in an article on what they called "state sponsored famine," but with less specific reference to current international law (Jappah and Smith 2012).)

Whatever international law and humanitarian practice may currently be, these four cases also highlight the central importance of civil and political rights and the rule of law to protection of the "economic" human right to food. In all four cases, rule of law either does not exist or, in the case of WBG, does not apply to the population enduring malnutrition. Similarly, as I show in Chapter 10, in all four cases either the population never enjoyed civil and political rights, or those rights were progressively undermined at the same time as food became scarcer. In some or all of the four cases, citizenship rights, mobility rights, property rights, and the right to work were also undermined; these rights are not as thoroughly examined in the literature on famine as are rights to vote or to press freedom. In the end, as I show in Chapter 11 on liberal democracy, it is internal human rights, not external law and practice, that protect citizens against state food crimes. Nevertheless, as I argue in Chapter 12, a new international treaty on the right to food might have some value in protecting citizens against rulers who create the conditions for famine or serious malnutrition.

The Rights to Adequate Food and Freedom from Hunger

I use the term "right to food" as shorthand for the rights to adequate food and freedom from hunger. The most basic document of the international law of human rights is the 1948 Universal Declaration of Human Rights (UDHR). Article 25,1 of the UDHR states that "Everyone has the right to a standard of living adequate for the health and well-being of himself and of his family, including food." This reflects the famous speech by US President Franklin Delano Roosevelt in 1941, proclaiming his "Four Freedoms," one of which was freedom from want (excerpted in Howard-Hassmann and Welch 2006, 211). The UDHR was followed by two international Covenants that codified its ideals into international law; namely, the 1976 International Covenant on Civil and Political Rights (ICCPR) and the 1976 International Covenant on Economic, Social and Cultural Rights (ICESCR). The ICESCR includes the rights to adequate food (Article 11,1) and freedom from hunger (Article 11,2). Scholars usually separate these two rights, noting that freedom from hunger is more urgent than the right to adequate food. Nevertheless, freedom from hunger is a minimalist approach to the human right to food, implying that a "minimum daily nutritional intake" is sufficient to fulfill it, rather than that both the quality and quantity of food should be such as to allow the individual to lead a productive life fitting with the principle of human dignity (Alston 1984, 167).

Article 1,2 of both the ICCPR and the ICESCR includes the sentence "In no case may a people be deprived of its own means of subsistence." This implies an international dimension to the right to food, suggesting that "a people" may not be deprived by outsiders of its means of subsistence, as I will argue was a consequence of Israeli policies in WBG. The meaning of "a people" is fluid, however, and might also refer to a minority group within a state, or indeed to the entire population, if the state imposes measures depriving it of its own means of subsistence, as occurred in both North Korea and Zimbabwe, as well as increasingly in Venezuela.

Article 2,1 of the ICESCR mandates that each state party to the Covenant (that is, each state that signs and ratifies the Covenant) is obliged to take steps "to the *maximum of its available resources*, with a view to achieving *progressively* the full realization of the rights recognized" in the ICESCR (my italics). This clause is usually interpreted to mean that developing states are not expected to fulfill all human rights immediately, but that they should do so progressively as the resources become available. However, the four cases I discuss in Part II are not instances in which developing states cannot provide enough food because they do not have the resources to do so. Rather, they are instances in which states deprive their citizens or those under their jurisdiction either directly of food or indirectly of the capacity to cultivate their own food; that is, they remove from the targeted populations resources that had been previously available.

Henry Shue argued in 1980 that for every basic right, states had three duties: to avoid depriving people of the right, to protect them from deprivation by others, and to aid those who were deprived of the right (Shue 1980, 52). This prescription has evolved into the idea that state responsibilities are first to respect human rights, second to protect them, and last to fulfill them. Fulfillment can be further divided into two steps: facilitating citizens' capacity to provide for themselves and actually providing the content of the right if citizens cannot do so (Eide 2006, 175). Regarding the rights to adequate food and freedom from hunger, this means that the state is obliged to protect access to food that already exists, prevent any undermining of this access, and fulfill the need for food when citizens cannot do so themselves, either by facilitating access to food, for example, by assisting farmers with fertilizer subsidies, or by directly providing food (or the means to purchase it) to citizens.

Food is a fundamental human biological need. Indeed, Alston notes that "the right to freedom from hunger is the only human right which the framers of the two international Human Rights Covenants specifically termed 'fundamental'" (Alston 1984, 162). Similarly, Shue argues that food is an aspect of minimal economic security. For Shue, food is a basic right: "Basic rights are the morality of the depths. They specify the line beneath which no one is to be allowed to sink." Basic rights, he maintains, must include "the provision of subsistence at least to those who cannot provide for themselves" (Shue 1980, 18, 24).

These opinions reflect a common-sense view that biological needs take priority over less biologically necessary wants or desires. If, for example, one were to ask people "What is it you cannot do without?" one would assume that the answer would be rooted in material needs (Felice 1996, 21), one of the most fundamental of which would be food. But contemporary interpretation of human rights stresses more than material needs; it stresses the need for human dignity. The starting point in understanding what are the core human rights that all individuals need lies, according to Beetham, "in identifying the grounds on which all humans deserve equal respect, or merit treating with equal dignity" (Beetham 1995, 46).

The preface to the UDHR states that "recognition of the inherent dignity and of the equal and inalienable rights of all members of the human family is the foundation of freedom, justice and peace in the world."

The rights to food and freedom from hunger are absolutely essential to human dignity. One essential aspect of human dignity is a sense of autonomy, a sense that an individual is in control of her life, yet a starving individual is incapable of enjoying or exercising any of her rights as an autonomous human being. The rights to adequate food and freedom from hunger are also essential to the wider meaning of human dignity, in which a dignified individual is one who enjoys other's concern and respect and who can participate in the community (Howard 1995, 16–17). Thus, the right to food has a much wider meaning than simply fulfillment of elementary biological need. A starving individual is preoccupied by her own hunger, too weak to take care of herself and family members, and certainly too weak to participate in any collective decision-making. Indeed, "individuals who do not know when (or even if) their next meal is coming are . . . reduced to a subhuman existence. There simply is no human dignity in suffering from starvation or malnutrition" (Carey et al. 2010, 91). By contrast, the properly fed individual, free from hunger and inadequate nutrition, is more likely to feel competent, empowered, and able in normal times to care for herself and her family and to participate in the wider community and polity.

In general, then, the right to food demonstrates the indivisibility and interdependence of civil and political and economic, social, and cultural human rights, as proclaimed at the 1993 United Nations' Vienna Conference on Human Rights; "All human rights are universal, indivisible and interdependent and interrelated" (United Nations 1993, Article 5). That is, to satisfy their economic human right to food, people also need to enjoy their civil and political human rights. An authoritarian government could keep its people alive, suggests Kent, merely by feeding everyone "prepackaged rations or capsules," but this would mean that people would have "no chance to influence what and how they are fed." It would also be undignified to be fed in such a manner rather than having the opportunity to provide for oneself (Kent 2009, 228).

The ICCPR and the ICESCR were followed by many other conventions, covenants, and declarations, some of which deal directly with the rights to adequate food and freedom from hunger. Indeed, the right to food is scattered all over international human rights law (Niada 2006–07), and many United Nations documents refer to it (Apodaca 2014): here I discuss only a few documents most relevant to state food crimes. The Universal Declaration on the Eradication of Hunger and Malnutrition was adopted by the World Food Conference and endorsed by the United Nations General Assembly (UNGA) in 1974 (World Food Conference 1974, December 17). This Declaration does not attribute any responsibility to states for depriving individuals of the right to food.

Rather, it refers to the histories of colonialism and apartheid and to the market economy as causes of food deprivation, insisting on the principle of non-interference in the domestic affairs of states and respect for national sovereignty and independence (World Food Conference 1974, December 17, articles c, d, and h). Such non-interference implies that under the principle of sovereignty states enjoy the legal right to deprive their own citizens of food; thus, when the Khmer Rouge took power in Cambodia only a year after the World Food Conference, there was no mechanism in the Declaration to penalize or even denounce it for starving its own people.

In 1996, a World Food Summit resulted in a request to the United Nations Committee on Economic, Social, and Cultural Rights (CESCR) to interpret the right to food: the CESCR complied by issuing General Comment 12 in 1999. According to this Comment, the "core content of the right to adequate food implies: The availability of food in a quantity and quality sufficient to satisfy the dietary needs of individuals, free from adverse substances, and acceptable within a given culture; [and] The accessibility of such food in ways that are sustainable and that do not interfere with the enjoyment of other human rights" (Committee on Economic Social and Cultural Rights 1999, Article 8). Referring to the consensus that human dignity is the basis of human rights, General Comment 12 also "affirms that the right to adequate food is indivisibly linked to the inherent dignity of the human person" (Committee on Economic Social and Cultural Rights 1999, Article 4). Perhaps in oblique reference to events since 1974, including mass starvation in Cambodia in the 1970s and North Korea in the 1990s, the General Comment also refers to "the use of food as a political weapon." It notes that "Violations of the right to food can occur through the direct action of States" (Committee on Economic Social and Cultural Rights 1999, Articles 5 and 19).

In 2004, voluntary guidelines on food security were drafted and adopted by the Food and Agriculture Organization (FAO) (Windfuhr 2010, 138). These guidelines are modeled on the content of General Comment 12, and note the importance of civil and political rights to the economic human right to food. However, all these guidelines are still voluntary; there is no obligatory code of conduct for states to follow regarding food (Kent 2005a, 58). Guideline 1.2 focuses on democracy, good governance, human rights, and the rule of law and specifically mentions the human rights to freedom of opinion, expression, information, press, and assembly/association as key to the right to food. It further states that "Food should not be used as a tool for political and economic pressure" (Food and Agriculture Organization 2005, 9).

Without referring to the human right to own property mentioned in Article 17 of the UDHR, which I will argue in Chapter 10 is essential to the right to food, the FAO guidelines also mandate in Article 8,1 that "states should . . . protect the assets that are important for people's livelihoods," especially "the rights of individuals with respect to resources such as land, water, forests, fisheries, and livestock" (Food and Agriculture Organization 2005, p. 16). In mentioning the importance of access to assets, the guidelines reflect Amartya Sen's thesis, discussed below, that deficits in asset entitlements are key causes of famines. States are also advised to ensure that humanitarian agencies have "safe and unimpeded access to the[ir] populations," a rule both North Korea and Zimbabwe violated (Food and Agriculture Organization 2005, Guideline 15.3, p. 27).

The FAO guidelines also refer to international obligations to protect the right to food, particularly relevant in this volume to WBG. Quoting from the pre-existing and obligatory 1949 Geneva Conventions, the guidelines state that in the event of war "it is prohibited to attack, destroy, remove or render useless objects indispensable to the survival of the civilian population, such as foodstuffs, agricultural areas for the production of foodstuffs, crops [and] livestock" (Food and Agriculture Organization 2005, Guideline 16.2, p. 28). In situations of occupation, moreover, the occupying power must ensure that the civilian population has the food it needs, even if that means importing food (Food and Agriculture Organization 2005, Guideline 16.3, p. 28). Outside of situations of international warfare, the guidelines suggest international responsibility to protect the right to food, grounding this in the principle that "developed countries should assist developing countries in attaining development goals" (Food and Agriculture Organization 2005, III, Article 4, p. 33).

Related to the human rights to adequate food and freedom from hunger is a developing right to water, again pertinent in this volume to WBG. This right is not mentioned in the UDHR or the ICESCR, but in the twenty-first century various United Nations agencies were involved in proposing it. In so doing they referred especially to the right to "an adequate standard of living" mentioned in Article 11,1 of the ICESCR, and the right to the "highest attainable standard of physical . . . health" mentioned in Article 12,1.

The right to water is most clearly elaborated in General Comment 15 of the CESCR, which states that "The human right to water is indispensable for leading a life in human dignity. It is a prerequisite for the realization of other human rights" (Committee on Economic Social and Cultural Rights 2002, para. 1). The General Comment also refers to Article 14,2, h of the Convention on the Elimination of All Forms of

Discrimination against Women, which stipulates that women must "enjoy adequate living conditions, particularly in relation to . . . water supply," and to Article 24,2, c of the Convention on the Rights of the Child, which requires states to provide clean drinking water for children (Committee on Economic Social and Cultural Rights 2002, para. 4).

General Comment 15 notes a core obligation of states to "ensure access to the minimum essential amount of water . . . on a non-discriminatory basis" and refers to the World Health Organization's (WHO) minimum standard of 20 liters of water per capita per day to ensure basic food and personal hygiene needs (World Health Organization 2013) (Committee on Economic Social and Cultural Rights 2002, para. 37, a and b, and fn.1); this does not, however, take account of agricultural needs. WHO's recommended daily amount of water for all needs is 100 liters per day (Howard and Bartram 2003, Table S1). General Comment 15 became the basis for resolutions on the right to water in the UNGA in 2010 (United Nations General Assembly 2010, August 3) and in the Human Rights Council that same year (Human Rights Council 2010, September 24).

Thus, although as of 2015 there was not yet an elaborated international law or covenant dealing only with the right to food (including the right to water), there were various documents that delineated states' responsibilities above and beyond the clauses in the UDHR and ICESCR. However, as Weissbrodt and de la Vega note, provisions for the right to food "are not so much a subject for lawyers and courts . . . Instead, the right to food is largely implemented by programs run by agronomists, biologists, doctors, engineers, farmers, managers, trade experts, and other technicians" (Weissbrodt and de la Vega 2007, 145). Yet the right to food ought to be a matter for lawyers and courts when states deliberately deprive their citizens or others for whom they are responsible of food. Individuals can be punished for egregious violations of civil and political rights such as genocide and crimes against humanity; they should also be punishable for what Jean Ziegler, the former United Nations Special Rapporteur on the Right to Food, calls "the daily massacre of hunger," noting that this hunger "is not a question of fate: it is the result of human decisions" (Jean Ziegler, "Foreword" in Kent 2005a, xv).

Civil/Political and Economic Human Rights

As the reference above to the two 1976 Covenants that succeeded the UDHR suggests, for some time there was an unfortunate split between advocacy of civil and political human rights and advocacy of economic, social, and cultural human rights. In the eyes of some "non-Western" and/or socialist critics, civil and political rights were merely a "Western construct with limited applicability," as two leftist American critics put it (Pollis and Schwab 1980). Some leaders of newly independent countries experimented with political systems in which civil and political rights were subordinated to what was then seen as an imperative to develop. For example, Julius Nyerere, the first president of independent Tanzania, said in 1969: "What freedom has our subsistence farmer? He scratches a bare living from the soil provided the rains do not fail; his children work at his side without schooling, medical care, or even good feeding . . . Only as his poverty is reduced will his existing political freedom become properly meaningful and his right to human dignity become a fact of human dignity" (quoted in Howard 1983, 467).

However, while Nyerere might honestly have believed that civil and political rights could be left in abeyance until economic human rights were achieved, his own policies proved him wrong. Between 1973 and 1976 he attempted a policy called "villagization," moving about five million peasants who had hitherto been scattered across the countryside into centralized villages where they had access to schools, clinics, and other services. This villagization was conducted without consultation with the peasants concerned, often in an arbitrary, if not brutal, fashion (Scott 1998, 223–61). Food production in Tanzania consequently declined, as peasants did not know how to cultivate in their new locations and did not have the resources to do so. Among many other problems, they were moved from lands that had water to lands that did not; they were moved to areas where the soil was unsuitable for the crops they were supposed to cultivate; and they were forced to live in villages rather than live close to their crops so that they could keep an eye on pests (Scott 1998, 246). Nor could they protest against their arbitrary removals from their original homesteads, as freedom of speech, assembly, and the press were significantly curtailed in Tanzania's one-party state (Howard 1986, 119–50).

By the early twenty-first century, it was clear that arguments such as Nyerere's that there was insufficient attention to the right to food as compared to civil and political rights were disingenuous. So also were arguments by non-Western leaders accusing Westerners who criticized their food policies of harboring colonialist or imperialist motives. Among the cases that are the focus of this book, Venezuela had been independent since 1811, North Korea since 1948, and Zimbabwe since 1980. Food policies in all three countries were of the governments' own making; comments by outsiders on their abuse of their citizens' rights attest to universal moral concerns, not to attempts to reassert colonial control.

In the past, some observers also criticized international non-governmental organizations (NGOs) for neglect of economic human rights such as the right to food, but such criticisms are no longer valid. Amnesty International (AI) changed its mission in 2001 to include concern with all the rights listed in the UDHR and adopted a particular focus on poverty (Khan 2009, 119, 121). Another major organization, Human Rights Watch (HRW) decided that it could not focus on all failures to fulfill economic human rights but could report on specific violations particularly if they were consequences of arbitrary or discriminatory judgments by states (Roth 2004, 69). Both AI and HRW have produced many reports relevant to the state food crimes with which this book is concerned.

The criticism that "Western" human rights scholars and practitioners neglect economic, social, and cultural human rights is also unfair because however much we might wish that similar policies might be used to ensure, for example, both the civil human right to be protected from torture and the economic human right to adequate nutrition, in practice the former is much more amenable to narrow policy objectives and formal laws than the latter. This is not to promote a distinction between "negative" rights that supposedly require no action by the state other than forbearance and "positive" rights than require action and resources. The state must devote resources to train police to ensure that they do not torture citizens, but it is still much more difficult to fulfill the right to adequate food than the right to protection against torture. For the state to provide food requires many material resources and many different types of policy interventions.

On the other hand, the state's obligation to protect access to food is partly a "negative" right; it requires that the state not prevent its citizens or others under its control from accessing food that is otherwise available to them: "It may well be that the state can avoid hunger better by being passive, by *not* interfering with the freedom of the individuals and with their control over their own resources" (Eide 1989, 38, italics in original). Some of the worst historical famines were caused by states' attacks on populations that previously had enjoyed adequate food, rather than states' inability to provide food to those who did not have access to it, as I will show in Chapter 2.

Above all, civil and political rights and economic rights such as the right to food are linked. The "full-belly thesis": that is, the belief that civil and political rights are irrelevant until an individual's belly is full, ignores the complexity of how access to food is protected or provided

(Howard 1983). As all four cases in Part II show, without civil and political rights citizens cannot protest policies that deprive them of food.

Food Security

By contrast to the concept of human rights, the concept of human security is relatively new, introduced into international discussion in the 1990s as a response to new (or more generalized) "downside risks" that could affect everyone (Howard-Hassmann 2012a). The United Nations Development Programme (UNDP) defined human security as both "safety from such chronic threats as hunger, disease and repression" and "protection from sudden and hurtful disruptions in the patterns of daily life" (United Nations Development Programme 1994, 23). Although the actual term, "human security," was first used by the UNDP in 1994, its origins can be traced to earlier UN commissions on the environment, development, and global governance (Oberleitner 2005, 185).

In 1974, the World Food Summit defined food security as the "availability at all times of adequate world food supplies of basic foodstuffs to sustain a steady expansion of food consumption and to offset fluctuations in production and prices" (Patel 2009, 664). This definition reflects concern at the time that there was simply not enough food in the world for everyone (Patel 2009, 664). Since then, the consensus has been that there is enough food, but that the problem is one of distribution. By 2001, the FAO definition had changed to focus on quality as well as quantity of food: "Food security [is] a situation that exists when all people, at all times, have physical, social and economic access to sufficient, safe and nutritious food that meets their dietary needs and food preferences for an active and healthy life" (Patel 2009, 664).

The human right to food is concerned with whether individuals have immediate access to the food they need; the concept of food security, however, requires analysis not only of whether people have access to sufficient food in the short run but also whether they can enjoy enough food in the long run. Both the human right to food and food security were extremely problematic in North Korea and Zimbabwe during the periods under study in this book. Individuals had no recourse against the state or its agents when they were malnourished or starving as a result of state policy; thus, their human right to food was violated. In both countries, moreover, the state disregarded long-run food security, persisting with agricultural and market policies that drastically reduced the amount of food that might otherwise have been produced. By contrast, in Venezuela, the short-run human right to food of some sectors of the population was fulfilled, but at the expense of the long-run food security of the entire population. In WBG, food security was constantly undermined by war, occupation, military rule, and corruption of local leaders.

Food security overlaps with, but is certainly not identical to, a newer term introduced by the international peasant movement Via Campesina, namely, food sovereignty. The underlying principle of food sovereignty is that distinct geographical areas (countries, regions) should be "sovereign" over their food both in the sense that the peoples of the area should decide how food is produced and distributed and that they should be (relatively) self-sufficient in food, not subjected to the vagaries of the world food market. Food sovereignty has many different definitions, but a minimal one is "the right of peoples and sovereign states to democratically determine their own agricultural and food policies," as opposed to being dependent on the international food market (Haugen 2009, 264). Many, although not all, aims of the food sovereignty movement are already subsumed under the international human right to food. Moreover, the food sovereignty moment focuses more on the international level, whereas this book is concerned mostly with the level of the state (Haugen 2009, 284). Thus, it is more in keeping with this book's focus to refer to the human right to food and food security, rather than to food sovereignty.

The concept of human security intersects with the principle of the Responsibility to Protect (R2P). According to R2P, international intervention is permissible when states fail to protect their citizens from large-scale loss of life that, *inter alia*, is a product of deliberate state action, neglect by the state, or inability of the state to act (International Commission on Intervention and State Sovereignty 2001, xii). If such principles actually inspired action, then it would seem that international humanitarian intervention should occur against any regime that either deliberately or by neglect deprives its citizens of food, thus endangering their lives. Yet as Chapter 9 will show, such intervention is subject to many obstacles.

Famine

In this book, I am concerned principally with crimes of commission: that is, crimes by states that actively deprive citizens of the food to which they previously had access. The principal form of such crime is state-induced famine, as in North Korea and Zimbabwe: these two countries directly violated Article 11,2 of the ICESCR, mandating that everyone has the right to freedom from hunger. Creation of malnutrition, a violation of Article 11,1 of the ICESCR mandating that everyone has the right to adequate food is a lesser, but still very serious, crime, in the moral if not in the legal sense. Food shortages in Venezuela and malnutrition in the WBG suggest violations of this right.

Amartya Sen defines famine as a "particularly virulent manifestation [of starvation] causing widespread death" (Sen 1981, 40). Famine, he argues, is not necessarily an outcome of starvation, but occurs principally as a result of the "*sudden collapse* of the level of food consumption," often as a consequence of market failures (Sen 1981, 41, italics in original). Similarly, Ó Gráda defines famine as "a shortage of food or purchasing power that leads directly to excess mortality from starvation or hunger-related diseases" (Ó Gráda 2009, 4). Thus both scholars note that famine can occur even when there is no shortage of food, if there is a shortage of the ability to purchase it.

According to Ó Gráda, common symptoms of famine include "rising prices [of food], food riots, an increase in crimes against property, a significant number of actual or imminent deaths from starvation, a rise in temporary migration, and frequently the fear and emergence of famine-induced infectious diseases" (Ó Gráda 2009, 7). These symptoms confirm Rangasami's view that famine is "a process during which pressure or force (economic, military, political, social, psychological) is exerted upon the victim community, gradually increasing in intensity until the stricken are deprived of all assets including the ability to labour." Rangasami maintains that famine is comprised of three stages: dearth, famishment, and morbidity (Rangasami 1985, 1749). If there is a dearth of food created by state policy, famishment may occur and mortality rise; we do not have to wait until widespread death occurs to identify the process of famine. In many cases, as in Zimbabwe, mass disease precedes or coincides with mass death. This is an indication of the process of famishment caused by a dearth of food, even if widespread death from starvation has not (yet) occurred. Thus, famine is as much a process as an event (Howe 2002, 21).

Sen's 1981 volume critiqued the then prevalent Food Availability Decline (FAD) approach to famine. FAD assumed that famines resulted from dramatic drops in the food supply, whereas Sen showed that famines could occur when there was a very mild drop – or indeed no drop at all – in supply. Rather, the cause of famine is rooted in what Sen called entitlement deficits. Entitlement refers to "the ability of people to command food through the legal means available in the society, including the use of production possibilities, trade opportunities, entitlements *vis-à-vis* the state, and other methods of acquiring food" (Sen 1981, 45). Deficits occur when citizens cannot use their direct entitlements to food grown on land they cultivate or their indirect entitlements to income with which they can purchase food or other goods that they can trade for food.

Sen showed, for example, how the war-inflated economy in the Indian state of Bengal in 1943 meant that landless groups such as agricultural laborers, fishermen, and artisans no longer had enough purchasing power to buy the food they needed (Sen 1981, 52–85). Similarly, pastoralists in Ethiopia during the 1973–74 famine could not sell their cattle at high enough prices to buy food, while agricultural laborers were left without jobs or income as the agricultural economy declined, causing them to migrate in search of food (Sen 1981, 86–112).

Sen's approach to the economics of famine is now accepted in its broad outlines: scholars no longer dispute that famines can occur even when there is no significant drop in the food supply, nor do they dispute that some sectors of the population suffer more than others when famine occurs. Some criticize specific aspects of Sen's theory; for example, that he emphasizes legal holding and transfers of assets but ignores the illegal transfers that often accompany famine (Sohlberg 2006, 362; Ravallion 1997, 1210). For example, the illegal informal market in North Korea was a significant source of food and income in the twenty-first century.

A more relevant comment for the present work is that Sen overlooks political famine; that is, famines that result from state policy. Sen deals mainly with entitlement failures caused by market conditions. By contrast, Stephen Devereux argues, "Contemporary famines are either caused deliberately (acts of commission) or they are not prevented when they could and should have been (acts of omission). Many recent famines are associated with catastrophic governance failures or collapses of the social order" (Devereux 2007a, 1). Devereux argues further that "Sen's characterization of famine as 'entitlement failure' excludes intentionality as a possible causal trigger, and ignores the reality that famine produces beneficiaries as well as victims" (Devereux 2007b, 80). Indeed, Devereux goes so far as to claim that "All contemporary famines are fundamentally political" (Devereux 2007a, 23). States lack either or both of political capacity or political will to prevent famine, undermining necessary democratic accountability and an "anti-famine contract" between governments and citizens (Devereux 2007a, 10).

Howe argues that the political roots of famine can be found in what he calls "priority regimes." Priority regimes are "the set of concerns that are privileged in the decision-making and actions of institutions and individuals." "Priority regimes that affect the famine process are often not formed around the specific topic of famine;" rather, "policies that create vulnerability to famine have their origins in other objectives." Famine can be a by-product of other priorities: It can be a trade-off, when the possibility of famine is accepted as a trade for realization of other policy goals, or it can be seen as a necessary means to another policy end.

Alternatively, famine can merely be a result of neglect, without malicious intent, as when a government fails to invest in marginalized areas (Howe 2007, 342–46).

The focus of the present volume is state food crimes and how they can be prevented and/or punished. This approach differs substantially from Sen's: it puts political conditions first and foremost, arguing that an important and often overlooked cause of famine is decisions taken by states, or more properly by the elites that govern them. Its focus is also different from that of Devereux, who mentions in passing what he calls "malevolent" policies (Devereux 2007a, 10) but concentrates mostly on political decisions that are meant to be benevolent or neutral yet can generate famine. This book investigates states' direct responsibilities for famines and for deprivation of food, leading to starvation or malnutrition.

Famines, says Edkins, ought to be considered not natural disasters but crimes caused by human agency (Edkins 2007, 57). International law should be revised to name this type of crime, prohibit it, and mandate punishments for it. An appropriate name for this crime, in my view, is state-induced famine. The agent causing famine, the state, is clear. "Induced" implies public policies that cause famine. Public policies by definition imply intent; some human agents must make the policy decisions. Not all state food crimes rise to the level of state-induced famine; some "merely" cause malnutrition or food shortages. While deprivation of food is currently subsumed in the Rome Statute of the ICC under the crimes against humanity category of extermination, state-induced famine itself is not explicitly named.

David Marcus coined the term "faminogenesis" to refer to state activities "creating or aiding in the creation of famine" (Marcus 2003, 245, fn. 9). He presented four degrees of faminogenic behavior. These four degrees are intentional famine, using famine as means of extermination; reckless famine, continuing policies despite evidence of famine; famine by indifference, turning a blind eye to mass hunger; and famine as a consequence of incompetence. In the first degree, "Governments deliberately use hunger as a tool of extermination to annihilate troublesome populations." In the second, governments "implement policies that . . . engender famine, then recklessly continue to pursue these policies despite learning that they are causing mass starvation." In the third degree, the government does not intend to create famine, but "turn[s] blind eyes to mass hunger," even though it might be able respond to the food crisis. In the fourth degree, the government simply cannot cope with food shortages that may be caused by exogenous variables such as weather conditions or price shocks (Marcus 2003, 246–47).

Marcus' categorization of faminogenesis specifies various degrees of public policy failures that Ravallion argues result from "faulty theories or misinformation." Ravallion discusses "public-action failures that arise when those in power may not share the objectives of avoiding or relieving famine," suggesting Marcus' category of indifference. Ravallion also mentions that "even when the famine is not itself the weapon, it can be an entirely predictable by-product of governmental policies," suggesting Marcus' recklessness. Finally, Ravallion points out the extreme cases in which "a government knowingly uses famine as a weapon against its (external and internal) enemies," a situation that Marcus would categorize as intentional famine. Ravallion discusses famines in the Ukraine (Soviet Union) in the 1930s, and China from 1959 to 1961, as consequences in part of "public-action failure through denial or obfuscation of the signs of famine" (Ravallion 1997, 1225–26): I discuss both these famines in Chapter 2.

Marcus' focus on intentional famine reflects Jonassohn's earlier observation that famine was often a result of "a planned campaign against a victim group" (Jonassohn 1992, 5). Jonassohn argued that there were two kinds of "man-made famines," the "unintended consequences of economic, political, and social processes that aggravate rather than ameliorate an existing shortage of food caused by natural events" and "intentional use of hunger as a means of conflict and warfare" (Jonassohn 1991, 2). The former might be considered analogous to Marcus' faminogenesis by incompetence, and the latter to his intentional faminogenesis. Jonassohn also mentioned "cases where the starvation was not intended, but once observed, was allowed to continue because it was perceived as the just punishment for the victims' perceived failure to make a success of the policy of the ruling group" (Jonassohn 1991, 4). This is analogous to Marcus' recklessness, though Jonassohn added the feature that the victims are blamed for starving when the government's policies cause them to do so, as in China (Jonassohn 1991, 14). After reviewing the historical use of famine in warfare, Jonassohn also noted the intentional use of mass hunger as a means of internal repression. As North Korea and Zimbabwe exemplify, "famine is a low cost and low technology method that is available even to the poorest and most underdeveloped state" (Jonassohn 1991, 10).

Marcus' four categories of intentional, reckless, indifferent, and incompetent creation of famine seemed when I began research for this volume to be a good way to categorize famines and creation of malnutrition. I originally thought of North Korea as an example of intentionality, Zimbabwe of recklessness, Venezuela of incompetence, and Israel of indifference. However, I came to the conclusion that these categories were

not discrete. Indifference and incompetence, when deliberately continued, suggest recklessness or intentionality. Moreover, in all four cases the
state denied civil and political rights to the population enduring hunger.
In that respect, starvation, malnutrition, and food shortages were always
consequences of intentional policies.

Plan of the Book

Chapters 2 and 3 provide historical background to debates about how
to implement the human rights to adequate food and freedom from
hunger. Chapter 2 discusses some well-known twentieth-century famines
under communist regimes, in Ukraine in the 1930s, China from 1958
to 1962, and Cambodia in the late 1970s. These cases illustrate by their
neglect the importance of civil and political rights to the protection of
the economic human right to food. Chapter 3 discusses Sen's thesis that
there is no famine in democracies. Using the examples of Britain and
Canada, it shows that while there may not be famines within democratic
countries, these countries sometimes induce or tolerate famine and/or
malnutrition in cases of colonialism and warfare. In the 1840s, Britain
neglected the starving people of Ireland, its colony. Between the armistice
that ended hostilities with Germany in November 1918 and the peace
treaty signed in June 1919, Britain's policy of blockade of Germany –
to force it to sign the peace treaty – caused an estimated quarter-million
Germans to die of starvation. In the late nineteenth century Canada took
advantage of famine among its Aboriginal population to open up the
western part of the country to European settlement, and later indulged
in policies that left Aboriginals near starvation or suffering from severe
malnutrition.

Chapter 4 discusses North Korea, whose pseudo-Communist government, actually a family dynasty, collectivized agriculture and prohibited
an open market in food, resulting in mass starvation in the 1990s, threatened again in the second decade of the twenty-first century. North Korea
is an excellent illustration of Sen's non-market "shortage economy" (Sen
1981, 155). As I show in Chapter 8, as of 2015 there were good reasons
that its then leader, Kim Jong Un, should be tried before the ICC for
crimes against humanity. However, North Korea presented a conundrum
regarding the use of both international criminal law and humanitarian
intervention, as its threat to develop nuclear weapons took precedence
over its citizens' right to food, as I discuss in Chapter 9.

Chapter 5 discusses Zimbabwe, ruled after independence in 1980 by
an increasingly authoritarian leader, Robert Mugabe. Mugabe's decision
in 2000 to arbitrarily strip white farm owners of their property caused

massive malnutrition in a country that had been self-sufficient in food. Zimbabwe's treatment of its white minority farmers illustrates the need to protect citizenship rights, property rights, and the right to work, as discussed in Chapter 10. Zimbabwe also illustrates the unwillingness of outside actors to become involved even when a state's policies cause its citizens to starve. The African Union and the Southern African Development Community were very reluctant to criticize Mugabe, as I discuss in Chapter 9.

Chapter 6 discusses Venezuela, where Hugo Chávez, the President from 1999 until his death in 2013, engaged in "twenty-first century socialist" policies that deprived food producers of their property and penalized food distributors for allegedly charging prices that were too high. Nicolás Maduro continued these policies through to 2015. Chávez's and Maduro's policies caused severe food shortages, and reports of malnutrition in Venezuela appeared shortly after I finished the research for this book. Neither leader may have intended to deprive his citizens of food, but both recklessly continued incompetent policies that caused food shortages and violated civil and political rights in order to continue those policies. Sometimes, famine results not from "a sudden and sizeable shock to food entitlements" but from "a past history of decline": "Sufficient destabilization of consumption over time will worsen or even produce a famine" (Ravallion 1997, 1217, 1216). One hopes that such a long-term decline in food supply will not result in endemic malnutrition or even starvation in Venezuela.

Chapter 7 discusses what is probably the most contentious case in this book, that of malnutrition among Palestinians. In WBG, as in the other three cases, violation of civil and political rights – not only by Israel but also by Palestinian authorities – is a major cause of malnutrition. So also is violation of property rights (by Israel and Israeli settlers in the West Bank) and Palestinians' general lack of citizenship and mobility rights. In this case, the international dimension is so complex that it is difficult to recommend what should be done, but at minimum, Israel should respect the international law of occupation, discussed in Chapter 8.

The four chapters in Part II present empirical descriptions of the state food crimes that create famine, induce significant malnutrition, or cause food shortages. I leave the legal and international dimensions of these cases to Part III, where the cases are discussed as a group, depending on which policies apply to each case, offering some lessons and recommendations for human rights law and practice. Chapter 8 considers international law, including the law of genocide, crimes against humanity, refugee law, the absence of law regulating what I call penal starvation, laws of occupation, and an emerging area of soft law. Chapter 9 deals with external obligations; that is, the obligations of states to protect the food rights of people who are not their own citizens or under their own political control, focusing on sanctions and food aid.

In Chapter 10, I revert to my argument that the economic human right to food cannot be protected without concomitant protection of civil and political rights. For citizens to enjoy their right to food, they require a democratic and accountable government operating under the rule of law. Citizens also require the political right to be treated as equal citizens, as the examples of discrimination against white land owners in Zimbabwe, and Palestinians' lack of citizenship rights, demonstrate. They need the mobility right to search for food within their own country or to flee their country to another where food is available, as North Korean refugees in China can attest. They need the right to own property, a right that has been neglected since its inclusion in the UDHR in 1948, yet which is essential to citizens' rights to produce or acquire their own food (Howard-Hassmann 2013). Finally, they need the right to work.

Chapter 11 considers why liberal democracies succeed in protecting the right to food. I discuss the needs for democracy and effective social institutions, as well as the need to protect markets and property rights. However, through the example of Aboriginal malnutrition in Canada, I also show that even democracies can create internal malnutrition. I then consider international obligations regarding the right to food. I end the book in Chapter 12 with a brief call for a new international treaty on the right to food.

2   Communist Famines

State-induced famine in its worst form is intentional and kills large numbers of people. In a moral sense, it is a state food crime of the highest order; in the legal sense, as will be discussed in Part III, it is not properly singled out as a crime. Reckless famine – continuing policies known to cause mass starvation – is also a serious moral crime that ought to be singled out for punishment under international law.

The famines I review in this chapter – in the Soviet Union in the 1930s, China from 1958 to 1962, and Cambodia in the 1970s – were induced by totalitarian communist states. Totalitarianism controls all aspects of people's lives, including how and by what means they can procure food. In the early twenty-first century very few totalitarian states existed, although one, North Korea, is the first case study in Part II. But non-totalitarian states that cause starvation and/or malnutrition follow a path of rights deprivation similar to the paths taken by these three historical examples, depriving their citizens of all civil and political rights, the rule of law, citizenship rights, mobility rights, property rights, and the right to work. They follow these paths of rights deprivation even if they were once democracies, such as Venezuela and perhaps Zimbabwe, or are democracies that colonize other people, as was Israel.

Famine in the Soviet Union 1932–33

The Bolsheviks took power in Russia in 1917 with the slogan "peace, land and bread," renaming the country the Soviet Union. Peasants all over the country reacted to the Bolshevik takeover with a mass movement to seize land; however, this caused productive and distributional difficulties, as much of the grain necessary to feed the cities and to export to foreign countries had come from the large landholdings that the peasants seized (Scott 1998, 206). A four-year civil war followed the Bolshevik Revolution. During this period, the government introduced "war communism," a "policy that repealed peasants' land seizures, forcibly stripped the countryside of grain to feed city dwellers, and suppressed private commerce"

(Jones 2006, 190). The result was a massive famine that swept several regions in 1921–22, especially in areas that had suffered most from food requisitions. Of twenty-nine million Soviet citizens affected by hunger in the early 1920s, five million are estimated to have died: about eleven million people relied on food aid (Werth 1999, 123).

Once the civil war was over, Soviet leader Vladimir Lenin introduced a New Economic Policy (NEP) that returned land to peasants and permitted private commerce and some private cultivation of food. During the NEP period, the government tried to buy grain from the peasantry, but offered only about a fifth of the market price (Scott 1998, 209). Thus the government was not able to purchase enough grain to feed urban centers or to export to the West in return for hard currency needed to buy machinery necessary for the Soviet program of rapid industrialization. Lenin's successor, Joseph Stalin, rescinded the NEP in the late 1920s, following it with a massive campaign of collectivization over the entire country: half the Soviet peasantry, or about 60 million people, were collectivized within the first two months of 1930 (Figes 2007, 85). At the same time, the small enterprises that had been allowed under the NEP were abolished, thus ruining rural distribution of consumer goods (Conquest 1986, 101).

One purpose of this collectivization campaign was to "break the back" of the despised kulak class by depriving them of land ownership (Naimark 2010, 51–69). Kulaks were supposedly village money-lenders and rich peasants who hired labor from others. Yet actual kulaks were wealthy only in comparison with even less wealthy neighbors: in 1927 the richest peasants normally possessed two or three cows and up to ten hectares of land that they could sow, for families of an average size of seven people, and their income was no more than 50–56 percent higher than the income of the poorest (Conquest 1986, 75). Even worse, the term *kulak* was eventually extended downward to refer to any peasant, however poor, who had even the tiniest bit of grain in his fields or household larder.

Soviet policy was not only to deprive the kulak class of its property, but also to oblige all peasants to engage in collective, as opposed to family based, farming. It was thought that collectivization would improve efficiency of food cultivation. Peasants were removed from their individual plots and forced to give up their land, livestock, and agricultural implements to collectives. Stalin literally conducted a class war against the peasantry: "dekulakization brigades" confiscated and looted all property of supposedly wealthy peasants, even their household implements and food (Werth 1999, 148).

The result of these policies was a "collectivization and procurement famine" in the early 1930s (Scott 1998, 212). Among the 5.5 million now estimated to have died during this famine were 3.3 million ethnic Ukrainians (three million in Ukraine and 300,000 elsewhere); one million people in Kazakhstan; and the remainder throughout the rest of the Soviet Union (Snyder 2010, 53). The Kazakhs were a nomadic people, but the Soviet rulers wanted to convert them to sedentary cultivation; authorities confiscated their livestock, leaving many who had relied on their animals for meat and milk to starve (Conquest 1986, 195).

Ukrainians were particularly hard hit by this famine. During the first four months of 1930 alone, Soviet authorities deported approximately 114,000 people from Ukraine to the barren Soviet east, as punishment for being kulaks or for resisting collectivization (Snyder 2010, 26). In total about 1.8 million people in the entire Soviet Union were deported as part of the dekulakization campaign (Werth 1999, 153), of whom perhaps 300,000 were Ukrainians (Snyder 2010, 27). These massive deportations had the added advantage to Soviet authorities of populating the slave-labor camps that were being set up to exploit natural resources in Russia's northern and easternmost regions (Werth 1999, 144), just as similar slave-labor camps were established in North Korea twenty years later. Many of those transported to the camps died en route from cold, disease, and lack of food (Werth 1999, 152). Ethnic Russians moved to Ukraine to settle in empty villages and to Kazakhstan to replace local inhabitants who had died of famine (Conquest 1986, 197, 263).

All of this preceded a poor harvest in Ukraine in 1932 (Tauger 2006, 974), so that peasants had far less food and seed after supplying their quotas of grain to the state than they might otherwise have had. Yet the state continued to requisition food, refusing to reduce the amount owed to it. The authorities sent activist cadres to Ukraine to enforce draconian collectivization measures: these cadres, many of whom were young people who had been raised since the 1917 revolution and had been subjected to massive communist propaganda in schools, were often very brutal. Houses and storage units were searched; rapes and other brutalities were common (Snyder 2010, 39).

Under the "ear law" (a law prohibiting the theft of "socialist property") 125,000 people over the entire country were sentenced to prison and 5,400 were sentenced to death, sometimes for stealing only a few ears of corn from a collective farm (Werth 1999, 162). 200,000 people were sentenced to five to seven years in prison, and over 10,000 were executed for stealing socialist property, presumably, in the majority of cases, food (Ó Gráda 2009, 55). Faced with these conditions, many Ukrainians resorted to "famine foods" similar to those eaten six decades later by North Koreans. The famine continued into 1933 as peasants were not permitted to hold back seed from the 1932 harvest for the 1933 sowing.

The famine was so severe that many people resorted to cannibalism (Snyder 2010, 50–52), as would occur in the 1990s and even later in North Korea. While the authorities punished those who engaged in this desperate practice, they made little effort to ensure that no one would be driven to it. That the government knew cannibalism was a major problem was evidenced by a poster it distributed saying "Eating your children is an act of barbarism" (Werth 1999, caption under top photograph, fifth page of photographs between pp. 202 and 203). "Amputators" cut the liver from the bodies of starvation victims and used them as filling for meat pies sold in the market (Werth 1999, 165). One memoir spoke of a couple who cut off their children's heads and then salted their bodies for meat (Totten et al. 1997, 95). Human beings were "decivilized:" violation *in extremis* of even the fundamental prohibition against cannibalism made it easier for the Soviet regime to kill the very people it had driven to this desperate practice (Naimark 2010, 62).

The Soviet famine was man-made in the sense that destruction of property, deportations, and requisitioning of the harvest were policy measures that severely exacerbated the grain shortage after the poor harvest in 1932. There appears to be no direct evidence that Stalin deliberately sought to starve the peasants (Davies and Wheatcroft 2006, 628), so that Marcus' category of intentional faminogenesis does not apply. Stalin was, however, certainly guilty of sins of commission, or what might be seen as reckless continuation of faminogenic policies. He was aware that there was famine in Ukraine (Snyder 2010, 34) but did not reverse or change his policies, although there is some evidence that in late 1932 he did somewhat reduce the quota of grain to be relinquished to the state and sent a little food to Ukraine, as well as some seed for the following year (Tauger 1991, 88; Wheatcroft 2004, 126). Nor did Stalin accept offers of foreign food aid or cease to export food (Naimark 2010, 75), suggesting indifference to the famine. Indeed, it may well have been that Stalin regarded starvation as a rational means of eliminating his class enemies, cheaper than deporting ever more hundreds of thousands to the East (Ellman 2005, 827).

Deprivation of property is an often overlooked violation of human rights that can result in malnutrition and/or famine, as I discuss in Chapter 10. Loss of their productive property was the most important precipitating factor causing Ukrainians to starve. Had peasants retained their land, livestock, and tools they would have been able to feed themselves and their families even during the reduced harvest of 1932, and they would have retained enough seed to plant for a better harvest in 1933. Like everyone in the Soviet Union, Ukrainians were also deprived of all civil and political rights: They had no free press that could publicize their plight, they were not permitted to assemble to demonstrate against the Soviet authorities, nor could they vote the Bolsheviks out of office. Finally, Ukrainians were deprived of all freedom of movement. In 1933 Stalin introduced internal passports prohibiting peasants from migrating to cities in search of food. If they did reach the cities they often lay dying and overlooked on the streets (Werth 1999, 164; Snyder 2010, 45). In 1933 alone authorities arrested 220,000 Ukrainians attempting to flee to other parts of the Soviet Union, sending 190,000 home to starve (Naimark 2010, 73).

The fact that such a disproportionately high percentage of ethnic Ukrainians died during the Soviet famine suggests a possible genocidal motive, perhaps to protect the Soviet Union from a nationalist Ukrainian uprising (Mace 1997, 80; Conquest 1986, 328). According to this view, the Soviets regarded Ukrainians as a threat because they had a distinct area of settlement and possibly might wish to join Western Ukraine, then German territory. In the mid to late nineteenth century, Ukrainian national interest in its language, literature, and music blossomed, continuing after the 1905 political liberalization in Russia and during the early 1920s when Lenin encouraged national minorities. Earlier researchers argued that one purpose of the Ukrainian famine was to end the existence of Ukraine as a cultural and national entity. Evidence for this thesis was that the Soviet authorities did not simply requisition grain from peasants; they also destroyed churches (Conquest 1986, 199–213), looted libraries, and banned the Ukrainian language from schools. Moreover, although the economic policy was supposed to be one of "dekulakization," in fact all Ukraine's peasants were targeted.

Nevertheless, Ó Gráda argues that this earlier research was mistaken in arguing for genocidal intent, and that later research showed that Stalin's purpose was to collectivize agriculture regardless of his victims' ethnicity (Ó Gráda 2009, 235–36). Werth argues that although Ukrainians suffered disproportionately in the 1930s and Stalin also targeted the supposedly nationalist Ukrainian intelligentsia, the famine was proportionately just as severe in other parts of the Soviet Union such as Kazakhstan. The richest, most agriculturally productive areas of the country suffered most from the famine: Ukraine happened to be one of those areas (Werth 1999, 168). Naimark, on the other hand, contends that the Ukrainian famine was genocide and that Stalin did want to destroy Ukraine as an enemy nation. He argues that the disproportionately high number of starvation deaths in Kazakhstan show that Kazakhs, too, suffered genocide, as Stalin was also purging their intellectual and cultural leaders in order to destroy them as a people (Naimark 2010, 76–79).

The debate about whether the Ukrainian famine was a result of genocidal intent as well as of brutal collectivization policies is a precursor to later debates about the possibly genocidal aspects of famine. That Ukrainians were deprived of all of human rights suggests genocidal intent, yet the measures were not confined to Ukraine alone: peasants (and everyone else) everywhere in the Soviet Union were similarly deprived of rights. Moreover, national symbols and languages were repressed all over the Soviet Union, not only in Ukraine.

Analysis of faminogenesis does not, however, require that a famine be genocide in order to characterize it as intentional. Whatever the reason, if a state deliberately starves its citizens the famine is intentional. At best, the famine in Ukraine and elsewhere in the Soviet Union was a result of second-degree reckless faminogenesis. Stalin may not have intended his victims to starve, but he refused to modify his collectivization policies when starvation occurred. On the other hand, the deliberate deprivation of all civil and political rights and the deliberate control of freedom of movement via internal passports suggest that Stalin did intend starvation. This is a problem that occurs in the cases I discuss in Part II, in which all victims of food deprivation and/or malnutrition were deprived of civil and political rights, and many of freedom of movement and property rights as well. The categories of reckless and intentional famine slide into one another. Reckless deprivation of civil and political rights in order to support totalitarian regimes or dictatorships suggests intent to deprive citizens of those means they need to avoid starvation. Analytically, this may not matter, but it does matter if international law is to be changed to prohibit state-induced famines.

China's Great Leap Forward 1958–62

One of the slogans and justifying policies of Communist-ruled China was the "iron rice bowl," the claim that no Chinese would starve under communism. Yet from 1958 to 1962 a government campaign known as the Great Leap Forward (GLF) caused massive starvation. Early studies suggested fifteen to twenty-five million people died in this famine (Ó Gráda 2009, 96). More recent research by Dikötter, who had access to many newly opened archives, suggests a minimum of forty-five million deaths (Dikötter 2010, 325) in a population at the time of about 650 million people: that is, almost 7 percent of China's population. However, Dikötter notes that of the forty-five million dead, perhaps 6 to 8 percent, or 2.5 million, were actually killed outright (Dikötter 2010, 298); thus, this was also one of the largest deliberate slaughters in human history. This violence was one way to keep down the demand for food; the more people were killed, the fewer ate.

The famine that hit China was a result of policies originally designed to institute a GLF in industrial production. Mao Zedong, China's dictator, had proclaimed in 1957 that just as the Soviet Union intended to catch up with American industrial production by 1972, so China would catch up with Great Britain, then a leading industrial power. The original plan was to catch up with Britain in fifteen years, but this was then reduced to two (Margolin 1999b, 488). This was voluntarist utopianism, the belief that any goal could be accomplished if only there were the will to do so, regardless of the actual material conditions. As one article in the government-controlled press in the state of Henan said in 1957, "The human will is the master of all things" (Margolin 1999b, 488).

After they took over China in 1949, the Communists redistributed land to the peasants, just as Soviet leaders had done after the 1917 Revolution. However, the authorities soon introduced agricultural "cooperatives" that eliminated peasants' rights to farm their private plots and market their produce as they saw fit (Porter 2011, 39). Agriculture was collectivized, with all farmers forced into communes to whom they had to relinquish all their land, livestock, and agricultural implements. Much of the livestock died for lack of food; peasants also slaughtered many animals rather than turn them over to the communes. The communes were then forced to give ever-increasing percentages of their crops to the state to feed urban workers and to earn income from food exports that in turn, as in the Soviet Union, could be used to buy the machines necessary for the GLF in industry. Working conditions on the collective farms resembled slavery.

As directives came down from the center to local areas to increase the amount of grain they sent to the state, a "wind of exaggeration of output" (Bernstein 2006, 423) affected the entire country. Local leaders feared detrimental repercussions if they did not claim to be able to increase production, thus they competed with each other to exaggerate the amounts they could produce. In turn, the central authorities believed the amounts reported to them and pressured for production goals to be raised even higher. Indeed, one of the major causes of the famine was that in 1958, influenced by falsified reports of an extremely good harvest, Mao actually ordered the peasants to eat as much as they could and cut back on the amount of land they cultivated (Article 19 1990, 43; Dikotter 2010, 136). The result was that there was not enough seed in 1959 and land was left uncultivated. Yet communes were still forced to give most of their grain to the state, leaving peasants with starvation rations, while Mao doubled grain exports (Glover 2001, 285). Grain was also turned into fuel for military equipment: each missile test used "10 million kilograms of grain, enough to radically deplete the food intake of 1–2 million people for a whole year" (Chang and Halliday 2005, 429).

Mao also ordered irrational cultivation techniques. One of the most dangerous was close-cropping of seeds (later copied by North Korea, with similar disastrous results), resulting in crowding of plants, which then could not grow. Demonstrating supreme ignorance of agriculture, Mao actually claimed that when seedlings were close-cropped they would have company and be able to grow better (Margolin 1999b, 489). Farmers were ordered to cultivate crops on previously wooded hillsides; the result was massive deforestation and susceptibility to floods when there were heavy rains. Farmers were also ordered to engage in "deep ploughing," (Dikötter 2010, 39) which was ostensibly to permit roots to grow further into the ground but in fact ruined the soil. A campaign to eliminate sparrows, considered to be pests, resulted in infestations of insects (Dikötter 2010, 187–88). Chinese scientists were also ordered to follow the discredited ideas of the Soviet geneticist, Trofim Lysenko, who thought that plant genetics could be rapidly changed by innovative farming methods (Margolin 1999b, 489).

All these orders came from party leaders who had little if no experience in or knowledge of agriculture. Meantime, in order to satisfy senior leaders and cadres that the policies were working, "Potemkin fields" were created so that visiting dignitaries could view them: Peasants transplanted ripe crops from several fields into one, where the plants often died after serving their purpose of satisfying leaders' wishful thinking about the harvest size (Chang and Halliday 2005, 427). Peasants were also forced to melt all their metal goods, including tools, pots and pans, doorknobs, and sewing needles, in "backyard furnaces" to supply steel to industry (Dikötter 2010, 58–59, 162). Most of the "steel" produced was of such poor quality that it could not be used, but in the meantime peasants lost the tools they needed to farm and cook. The farming population was also reduced as many peasants were forced to leave their land to work on gigantic irrigation projects, most of which were so hastily conceived that they did more damage than good (Dikötter 2010, 25–33). Other agricultural laborers were forced to leave the countryside for industrial work (Ó Gráda 2009, 243), while some voluntarily migrated to cities because there was no food for them at home.

To fuel the drive for collectivization, houses were destroyed, stripped of wood and any other usable parts to build new communal facilities such as kitchens. Peasants were even deprived of their clothing; the cotton was used in industrial production of clothes for export (Dikötter 2010, 140). It was not uncommon for travelers, including officials occasionally sent out to report on the most egregious abuses, to see naked, emaciated people by the roadside in the middle of winter. In some places money was eliminated and citizens were issued with ration books; these books tied them to the places where they lived even when no food was available (Article 19 1990, 23). Without housing, tools, and household implements, peasants had no choice but to move into shoddy, crowded dormitories and eat in communal kitchens, where cooks and servers abused their powers to deny people even the meager, less than subsistence rations to which they were formally entitled.

All over China, peasants starved, though in some regions more than others. Grain rations were reduced to far below subsistence levels; peasants turned to turnips or sweet potatoes as their staple foods, as the state could not easily store these root crops. Yet at the same time, much food was wasted (Dikötter 2010, 138) as the transportation system could not keep up with the Party's demands to move food to cities, or to requisition grain and then sell it back to the peasants, rather than simply leave more grain with them in the first place. As was to occur forty years later in North Korea, peasants resorted to foraging, eating insects, bird droppings and rats, consuming bark and mud (Dikötter 2010, 169, 311), even eating the thatch and plaster from their own houses and cotton from their own bedding (Chang 1991, 233). Women prostituted themselves in return for food (Dikötter 2010, 234). Children were abandoned or sold to strangers by parents who could not feed them (Dikötter 2010, 67, 206–07): at one terminal in Sichuan, children congregated to eat the vomit from bus passengers (Ó Gráda 2009, 75). As in Ukraine, some resorted to cannibalism, eating the flesh of newly buried people (Dikötter 2010, 320–23). Some individuals actually killed others, either to eat the human flesh themselves or sell it in the market. As a child in Chengdu, Jung Chang heard of a couple who were stealing babies, killing them, and then selling their flesh as rabbit meat (Chang 1991, 234).

As this was happening, the government promoted the irrational slogan, "Capable women can make a meal without food," reversing the traditional Chinese saying, "No matter how capable, a woman cannot make a meal without food" (Chang 1991, 223). Babies born during the famine and small children who grew up during it suffered serious health problems for the rest of their lives (Chen and Zhou 2007). Yet party officials enjoyed larger rations than ordinary people; the higher the rank, the more food the individual received (Chang 1991, 232).

Those who protested against either government policies or the actions of cadres were subjected to brutal, sadistic tortures. In one commune in 1960, four peasants died after they were tied up and hanged, allegedly for concealing grain; another thirty-six survived this torture (Article 19 1990, 61). Even children were tortured; one child had four fingers chopped off for stealing food, while elsewhere two children were hanged by wires strung through their ears: These punishments were common, not unusual

(Chang and Halliday 2005, 436). A father in Hunan was forced to bury his own son alive after he stole a handful of grain (Dikötter 2010, 248). Ralph Thaxton published a detailed oral and documentary history of one village during the GLF, Da Fo in the state of Hebei. In 1959 Da Fo villagers survived by eating turnips and carrots and by "secretly eating green corn prior to the fall harvest" (Thaxton 2008, 130). By 1960 the grain ration was one quarter of that promised in 1958 (Thaxton 2008, 125). The entire village was, in effect, a "communal penal colony" (Thaxton 2008, 146). Even the blind were obliged to work, pulling the millstones used for grinding wheat (a job previously done by animals) in order to justify their consumption of food. Children were left without care as their parents worked in the fields in "endless corvée labor": Between work and compulsory propaganda meetings, peasants were often left with only two hours' sleep a night (Thaxton 2008, 133–38).

Da Fo's villagers were forced to give up grain to the state without any payment for it whatsoever, while cadres withheld food coupons from those who did not work hard enough in irrigation or other projects (Thaxton 2008, 131, 135). People who were unable to work as hard as the cadres demanded were subject to public criticism sessions where they were often beaten, as also were lower-level Party officials who tried to tell the truth about crop sizes instead of conforming to the Maoist wind of exaggeration (Thaxton 2008, 146–47). Pregnant women were forced to work in the fields until a few hours before birth and return to work a few days later: suffering from malnutrition and exhaustion, many lost their babies (Thaxton 2008, 141).

There was bad weather during the GLF, but according to one study it was responsible for only about 13 percent of the decline in agricultural output, while diversion of resources from agriculture was responsible for about 33 percent and excessive procurement for another 28 percent, as without food rural workers were too weak to work in agriculture (Li and Yang 2005, 872–73). The Maoist "überleftist policies" (Ó Gráda 2009, 243) were exacerbated by floods and droughts, so that the Chinese premier Liu Sha-ch'i later said the famine was "three parts nature and seven parts man" (Ó Gráda 2009, 244). Another explanation of the GLF is that the country had to increase grain exports in order to pay accumulated debts to the Soviet Union after the Sino-Soviet split, but Nikita Krushchev, the leader of the Soviet Union, offered very easy loan repayment terms to China, which did not require a massive export drive (Dikötter 2010, 104–07).

The GLF illustrates Sen's proposition (Sen 1999), discussed further in Chapter 3, about the importance of a free press and freedom of speech to avert famine. China was characterized by "totalitarian intolerance of debate, criticism, and empirical facts ... it tolerated a disorganized information system based on wrong reporting" (Jonassohn 1991, 13). No one, including high members of the Communist Party, regional and local leaders, and peasants and ordinary citizens could speak out without fear of extreme penalties, including torture, imprisonment, and death. No free press existed; only Communist Party newspapers were permitted, which at best could report specific localized abuses in a very roundabout manner. Like Stalin before him and Pol Pot of Cambodia afterwards, Mao made conscious decisions to deny citizens the civil and political rights necessary to ensure their rights to food. There was no democracy and no way to overthrow either the central party leaders or local cadres. There was no rule of law, nor were citizens allowed freedom of movement in order to seek food outside their own collectives. As had occurred in the Soviet Union during the famine period of the 1930s, comprehensive internal passports were introduced in 1958 (Torpey 1997, 856).

The question arises whether Mao had faminogenic intent. It appears not; rather, he believed his own and others' propaganda about increased agricultural yields, so that without concern he ordered increased quotas of grain to be paid to the state. He also believed it was absolutely essential to industrialize, especially after China's split with the Soviet Union resulted in withdrawal of Soviet technical assistance, just as withdrawal of Soviet and Chinese support would be one cause of famine in North Korea forty years later.

However, one can certainly indict Mao for reckless faminogenesis. Information did reach him that peasants were starving; sometimes he waved it aside, while at others he ordered investigations and occasionally punishment of abusive cadres. In general, however, he not only supported but intensified the GLF policies until finally halting them in 1962, when peasants were once again allowed small private plots of land and peasant markets were reopened, although agriculture remained collectivized. Mao ignored warnings about famine from senior Party figures as early as 1958, accusing them of being "right deviationists," and treated the occasional reports of abuse and starvation that he actually believed as isolated cases requiring "cadre rectification" (Bernstein 2006, 439), rather than as evidence of systematic policy errors.

Bernstein argues that Mao easily accepted "mass death as the price of progress" (Bernstein 2006, 443). This is also the position of Jung and Halliday, who argue that as early as 1958 "Mao knew that in many places people were reduced to eating compounds of earth. In some cases, whole villages died as a result, when people's intestines became blocked" (Chang and Halliday 2005, 428). Indeed, Chang and Halliday quote Mao as having said in 1957, "We are prepared to sacrifice 300 million Chinese [about half of the population] for the victory of the world revolution." They further repeat a statement he made about the GLF to senior leaders in November 1958; "Working like this, with all these projects, half of China may well have to die" (Chang and Halliday 2005, 439). Another famous quote from Mao was "It is better to let half of the people die so that the other half can eat their fill" (Dikötter 2010, 88).

Thaxton agrees with Chang and Halliday that "Mao Zedong himself was substantially responsible for the misinformation crisis of the Great Leap," suppressing and ignoring complaints that were addressed to him (Thaxton 2008, 3). However, Bernstein argues that "the accusation that Mao deliberately exposed China's peasants to mass death during the GLF is not . . . plausible." Bernstein believes that large-scale famine undercut Mao's core claim to legitimacy, which was that Chinese would no longer suffer famine: therefore, he did support corrective measures after 1960 (Bernstein 2006, 444). This is an argument for reckless rather than deliberate faminogenesis. Nevertheless, Bernstein argues that Mao could have stopped the faminogenic policies much earlier than he did, rather than continuing them after warnings about their catastrophic impact in 1958. "This act of willful abdication of his duty as the country's undisputed leader makes him directly responsible for the immense catastrophe that ensued" (Bernstein 2006, 445). Margolin agrees that "Undoubtedly it was not Mao's intention to kill so many of his compatriots. But the least one can say is that he seemed little concerned about the death of millions from hunger." Mao, says Margolin, "displayed economic incompetence, wholesale ignorance, and ivory-tower utopianism" (Margolin 1999b, 487). These descriptions fit the criteria for reckless faminogenesis, the refusal to change policies known to cause famine.

Cambodia 1975–79

From 1975 to 1979 Cambodia (then Democratic Kampuchea) was ruled by a militant group called the Khmer Rouge (KR), or red Khmer, referring to Cambodia's major ethnic group. Led by Pol Pot, the KR was originally a guerilla group fighting the corrupt military dictatorship of General Lon Nol that had taken power from King Sihanouk in 1970.

In the early 1970s parts of Cambodia were under heavy and illegal bombardment by the US, which was trying to stymie the flow of North Vietnamese troops via Cambodia to South Vietnam during the Vietnamese war. The US dropped three times as many bombs on Cambodia between 1970 and 1973 as it had dropped on Japan during all of WWII (Staub 1989, 190). Estimates of the numbers killed by US bombing in

Cambodia vary from a low of about 50,000 to 150,000 (Marchak 2008, 102) to the 600,000 that Pol Pot claimed were killed (Margolin 1999a, 590); Margolin cites a demographer's estimate of 240,000 as a reasonable figure (Margolin 1999a, 590). The bombing caused chaos in the countryside and many peasants fled to Phnom Penh, the capital. As a result of the bombings and population movements, the amount of land under cultivation for rice, the staple food, drastically declined from six million to one million acres; American charities sent food aid to avert starvation although malnutrition was rampant (Jones 2006, 287). Under these conditions, rural hatred of the US and Lon Nol grew, as did concomitant support for the guerilla KR forces. When the Vietnamese war ended and the US withdrew from South Vietnam in 1975, the Lon Nol government fell to the KR.

Several experts agree that between 1.5 and 1.7 million people, of a total of 7.9 million Cambodians, died during KR rule, or about 19 to 21 percent of the population (Weitz 2003, 186; Kiernan 1997, 343). A survey of refugees in Thailand in 1980 suggested that about a quarter of the lost population died directly of starvation and a quarter of disease, much of which had been caused or exacerbated by starvation (Fein 1993, 19). More would have died had not the KR been driven out of Cambodia in 1979 by Vietnam, which was both protecting itself against incursion by the KR and trying to protect those ethnic Vietnamese who still lived in Cambodia. Vietnam was also motivated by its regional rivalry with China, which had backed the KR.

The KR believed in autarky, "self-reliance," and complete independence from the world market, to the point that they even refused offers of aid, for example from UNICEF, after they took over Cambodia in 1975 (Chalk and Jonassohn 1990, 403). The KR's agricultural policy was, in effect, a "Super Great Leap Forward," intended to surpass China's disastrous policies (Kiernan 1997, 351). Some KR leaders, including Pol Pot, had been educated in Paris and joined the French Communist Party, where they apparently were influenced by Marxist and Maoist thought (Weitz 2003, 146; Staub 1989, 202). They were also influenced by the French revolutionary tradition: One leader especially admired Robespierre, initiator of the terror that followed the 1789 revolution (Margolin 1999a, 624).

In Paris, these KR leaders also acquired the voluntarist belief that as long as there was enough commitment to a cause it could succeed, regardless of the material situation. Indeed, the KR view was that neither the Soviet Union nor China had applied its policies with enough rigor: had they been more committed to the cause, agricultural collectivization could have succeeded (Weitz 2003, 145). Thus, the KR ideology was one of fanatical utopianism. Utopianism is often accompanied by mass destruction of any social institutions and values which appear to compete with the ideology and practice of the rulers, such as family and religion. It is also characterized by a perceived necessity to physically "cleanse" or purge the population. The KR's ideology of purification demanded the elimination of the urban population, intellectuals and professionals, groups who were not ethnic Khmers, and those connected to the former corrupt regimes. The KR view was "What is infected must be cut out" and "what is rotten must be removed" (Chalk and Jonassohn 1990, 404).

There was, however, one crucial difference between Cambodia and its predecessors: whereas Stalin and Mao exploited the peasantry in their quest for industrialization, Pol Pot extolled the peasantry and despised urbanites. Within a week of their takeover, the KR expelled two to three million people from the capital, many of them actually refugees from the earlier warfare in the countryside. The expellees included the old, the sick, and even those in hospitals: Hospital patients who could not walk were simply shot (Criddle and Mam 1996, 451). Many refugees spent several weeks on the road without food or medical assistance (Margolin 1999a, 583). This was, in effect, "urbicide": the KR's fanatical view was that cities were "cesspools of corruption and of foreign-affiliated cliques, requiring 'cleansing' and 'purification' by genocidal agents" (Jones 2006, 291).

In contrast to urban sophistication, the KR adopted a form of "primitivism," in part influenced by its years in hiding among the mountain tribal people of Cambodia (Jones 2006, 289–90). The perceived innocence and communalism of these tribal peoples, as opposed to the individualism and modernity of the cities, influenced the KR to eliminate cities entirely, as opposed to Stalin and Mao, who exploited the peasantry to feed the cities. Moreover, everything perceived to emanate from the West, including all forms of modern transportation and communication, was outlawed (Criddle and Mam 1996, 454).

Just as North Korea was later to do in dividing its population into loyal, wavering, or hostile classes (discussed in Chapter 4), so the KR divided its population into immutable social groups, including so-called base people, who had full rights (in so far as anyone actually had rights in Cambodia); candidates, who might become as loyal as base people; and "depositees," who had no rights (Weitz 2003, 160) and were sometimes called "subpeople" (Chalk and Jonassohn 1990, 405). Sometimes, the divisions were simply between strong and weak (Weitz 2003, 160), or between "old" people in rural areas who had been under KR rule before 1975, and "new," predominantly urban, people, who had not (Fein 1990, 78). Old or base people could stay in their villages and their own homes and received more food than new people (Weitz 2003, 160). Old people were permitted hard rice and some fruit, sugar, and meat, whereas new people were fed clear rice soup, "a symbol of famine" (Margolin 1999a, 591). The half-French memoirist Denise Affonço recalled that the "old people" in the village to which she was assigned received twice as much food as the new people (Affonço 2007, 56). The enslaved population was not allowed to pick fruit, to fish, or to forage after work.

The result of this difference in distribution of food was that about 25 percent of urban Khmers died, as opposed to 15 percent of the rural population (Midlarsky 2005, 312). As one survivor testified "There were eleven people in my family. None were killed, but ten died of starvation in 1977–78, and only I survived" (eyewitness Ang Ngeck Teang in Totten et al. 1997, 365). Not surprisingly, as in the Soviet Union and China, there were acts of cannibalism, although mainly of eating those already dead (Margolin 1999a, 603).

As in China, people were fed according to how much they could work; thus, healthy men ate the most, while the old, very young children, and the disabled were called "useless mouths" (Margolin 1999a, 585). Children who could not work were killed: in one group of one hundred boys aged eleven or older whose job was to plant rice, twenty were executed for not working hard enough or playing games (eyewitness Sat, in Totten et al. 1997, 368). Disabled people were considered lazy and executed (Margolin 1999a, 598). Affonço's nine-year-old daughter starved to death and a nine-year-old nephew was executed for stealing food, while her somewhat older and stronger son survived because he was allowed more rations, although his growth was severely stunted (Affonço 2007, 84, 115, 123).

Like the Chinese before them, the KR directed agriculture from the center, giving detailed instructions to peasants without considering local conditions or agricultural knowledge. Just as Mao had stated he wanted to surpass Britain within fifteen years, Pol Pot wanted Cambodia's agricultural yield to be higher than Japan's (Midlarsky 2005, 315). The ideological core of KR agricultural policy was that rice alone would be enough to feed everyone who deserved to be fed, leaving enough for export to earn hard cash for such industrial products as were needed. Yet although the KR ordered peasants to uproot banana trees to make room for rice, its production fell abysmally (Margolin 1999a, 602). At the same time, as in China, massive irrigation projects brought death to workers and destruction to the land; following the extreme voluntarist ideology, hydraulic engineers were ignored and their criticisms considered acts of political treason (Margolin 1999a, 601). In reality, the KR was completely uninterested in providing enough food; just as Mao stated that millions could die without any concern to the Chinese Communist Party, so the

KR slogan was "If you die, it is no loss. If you remain alive, it is no matter" (Weitz 2003, 167). Such rice as was produced was distributed to KR cadres, sold to China in exchange for weapons, or merely left to rot in storage, even though so many were starving (Glover 2001, 302).

Many people died in Cambodia from causes other than famine. Former officers of the previous military regimes, civil servants, and members of former governments were purged. So-called class enemies, including all intellectuals, teachers, professionals, anyone defined as "petty bourgeois," anyone who was wealthy, indeed anyone who wore glasses were also killed. "Old" KR officers who disliked the post-1975 policies were purged, as were any regional KR leaders seen to be threatening central control: In their turn, regional leaders purged anyone threatening control of their territory.

Aside from these purges, some groups were victims of genocide in the classic sense of mass murder of members of racial, ethnic, national, or religious groups, as discussed in Chapter 8. These included 40 to 60 percent of the minority Muslim Cham group: In a country in which almost everyone was starving, the Cham were forced to eat pork and were killed if they refused (Weitz 2003, 172). About 100,000 ethnic Vietnamese were killed and the rest driven out of the country: Vietnam was a traditional enemy of Cambodia as it was a stronger south-east Asian power. About 225,000 of 425,000 ethnic Chinese, also heavily urban, were killed (Kiernan 1997, 341). In the case of these groups, starvation was but one means of genocide, as opposed to the starvation of ethnic Khmer, whose deaths were attributable to fanatical ideology.

Finally, the question of intent arises: was the famine deliberate? Scholars debate whether Pol Pot and his clique intended to kill so many people, either directly or by starvation and disease, or whether they lost control as regional and local commanders did as they wished. Kiernan contends that the KR was a centralized organization that "was able to plan such mass murders precisely because of its concentrated power" (Kiernan 1997, 353). It is difficult to determine how much starvation was a consequence of intentional policy and how much was a consequence of the reckless continuation of ideologically based economic policy, but the deaths from famine, as well as executions and massacres of former elites, professionals, urbanites, perceived dissidents, "useless mouths," and minority groups suggests that the central authorities knew full well what was occurring. That they did nothing to check the atrocities but instead encouraged them through their orders, policies, and extreme dehumanizing language suggests intentional faminogenesis.

Moreover, imitating their predecessors in the Soviet Union and China, the KR denied Cambodians all civil and political rights. There was no democracy, no rule of law, no free press or speech, no mobility rights, no private property. Hundreds of thousands of people perceived to challenge KR rule were murdered in exceptionally brutal ways. Perceived enemies were completely dehumanized, called "microbes" who caused illness in the ruling party (Weitz 2003, 155). The KR leaders' conscious decisions to ignore the evidence of their own eyes as their citizens (if they can be called that) starved, and to deny even the most fundamental right to life, is clear evidence of reckless continuation of their policies.

Famine as a Process of Rights Deprivation

Jones describes the famines under Stalin and Mao as "manipulated famines," which "were not planned as such, but . . . were the predictable result of regime policies, exacerbated by leaders' conscious refusal to intervene and ameliorate them" (Jones 2006, 189). Manipulated famine suggests, at minimum, reckless faminogenesis, which characterizes the Cambodian as well as the Soviet and Chinese famine.

Jonassohn points out the advantages to political elites of intentional famine.

Its appeal to the perpetrators is manifold. It conserves food resources that may already be in short supply. It allows the perpetrators to hide their real motives behind an apparent natural disaster. Because it is a method that requires neither an advanced technology nor a highly developed bureaucracy it can be applied by even the poorest country. It weakens the victims physically and lowers their resistance to epidemics, while at the same time it undermines their morale and their ability to resist. And eventually it kills (Jonassohn 1992, 5–6).

The cases discussed in this chapter illustrate Jonassohn's analysis. Perpetrators of famine conserved food for themselves while denying it to others; they claimed that food shortages were caused by natural disasters when they were actually caused by government policies; they managed to generate famine without highly developed bureaucracies; and they weakened and killed their real or perceived opponents. All three cases, moreover, were based on voluntarist ideologies. Stalin, Mao, and Pol Pot all believed that their agricultural policies would increase crop sizes, when the result was the opposite. They also believed that ideological enthusiasm would permit them to dispense with technical expertise. All three were willing to exterminate substantial proportions of their populations, as long as those who remained adhered to the ideological line and fulfilled the criteria of people worthy of life.

Ó Gráda claims that "Stalin, Hitler, and Mao, three totalitarian despots linked to some of the greatest famines of all time, have left no important heirs," as famines are now less frequent and are smaller in scope and famine relief reaches victims more easily (Ó Gráda 2009, 261–62). Nevertheless, Stalin and Mao had their heirs in the political leaders who in the twenty-first century still used food as a weapon against their own and other people. The Kim dynasty in North Korea was a direct heir of Stalin and Mao. While North Korea is the only one of the four cases discussed in Part II to be a totalitarian regime, traces of voluntarism could also be found in Chávez's and Maduro's economic policies in Venezuela.

The ruling elites of all three cases described in this chapter used dehumanizing vocabulary to describe their victims. Stalin referred to Soviet deportees as vermin, filth, pollution, or weeds (Applebaum 2003, 102). Similar terms were used to describe victims in China and Cambodia. Having transformed human beings into sub or non-humans, vermin, and the like, it was easy to exclude them from the universe of obligation, that narrow band of people to whom the leaders of these ideological movements felt some obligation (Fein 1979, 4). We will see this again in the contemporary cases on which this book focuses, especially North Korea and Zimbabwe.

Moreover, all three historical cases exemplify the human rights abuses that characterize the contemporary cases discussed in Part II. Civil and political rights either never existed or were abrogated in the Soviet Union, China, and Cambodia. In none of the three countries was there rule of law, free elections, a free press, or a right to organize against the regime. Nor was freedom of movement permitted in any of the three cases; rather, they were characterized by internal passports and forced migrations. All three regimes abrogated both large landowners' and small peasants' rights to own property, forcing them instead into state-run collectivized enterprises or, in Cambodia, into agricultural slave-labor camps. All tried forms of autarky, ignoring the rules of internal and international market economies. And in none was there any active citizenship, by which individuals could participate in the decisions made by their governors. All three refused foreign food aid. Thus, it can be argued that at best, all three experienced famines by recklessness; at worst, some of the dehumanizing language suggests intentionality.

While one might hope that only totalitarian regimes are responsible for state-induced famine, Chapter 3 shows that democratic governments are willing to tolerate famine in their colonies, and even induce it against their enemies. These famines may not be intentional, but they certainly illustrate indifference, and possibly recklessness.

3   Democracies and Famines

Democracies and Famines

Sen argues that "there has never been a famine in a functioning multiparty democracy" (Sen 1999, 178). In democracies, he argues, a free press can alert citizens, governments, and outsiders to famine conditions; opposition politicians can criticize the government; and citizens can vote governments out of office if they do nothing to avert the famine or feed those who face starvation. These same groups can criticize the government's impending or implemented social policies if they are likely to result in famine (Sen 1999, 178–86). "Transparency freedom" (Sen 1999, 185) lets citizens and the opposition know what the government is doing before it is too late to remedy its policies. Sen particularly mentions that "the positive role of political and civil rights applies to the prevention of economic and social disasters in general" (Sen 1999, 184), an argument I also make throughout this volume. In all four cases discussed in Part II, governments denied the right to vote, media freedom, and other civil and political rights to the people who became victims of famine and malnutrition.

Other studies also mention the relationship between violations of civil and political rights and famine. *Article 19*, a non-governmental organization named for Article 19 of the Universal Declaration of Human Rights, focuses on freedom of opinion and expression. It reported on the connection between famine and censorship as early as 1990. Using studies of China's Great Leap Forward (authored by an anonymous scholar of China), and famine in Ethiopia and Sudan in the 1980s (authored by Alex de Waal), *Article 19* showed that, as Sen later argued, "censorship [is] a cause of famine" (D'Souza 1990, 3): Citizens lacking the right and capacity to protest against government policies endured faminogenesis.

Ó Gráda proposes other advantages of democracy that lessen the likelihood of famine. He argues that "Effective and compassionate governance might lead to competitive [food] markets, sanctions against corruption, and well-directed relief" (Ó Gráda 2009, 13). As Part II shows, competitive market economies were prohibited in North Korea and undermined in Zimbabwe and Venezuela. "Well-directed relief" suggests not only national governments' responsibilities to provide relief to the starving and malnourished but also their obligation to accept foreign food aid and distribute it equitably. North Korea and Zimbabwe erected barriers to the efficient relief of the people under their control, as will be discussed in Chapter 9.

Sen's argument is one with which, on the whole, I agree. As the four cases in Part II show, twenty-first century famines and severe malnutrition occurred in countries that either never had democracies (North Korea), or that changed from formal democracy to authoritarian dictatorship (Zimbabwe and Venezuela). It seems, however, that democracy itself is not sufficient to prevent famine. A formal democratic system, permitting elections, a free press, and opposition political parties might still be one in which there is political corruption, clientelism, and other such impediments to concern for citizens' right to food. The democracy might simply be too new and unconsolidated to prevent famine, lacking institutional capacity even if it possesses political will (Rubin 2011). And those most in need of protection or fulfillment of their right to adequate nutrition may be those least likely to have influence over the government, hence the food insecurity of many households in Canada and the US, especially Aboriginal households, which I discuss in Chapter 11. Finally, as Israel shows, Sen's maxim must also be modified by attention to democracies' practices of warfare, conquest, and colonialism. Israel was a democracy, but it was an occupying power in the West Bank and exercised effective control over Gaza: Significant malnutrition pervaded both territories.

In this chapter I discuss three cases in which Britain and Canada, both formal democracies, nevertheless ignored, caused, or tolerated famines in countries they conquered and/or colonized. The three cases are the Irish famine of the 1840s, starvation in Germany after WWI, and starvation and malnutrition among Canada's Aboriginal population in the 1870s. The debate on the Irish famine of the 1840s focuses, in Marcus' terms, on whether it was a consequence of intentional or reckless behavior by the British government, or whether it was significantly exacerbated by British indifference (Marcus 2003). After the November 11, 1918 armistice, the democratic British government imposed policies on Germany that resulted in the starvation of an estimated quarter-million civilians: This was intentional faminogenesis for the purpose of forcing Germany to sign a peace treaty. Finally, Canada recklessly capitalized on famine among Aboriginal people in order to settle its Western region with Europeans.

These cases show that democracies can perpetrate state food crimes. Within a democratic state, those who have or can garner political influence can protect themselves against such crimes while those in conquered territories and colonies or those denied political influence cannot. It is not the fact of democracy itself that prevents state food crimes; it is the capacity of those subject to such crimes to react politically against their governors that prevents their starvation or nutritional insecurity. Democracies sometimes induce famine or at minimum are indifferent to it, in cases of warfare, conquest, and colonialism.

Colonialism: The Irish Famine

Ó Gráda notes that there are some "half exceptions to Sen's claim," including "perhaps Ireland in the 1840s (a free and sometimes vocal press, but only a middle-class franchise)" (Ó Gráda 2009, 231). A standard estimate is that 1.1 million of Ireland's 8.2 million people starved or died of disease between 1845 and 1855, while another two million emigrated, many hundreds of thousands to England and the rest to Canada and the United States (Kelly 2012, 2). Revisionist historians think that the figure of one million dead is too high, while Irish nationalists think it too low (Ó Gráda 2009, 93). Sen's estimate is that famine killed one fifth of Ireland's total population and forced another fifth to emigrate: This was the highest proportion of a population ever killed in a famine (Sen 1999, 39, 170). At the time, Ireland was officially part of the United Kingdom but was actually a colony of Britain, which at the time was a quasi-democracy, universal suffrage for males not being introduced there until 1918. Ireland was ruled from London and did not have its own democratic political structure, although some Irish males could vote.

Writing in the early 1840s, before the famine had taken hold, Frederick Engels described the terrible poverty in which Irish peasants already lived.

The Irish people is . . . held in crushing poverty . . . These people live in the most wretched clay huts, scarcely good enough for cattle-pens, have scant food all winter long . . . [T]hey have potatoes half enough for thirty weeks in the year, and the rest of the year nothing. When the time comes in the spring at which this provision reaches its end . . . wife and children go forth to beg and tramp the country . . . Meanwhile, the husband, after planting potatoes for the next year, goes in search of work . . . This is the condition in which nine-tenths of the Irish country folks live. They are poor as church mice, wear the most wretched rags . . . [T]here are in Ireland 2,300,000 persons who could not live without public or private assistance – or 27 percent of the whole population paupers! (Engels 1969 [first English edition 1892: first German edition 1845], 296–97)

Engels was describing "normal" Irish poverty, before the actual famine. But this "normal" poverty had been created by factors that predisposed the Irish poor to famine, especially expulsion from their lands by English and Scottish landlords (Butterly and Shepherd 2010, 46). This resulted in turn in over-reliance on the potato for food, as peasants no longer had enough land to grow the various crops that had sustained them in earlier centuries.

The famine itself was caused in the first instance by the potato blight, a disease that wiped out Ireland's staple food; one-third of the population was dependent on the potato on the eve of the famine (Ó Gráda 2009, 77). The Irish turned to imported maize (corn), not their preferred food, as well as "famine foods... leaves, shoots, pods, seeds, fruits, meats, or vegetables not usually consumed" (Ó Gráda 2009, 73). The fishing industry was underdeveloped, so the Irish could not adopt fish as a staple food (Ó Gráda 2009, 76). During the famine there were food riots in which shops, warehouses, and bakeries were looted; the incidence of burglary and robbery quintupled; and many of those who were arrested died of hunger in jail (Ó Gráda 2009, 53). First to die were vagrants, followed by landless laborers, and then small farmers (Ó Gráda 2009, 90); eventually, even some of the wealthier farmers and landed gentry died (Kelly 2012, 325). Like all famines, the Irish one had a class dimension: Those who lacked Sen's entitlements, as discussed in Chapter 1 (Sen 1981), and could neither produce their food nor buy it died first.

The Irish famine was not state-induced, as the Ukrainian, Chinese, and Cambodian famines discussed in Chapter 2 were. No one planned it or instituted policies that would cause it. Instead, potato blight ruined the 1845 and 1846 crops. At the same time, though, some of Ireland's higher quality food was exported to England; Sen calls this a "food countermovement" noting that such counter-movements are not uncommon when the local food supply slumps but the food that does exist can sell at higher prices elsewhere. "Ship after ship – laden with wheat, oats, cattle, pigs, eggs, and butter – sailed down the Shannon [river] bound for well-fed England from famine-stricken Ireland" (Sen 1999, 172). On the other hand, the British colonial rulers eventually did try to buy food for Ireland from America, but there was a worldwide shortage at the time and other famine-stricken European countries such as Belgium, France, and Germany were also trying to buy food (Kelly 2012, 129). In Marcus' terms, then, this was perhaps famine by indifference in the early stages when the British did little to alleviate it, and famine by incompetence when the British tried to alleviate it but took measures that did not provide enough food. In neither case did the British rulers intend that the Irish should starve.

An important cause of the Irish famine was alienation of the English rulers from their Irish subjects (Sen 1999, 173). An example of such cultural alienation was the philosophy to which a small group of influential men in the British cabinet and bureaucracy adhered at the time. Called "Moralism," this philosophy taught that people should work hard and take responsibility for themselves. The Moralists thought that famine would teach the "lazy" and "indolent" Irish a lesson, so that they would avoid what the Moralists considered to be the causes of their poverty – sexual promiscuity (resulting in large numbers of children needing to be fed) and alcoholism as well as laziness. They thought that it was too easy to cultivate potatoes, so the Irish had never learned to work hard (Kelly 2012, 91, 25).

Moralist ideology was supplemented by another ideology, that of market fundamentalism. The influential business journal, *The Economist,* said "It is no man's business to provide for another," noting that "[for] the government to supply the people with work is just as injurious as . . . to supply them with food" (Kelly 2012, 156). Food relief for the Irish, *The Economist* believed, would shift resources from "the more meritorious to the less" (Ó Gráda 2009, 204–05). The Prime Minister at the time, Lord John Russell, worried that if the British were to distribute free food, it would upset the Irish markets and purveyors of food would be unable to make a profit; this was an early example of the difficulties of providing food aid. Russell thought the peasants should work for their food, so for the first two years of the famine he established "public works" projects (breaking rocks to build useless roads) to provide employment. "Lazy" Irish men, starving and half-naked (as they had sold their clothes to buy food) marched miles every day to earn a pittance to buy food for themselves and their families, many dying en route (Kelly 2012, 173, 178).

Ó Gráda comments that the Irish starved in part because of "a dogmatic faith on the part of the ruling elite in markets as a mechanism for relieving famine." As an Irish commentator said at the time, the Irish "died of political economy" (Ó Gráda 2009, 158, 205). Political economy also permitted massive land clearances in 1848–49, evicting peasants from their homes, which they were too sick and weak to protest (Ó Gráda 2009, 55). All this took place under embryonic democratic rule in Britain, in which very limited suffrage (about 18 percent of adult males) had just been introduced under the 1832 Reform Act (British Library undated), it was possible to vote the ruling party out of power, and there was freedom of the press.

Self-interest – what we would now call corruption – also played a part in British government policy. Several members of Cabinet were landowners in Ireland. They thought the famine would enable them to remove peasants from their properties so that they could convert the small-scale peasant farms to large-scale commercial farming; thus, they took the opportunity of the famine to engage in mass evictions of peasants who could not pay their rent. These clearances also relieved them of their formal obligation to provide food for their own tenants, an obligation that had been imposed on them by the Poor Law Extension Act of 1845 (Butterly and Shepherd 2010, 45). Landlords also wanted to get rid of peasants because, as landlords, they had to pay a "poor rate" (or tax) that steadily increased as the famine progressed, and they were also responsible to pay the rate on behalf of their tenant peasants. The fewer the peasants on their land, the less tax they had to pay (Kelly 2012, 212, 326).

Another hypothesis about the famine is that one of its causes was outright racism. The British viewed the Irish as a separate race, Celts, inferior to British Anglo-Saxons; the influential essayist Thomas Carlyle referred to them as "human swinery" (Painter 2010, 133–35, 163); other referred to them as "white negroes," "apes," and "human chimpanzees" (Butterly and Shepherd 2010, 182). Far from being a liberal counter-weight to these views, the free English press reinforced them throughout the famine, portraying the Irish as thuggish, lazy, and dirty, in effect the "undeserving poor," as opposed to the deserving, hard-working English industrial classes (De Nie 1998). It might be difficult for contemporary readers to understand the extent of racism against the Irish in the nine-teenth century, yet the stereotype that the Irish were brutal, ignorant, lazy people who lived with pigs was widespread.

Such stereotypes justified both colonialism and famine; if such infe-rior people starved, it was largely because of their own laziness. Racism interacted with the Malthusian philosophical position that there were too many people in the world and that periodic culling of the population, for example via famine, would keep the number of people and the food supply in balance (Butterly and Shepherd 2010, 35–36). These "too many" were of course in Ireland where, it was thought, Catholicism was responsible for the irresponsibly large numbers of children in Irish fam-ilies (Butterly and Shepherd 2010, 42). The Irish were also blamed for their tendency to eat potatoes, as if this were a cultural choice rather than the result of necessity (Sen 1999, 174–75).

Although the British did make some efforts to assist the Irish, their orig-inal priority was to alleviate famine in Scotland (Kelly 2012, 168) where more men could vote, confirming Sen's argument that in democracies voters can remove governments that do not alleviate famine. Moreover, the Irish system of poor relief was not used much during the first years of the famine. Unlike in Britain proper, there was no tradition of relief (Kelly 2012, 51). The poor relief system required that entire families enter a workhouse as a unit, although they were then split up so that husbands and wives, parents and children, and brothers and sisters would never see each other again; thus, families were very hesitant to avail themselves of it. By the end of the famine, however, the workhouses were overcrowded with people who had entered in desperation to obtain food.

There was at first much official resistance to "outdoor relief" (Kelly 2012, 180); that is, to the establishment of soup kitchens to feed the starving without obliging them to enter the workhouse: The British finally agreed to soup kitchens. At one point in 1847 soup kitchens fed three million people a day (Kelly 2012, 316), but they were not continued through later famine years. The British also insisted that the Irish themselves finance famine relief, but even if Irish landlords and gentry had all cooperated to pay the poor rate, there was not enough money in Ireland to pay for all the food that was needed (Kelly 2012, 50, 124, 328, passim).

Not everyone was indifferent to the plight of the starving Irish. Kelly (Kelly 2012) uses memoirs and diaries of observers and relief officials who described the horrible conditions in which the Irish lived and died. Some were so upset at their inability to do anything to help that they killed themselves. Whatever internal opposition to British policies in Ireland was manifested by voters and a free press, this was enough to focus attention on the Irish but not to alleviate their plight. While Britain may have been a partial democracy in the 1840s, Ireland was a colony whose landlords and officials may have had the right to vote in British elections, but the mass of whose inhabitants had no such rights.

Warfare: The WWI British Blockade of Germany

In the past, democracies were not averse to starving their enemies. By definition, enemy populations had no votes or other capacities to formally influence government policies. The British treatment of German civilians between the Armistice of November 11, 1918, and the Treaty of Versailles that formally ended WWI on June 28, 1919, was an example of such utter disregard of enemy civilians.

During the war, the British had imposed an effective blockade on food exports to Germany, preventing it from importing food not only from its actual enemies but also from neutral countries. Britain's allies joined the blockade, including the US as of 1917. Instead of ending it in November 1918, though, Britain and its allies forced Germany to agree to an extended food blockade as a condition of armistice: The blockade was not terminated until July 12, 1919, after the peace treaty was signed (Vincent 1985, 50, 71). Prewar Germany had imported a third of its food supply, which the wartime blockade cut off; the German army had priority access to the food that remained (Vincent 1985, 20). German mismanagement, caused in part by officials' initial optimism that the war would not last long, combined with a failure of the potato crop to cause famine in 1916–17 (Vincent 1985, 126), although there were regional disparities in food shortages (Offer 2000, 177) and some places, such as Berlin, managed a rationing system that protected their citizens from starvation (Allen 1998). Food riots occurred daily as of late 1915 (Jackson 1996, 568).

The Germans were short of fertilizer, which was also blockaded by the British (Van der Kloot 2003, 187–88). Moreover, they were as short of food for livestock as they were of food for humans; thus, the supply of livestock deteriorated. Nevertheless, many farmers preferred to sell meat, the price of which was not regulated, over grains, whose price was regulated; thus, they fed scarce grains to animals (Jackson 1996, 567). Workhorses were taken over by the military, to whom farm tools also had to be surrendered (Vincent 1985, 129). Despite the use of captive Belgians, Frenchmen and Poles as substitute laborers (Loewenberg 1996, 555) farms also suffered from a severe shortage of workers, as many farm workers were drafted (Jackson 1996, 569).

The Germans turned to turnips as their staple food and malnutrition and starvation became common, especially in institutions such as jails and asylums. German women, already overburdened by the addition of war work to the normal work of caring for their children, wasted much energy standing in line for hours for food. By 1918 the German diet consisted of only about 1,000 calories per day: Fats and meats were 12 and 18 percent respectively of the prewar diet (Vincent 1985, 49). Children ate rotting food and drank unsanitary milk (Vincent 1985, 143). Many children starved to death, tuberculosis was rampant, and adults lived on rations that hardly began to cover their basic nutritional needs. An American report stated that by 1918 the German population as a whole was 20 percent below normal weight, and that child mortality had risen 30 percent over 1913 (Vincent 1985, 81).

At the time, it appears, a complete food blockade might have violated customary international law. The law of blockade had a long history, starting after the Dutch blockaded Flanders in 1584: Traditionally, the principles governing blockade included respect for the rights of neutral countries to continue trading. In 1909 the world's major maritime powers met in London to issue a formal Protocol on the law of blockade, but the British House of Lords did not ratify it; thus, when WWI began, the

British had not signed any law limiting their right to blockade Germany (Fraunces 1992, 895–96). In any event, the Protocol permitted complete blockade of enemy ports, including blockade of ships from neutral nations. It also permitted foodstuffs and grain and forage (for animals) to be treated as "contraband of war" as they were "susceptible of use in war as well as for purposes of peace" (Naval Conference of London 1909, Articles 5, 24, 1 and 2).

Engaged as they were in a total war, defined as "wartime conditions in which both belligerents expend most of their available resources to win the war" (Fraunces 1992, 909, note 89), by 1916 the British no longer distinguished between the German military and civilians (McDermott 1986, 70). For its part, Germany also tried less successfully to blockade Britain (Fraunces 1992, 900). The British had also endured a shortage of food, and death and disease increased at home as tuberculosis rates rose, resulting in rationing in 1917. This was in part because of a worldwide drought, but the average British citizen blamed Germany for food shortages; thus, it was easy in revenge to justify blockading Germans' access to food (Vincent 1985, 9–12).

The post-Armistice blockade was even worse than the one during the war, as the British now prevented German ships from travelling from one German port to another to transfer food from surplus to deficit areas. The British also demanded that Germany surrender its rolling stock, so that it could not transport food over land (Vincent 1985, 134), and they prohibited fishing in the North Sea and Baltic (Van der Kloot 2003, 191). Food from other countries meant for Germany was still blockaded: Shiploads of food from the US spoiled in Dutch ports awaiting permission to enter Germany (Ó Gráda 2009, 230).

As a result of the tightening of the food blockade, slaughter of animals in Germany increased during the Armistice-Peace Treaty interlude: between April 1918 and April 1919 approximately 250,000 milk cows were slaughtered (Vincent 1985, 135). The malnutrition already suffered during the war undermined Germans' resistance to diseases such as "tuberculosis, rickets, influenza, dysentery, scurvy, . . . and hunger edema" (Vincent 1985, 137), also contributing to Germany's high mortality rate during the Spanish flu epidemic of 1918–19. At the end of the war, Germany's health office calculated that 763,000 civilian deaths were a result of the blockade since 1914, not including the 150,000 deaths from flu (Vincent 1985, 141), although Offer questions this, estimating the excess deaths at 424,000, plus 209,000 from flu (Offer 1989, 34, cited in Jackson, 571). Howard concluded that the post-armistice food blockade alone caused about a quarter of a million civilian deaths (Howard 1993, 162). The normal post-war surge in births did not occur:

The 1924 birth rate was still 23.9 percent lower than 1914 birth rate (Vincent 1985, 146).

The US was less intransigent than Britain about maintaining the blockade. Herbert Hoover, then Chairman of the American Food Administration, worked to supply the starving Germans with food: The Americans feared that starvation would result in anarchy, or support of the Bolshevism that was sweeping Germany at the time (Vincent 1985, 65, 81). The British, by contrast, deliberately continued their blockade as a way to force the post-war German government to reduce the influence of the Soldiers' and Workers' Councils that had spontaneously formed at the end of the war and that, in British eyes, threatened a Bolshevik takeover (Jackson 1996, 573; Howard 1993, 170). Meantime, some Europeans supported the blockade: Prime Minister Clemençeau of France said there were "twenty million Germans too many," according to notes taken by a German diplomat. The French and British also prevented Germany from buying food with gold, claiming that it was needed for reparations (Vincent 1985, 85–86).

Nor was this terrible famine without long-term consequences, as the American president, Woodrow Wilson, foresaw. On Armistice Day in a speech to Congress, Wilson said "hunger does not breed reform: it breeds madness and all the ugly distempers that make an ordered life impossible" (Vincent 1985, 72). Indeed, the famine may have contributed to the rise of Nazism, as young men who had starved as children joined the Nazi party in the 1920s and 1930s, seeking a nationalist solution to the problems they had faced both as children and later as unemployed youths (Loewenberg 1971, 1465). Moreover, having been blockaded from the west during WWI, German decision-makers decided to take over land in the east that would provide them with food (Vincent 1985, 150).

The relevance of the British blockade to this work lies in its using starvation as a weapon of war despite being a formal democracy itself. One reason for this might have been the underdeveloped state of British democracy in the early twentieth century. Another may have been that during periods of war, the press is constrained, as under the 1914 Defense of the Realm Act (Government of the United Kingdom 1914), and patriotism becomes a higher value than usual. Indeed, in 1919 a campaigner trying to bring attention to the starvation in Germany was fined £5 for distributing a pamphlet entitled "A Starving Baby" in Trafalgar Square (Girling 2006, July 2). In any event, while democratic states may not deliberately starve those whom they consider their own citizens, they seem willing to starve or to tolerate starvation among others, as the treatment of nineteenth-century Aboriginal populations in Canada also shows.

Settler Colonialism: Canada

Settler colonialism, in which settlers from colonial powers take over land from colonized peoples, is a particularly intransigent type of colonialism, as the individuals who take over the land do not wish to give it up. Chapter 5 discusses the aftermath of European settler colonialism in Zimbabwe, where Africans were pushed off their land by whites during the colonial period. In North America, the demographic predominance of settlers over Aboriginal peoples by the nineteenth century meant that independence for the colonized was not a possibility: rather, they were marginalized and sometimes almost exterminated during the period of settlement. Such was the case in Canada's west, where famine among Aboriginal peoples – exacerbated by central government unwillingness to aid its victims – facilitated European settlement. In the 1870s one-third of the original Aboriginal population of the west was estimated to have died in a period of six years, leaving about 15,000 people, as a brilliant book by James Daschuk, on which this section is largely based, documents (Daschuk 2013, 172). This was a period during which many other populations worldwide also starved, as both colonizers and independent governments either ignored or were incapable of compensating for the effects of extremely adverse weather on food production (Davis 2002).

This relatively small famine was nevertheless an intrinsic part of Canada's history. It was instrumental to Canada's conquest of the Aboriginal peoples of its west, facilitating the opening up of that vast territory to settlement by European immigrants and the linking of the country "from sea to shining sea" via the Canadian Pacific Railway. Aboriginal societies in the west had previously been relatively self-sufficient hunters and had been able to negotiate economic and political relations with incoming Europeans on relatively equal terms. While they had periodically suffered famine since European fur traders first penetrated their territories in the seventeenth century, Europeans had also been victims of these famines, which were usually caused by adverse climatic conditions or by over-hunting of game (Daschuk 2013, 53). The famine of the 1870s and 1880s, however, was partially caused by political decisions, while its amelioration – or lack thereof – was certainly a political matter.

The immediate cause of this famine was the destruction of the Aboriginal peoples' staple food, the bison. This food was so healthy that anthropologists have concluded that nineteenth-century bison hunters were the tallest people in the world (Daschuk 2013, 8). It is unclear what caused the bison's destruction. One cause appears to have been over-hunting by Aboriginal people, while another was that as (European-owned) commercial cattle-ranching developed, bison were driven out by competition for forage. High European demand for bison skins and meat might also have been a cause (Walton 2007, July 31). Yet another cause may have been the expansion of the railroad in the northwest United States (Daschuk 2013, 102), but all this may also have been affected by environmental factors.

The spread of tuberculosis exacerbated the detrimental effects of food shortages. This was not deliberate, but it contributed to a famine/disease nexus similar to the HIV/AIDS "new variant famine" in Zimbabwe in the 2000s, discussed in Chapter 5. In the Canadian case, medical authorities first did not know how tuberculosis was spread among humans. Later, they did not know that bovine tuberculosis, rampant among bison in the late nineteenth century and then transmitted to cattle, was also transmittable to human beings (Daschuk 2013, 102). Thus, tragically, the very bison and cattle that Aboriginal peoples needed to eat caused their illnesses. Diseases first contracted from Europeans and then from bison and cattle meant that there were fewer hunters available to find food.

In the 1870s and 80s the Aboriginal peoples of western Canada were reduced to eating their horses and dogs, the carcasses of wolves, and wild roots (Daschuk 2013, 109–11). With few if any substitutes for bison meat, they became dependent on the government, which threatened to withdraw rations in order to force the Aboriginal peoples to accept treaties (Daschuk 2013, 114). In these treaties they gave up substantial portions of their traditional lands in return for small areas of reserved lands, food, and sometimes other goods such as "medicine chests." At one point, the government ordered that food would only be given to Aboriginal people on reserves, then forbade those living on reserves from providing food to those still living off-reserve; that is, to those who had not yet surrendered their traditional sovereignty to the Canadian state (Daschuk 2013, 122).

The Aboriginal people were supposed to learn to farm on their reserves under the watchful eyes of "Indian agents" (government bureaucrats), eventually to become self-sufficient agriculturalists. Yet they were also confined to their reserves against their will, only permitted to leave if they had an official pass. The pass system meant that they could not look for work off the reserve which might enable them to buy food: it also meant that Aboriginal traders could no longer participate in the emerging capitalist economy of the west (Daschuk 2013, 159–61). Thus, the Aboriginal peoples of the west were now safely (from the point of view of white authorities) confined to reserves, no longer roaming the countryside for game or interfering with plans for European settlements. Meantime, famine continued. As Daschuk concludes, "Communities that entered into treaties assumed that the state would protect them from famine and socioeconomic catastrophe, yet in less than a decade the 'protections' afforded by treaties became the means by which the state subjugated the treaty Indian population" (Daschuk 2013, 125).

The official Canadian response to this famine was paltry. As in the case of the Irish famine, officials debated how much food Aboriginal people should be given. Some worried about "lazy Indians" (as Aboriginal peoples were then called) and argued that food should be given in exchange for work except for those who were "really starving" (Daschuk 2013, 111), but the Indians were so weakened that work was impossible. In the cold Canadian climate Aboriginal women and children were often completely naked, having sold their clothes for food; many women submitted to rape by white men as the only means to acquire food (Daschuk 2013, 153). Yet food lay rotting in storage on reserves until officials decided that their inhabitants were sick and starving enough that some food should be distributed (Daschuk 2013, 185). Officials actually in the Canadian West who witnessed this starvation tried without success to persuade bureaucrats and politicians in the capital city, Ottawa, thousands of miles away, of the severity of the famine, just as officials on the ground in Ireland had tried to persuade bureaucrats and politicians in London to provide more relief. Meanwhile, corruption and fraud deprived Aboriginal people of food meant for them (Daschuk 2013, 140). After a rebellion by some of the remaining Aboriginal peoples in the West in the early 1880s, the government retaliated by cutting off even more food rations (Daschuk 2013, xxii, 163).

The general viewpoint of government officials was that Aboriginals should be given just enough food to prevent their actual death by starvation, but no more. In 1880 Prime Minister Sir John A. Macdonald assured Parliament that the government would be "rigid, even stingy" in distributing food, refusing it "until the Indians were on the verge of starvation, to reduce the expense" (Daschuk 2013, 134). The willingness to provide food when Aboriginals were on the verge of starvation was driven by fear of scandal in eastern Canada, if the government actually tolerated starvation (Daschuk 2013, 136). A free press among the white Canadian male elite acted as a brake on the worst form of neglect.

Daschuk describes the Canadian government's attitude as "indifference" (Daschuk 2013, 105). This is a generous interpretation of the government's actions and decisions. Although the famine was not caused by any actions it intentionally took, Ottawa did contribute to the famine's prolongation, choosing to reduce rations because, in the perception of some officials, Aboriginals were refusing to work for food. It also chose to reduce or suspend rations in order to force Aboriginals to accept treaties and move onto reserves, thus vacating their traditional lands in favor of the railroad and European settlement. Faced with overwhelming evidence of starvation relayed to it by missionaries, traders, doctors, and government officials, the central government nevertheless permitted Aboriginal people to starve.

Nor did Aboriginals starve only in the west. A "widespread pattern of Indian famine" also occurred in the 1870s in the eastern parts of the country; for example, among Aboriginals at Ungava Bay, just east of Hudson Bay (Shewell 2004, 75). These Aboriginals had no treaty with the Canadian government and as one official claimed, "the Government is under no obligation except on humanitarian grounds . . . to supply Indians with food": this official also claimed that "the Indians are prone to greatly exaggerate their condition at times" (Shewell 2004, 76). Canadian officials witnessed horrendous starvation with little compassion but with an attentive eye to national accounts. No doubt the logistics of predicting famine and delivering relief were very difficult in a new country lacking adequate transportation to the north and to remote Aboriginal settlements. The difference, however, was that Aboriginal peoples were subjects of – but in no way citizens participating in – the Canadian state. However recently formed that state and however difficult nineteenth century logistics, it possessed some capacity to fulfill the nutritional needs of its subject population, yet did not do so. Canadian officials were adamant that relief was a privilege, not a right. As one member of Parliament advocated in 1886, the best policy was to give Aboriginal peoples only "enough [food] to keep them alive" (Shewell 2004, 41).

Various Canadian treaties with Aboriginal bands supposedly guaranteed that in return for giving up land, Aboriginals would be ensured adequate nutrition, but parsimonious government officials were reluctant to spend money on food. Moreover, officials worried that Aboriginal people would never become self-reliant if they could rely on relief. Stereotypes of Aboriginals as "lazy," "shiftless," and "alcoholic" convinced these officials that Aboriginals preferred not to support themselves, notwithstanding their knowledge that traditional ways of life based on hunting, fishing, and some agriculture had been eroded by the encroachment of Euro-Canadian settlers. Able-bodied Aboriginals were expected to contribute to their own and their families' support via hunting and fishing even in the face of ever increasing restrictions on these activities, restrictions that in some cases were not lifted until late twentieth century legal decisions forced the state to adhere to long-ago treaty provisions.

Until well into the twentieth century, policy debates about "relief" for Aboriginals were confined to responsibilities to Aboriginal widows, children, the disabled, and the aged. To be fair, this was also the focus of relief for Canadians as a whole, conforming to the principle that able-bodied men should be able to support themselves and their families (Shewell 2004, 90). Nevertheless, policy-makers argued over whether government was responsible to allocate Aboriginal people the same level of relief as Euro-Canadians; municipalities, provinces, and the federal government argued over who was responsible to provide what while Aboriginals, if no longer starving, were suffering from malnutrition and severe nutritional insecurity.

Meantime, diseases related to nutritional deficiencies increased Aboriginals' death rates, as they had ever since Europeans began to infiltrate what later became Canada. As Shewell put it, in a perhaps unintentional reference to the Irish famine, reserves became "workhouses defined by geography rather than by walls" (Shewell 2004, 167). As late as 1947, a welfare official stated that "the scale of relief supplied to able-bodied Indians must err on the parsimonious rather than on the generous side . . . relief is not the right of any Indian . . . in no instance are the quantities of relief allowed to be sufficient to remove the incentive to obtain employment" (Shewell 2004, 231). Paternalistic debates discussed whether cash benefits, rather than benefits in kind, might discourage proper nutrition among Aboriginals because they might make poor decisions about how to spend their money (Shewell 2004, 245).

Some scholars think that human rights are a "Western" invention that does not, and should not, pertain to Aboriginal peoples because human rights are individualistic and anti-communitarian, undermining Aboriginal collectivities (Kulchyski 2013). But it is precisely the lack of human rights – especially civil and political rights – that enabled the Canadian state to treat Aboriginal people so badly for so long, a fact that was noted by Britain's Aborigines Protection Society as long ago as 1846: "their [Indians'] position is anomalous, inasmuch as they do not participate in some of the most important rights of British subjects – . . . they take no part in elections or other public affairs . . . in which respect their position is far worse than that of any foreign emigrant" (quoted in Dickinson and Wotherspoon 1992, 410).

For many decades after Canada became a country in 1867, Indians were legal minors, subjected to "paternal supervision" by the state and the local white officials responsible for them (Shewell 2004, 36). By 1898 almost all white males could vote in provincial elections, a prerequisite to the right to vote in federal elections, but most provinces specifically barred Indians living on reserves from voting (Satzewich and

Wotherspoon 1993, 220–23); thus, to vote, they had to abandon their communities. In 1920 the federal government made the franchise universal except for Aboriginal peoples and "racial" minorities such as Chinese and Japanese Canadians. Not until the Canadian Bill of Rights was introduced in 1960 could all Aboriginals, including those living on reserves, vote in federal elections (Satzewich and Wotherspoon 1993, 221).

Aboriginals were also denied freedom of association. In 1927 the government passed an amendment to the 1876 Indian Act that prohibited Indians from collecting funds for advancement of land claims (Berger 1981, 235). This prohibition was introduced after the Allied Indian Tribes of British Columbia presented a list of demands for land and hunting rights to the federal government in 1923 (Frideres 1988, 103, 260; Shewell 2004, 157). At the same time, Indians in Ontario attempted to form a League of Indians of Canada (Satzewich and Wotherspoon 1993, 228), whose objectives included hunting rights and economic development on reserves, as well as greater freedom from government supervision and the right to vote (York 1989, 246). The 1927 Act also included an amendment that prohibited all national organization by Indians (Satzewich and Wotherspoon 1993, 226) and was exacerbated by the refusal of the Department of Indian Affairs – which controlled Indian bands' finances – to release funds for travel to meetings (York 1989, 246). When hereditary Iroquois Chief Deskeheh petitioned the League of Nations for sovereignty, the government stationed a permanent police presence on his reserve and deprived hereditary chiefs and councilors of their positions (York 1989, 249). The ban on Aboriginal political activism was not removed until 1951 (Kulchyski 2013, 82).

Meantime, the pass system, never implemented legally, nevertheless was rigidly enforced, prohibiting Aboriginal freedom of movement (York 1989, 248), while restrictions on commerce meant that Aboriginals could not participate as equals in Canada's evolving capitalist economy (Satzewich and Wotherspoon 1993, 222). Even service in Canada's armed forces – generally a path to citizenship for males – did not mean that Aboriginals accrued equal rights compared to other veterans. Despite their WWII military service, Micmac Indians in Nova Scotia were pleading for rations in 1953, in part because they did not receive the land grants available to non-Aboriginal veterans (York 1989, 67).

Thus, Aboriginal Canadians have been formally entitled to the full range of civil and political rights for only fifty-five years. Canada's democracy until 1960 resembled that of apartheid South Africa, but with proportions reversed. In South Africa, a small minority of whites ruled over a large majority of blacks, while in Canada the large majority of whites ruled over the small Aboriginal population. It is difficult to avoid the conclusion that for most of its existence, the government of Canada considered Aboriginal peoples to be "superfluous" (Dickinson and Wotherspoon 1992, 411). Canada's functioning democracy, Sen's criterion for avoiding famine, excluded Aboriginal Canadians.

Conclusion

As Chapter 2 showed, the most well-known state-induced famines of the twentieth century took place in communist countries, the Soviet Union, China, and Cambodia. These three famines are negative cases confirming Sen's thesis that famines do not take place in democracies; none of these countries was remotely democratic. Of the four contemporary cases I discuss in Part II, three were not democracies at the time of their food crises. North Korea was a totalitarian state heavily influenced by the communist ideology of Stalinist Soviet Union and Maoist China. Venezuela and Zimbabwe had been formal electoral democracies, but they deteriorated into dictatorship (Zimbabwe) and quasi-dictatorship (Venezuela).

Nevertheless, as the British and Canadian case studies in this chapter show, democracies are not exempt from the charge that they too ignore the food needs of those under their control or over whom they have temporary power. Democracies can cause, ignore, or tolerate famines in countries that they conquer or colonize. Although it did make some attempts to provide relief to the Irish, on the whole Britain tolerated famine in Ireland. It actually caused famine in post-WWI Germany, a country for which it had no responsibility and whose citizens had no say in British affairs. Ireland was a colony at the time of the famine; Germany had just been defeated in war.

Recognizing, presumably, that famines could occur in territories colonized by democracies, Sen noted that "there is hardly any case in which a famine has occurred in a country that is *independent* and democratic" (Sen 1995, 217, italics added). But despite being independent and democratic, Canada tolerated and ignored starvation among its Aboriginal peoples. Similarly, as Chapter 7 will show, Israel was a democracy, but its democracy did not extend to electoral rights for the West Bank Palestinians whom it conquered in 1967 and whose land it had since colonized. In that sense and others, the situation of Palestinians resembled that of Aboriginal Canadians in the past and present: in both cases, colonial powers stripped colonized populations of their land, undermining their abilities to support themselves, and simultaneously denying them the civil and political rights that they needed to defend themselves.

Democracy, political opposition, and free media are not sufficient to prevent famine; human rights other than those Sen mentions are also necessary. I do not question Sen's theory of entitlement failure, which appears to be a sufficient description of what happens in some famines, whether or not politically caused. My focus is the political decisions themselves, the policies that flow from them, and the human rights that individuals need to resist these policies. While it appears that full protection of human rights requires a democratic political system, democracies do not necessarily promote the full range of human rights, nor do they do so for everyone, often leaving rightless a subset of citizens. Neither the starving Irish nor Aboriginal Canadians possessed the full range of human rights at the time that they were suffering from severe malnutrition. And the Germans who starved during and after WWI were under assault by a democracy carrying out a total war, with no regard whatsoever for its enemies' nutritional needs.

Landman distinguishes between "thin" and "thick" democracy. Thin democracy is merely procedural, allowing contested elections with political participation (Landman 2013, 26–27). Britain and Canada were not even thin democracies when some of their colonial subjects and enemies suffered massive malnutrition and starvation. Even if some propertied males could vote in Britain in the 1840s and in Canada after 1867, the famine victims themselves, living in colonies, had no vote. Landman's next level of democracy is liberal, including civil and political rights, the rule of law, and the right to property (Landman 2013, 27–29). In warfare and under colonialism, famine victims do not enjoy liberal democracy. Finally, the "thickest" kind of democracy is social democracy, in which a state endeavors to protect economic human rights, including the right to food (Landman 2013, 29–31). In effect, Landman categorizes the thinness or thickness of democracy according to the kinds and number of human rights it protects.

Sen's conception of democracy appears to be Landman's thin procedural type, allowing contestation and political participation. However, as I will show in Chapter 10, even if freedom of the press and freedom of association are included as aspects of procedural democracy, this is not sufficient to guard against food crises. While a free press is required, unless significant parts of it perceive the starving as members of the community deserving of compassion and assistance the press may reinforce, rather than undermine, faminogenic policies, as Ireland shows. The rule of law is also necessary but requires judges imbued with liberal rights principles, not merely judges willing to uphold illiberal laws. Depending on its type and to whom it is extended democracy may provide a partial defense against famine but not a sufficient one.

Other human rights are also important as defenses against famine and malnutrition. They include the right to citizenship, to be seen as an equal citizen in society; the right to own property, a right necessary to outsiders and the poor as well as rich insiders; the right to work; and freedom of mobility. Neither the Irish nor aboriginal Canadians were citizens of Britain or Canada; Germans civilians were enemies of the country that starved them. Irish peasants had lost much of their property before the famine began and were heavily dependent on English landowners; Aboriginals in Canada lost their territorial rights to hunting, fishing, and agricultural grounds before and during the famines that led to their confinement on reserves. The Irish were comparatively fortunate in that those who had enough money to pay for passage could emigrate relatively easily to England, Canada, and the United States, though the very poor had to stay home and starve. By contrast, Aboriginal Canadians were confined to reserves, and Germans immediately after WWI were confined to their own country, unable to move elsewhere. Without access to land, neither the Irish nor Aboriginal Canadians could work; confined for decades after the famine of the 1870s to their reserves, Aboriginals were also precluded from taking part in Canada's emerging capitalist economy. Mobility rights, property rights, citizenship rights, and the right to work are all necessary to prevent state food crimes.

The cases in Part II variously illustrate the importance of these human rights to famine prevention. Their enjoyment lessens the possibility of state-induced famine, as in North Korea and possibly Zimbabwe; malnutrition, as in the West Bank and Gaza; and nutritional insecurity, as in Venezuela. Freedom from hunger, though, also requires a global sense of responsibility. Yet as Chapters 8 and 9 show, this global sense of responsibility is weak and fragmented. Neither international law nor the principles of humanitarian intervention are strong enough to ameliorate famines, in the face of political resistance from the governors of famine or food-deficient areas. The major protections against famine are internal: countries must develop both real commitment to human rights for all citizens, and the institutional capacity necessary to guard against malnutrition and nutritional insecurity, as Chapters 10 and 11 explain. These long-term moral, ideological, political, and economic developments may be assisted by a new international treaty on the right to food, as I suggest in Chapter 12, but such a treaty will hardly be sufficient in the absence of serious internal developments.

Part II

Contemporary Case Studies

4 North Korea

One purpose of the case studies chosen for this book is to illustrate the degrees of faminogenesis proposed by Marcus. Some regimes, Marcus argues, intentionally impose famine and malnutrition, while others recklessly continue policies that undermine their population's access to food, and yet others are indifferent to starvation and malnutrition or incompetent to correct such problems (Marcus 2003, 246–47). North Korea is an example of state-induced famine, at best recklessly but possibly intentionally caused and perpetuated. From the 1990s through the early years of the twenty-first century, government policies caused hundreds of thousands, if not over a million North Koreans to die of starvation, while many others suffered severe malnutrition. A subset of North Koreans, those imprisoned in a network of prison camps, was even more likely to starve than the general population. This chapter explains the policies behind the famine and malnutrition.

Theoretically, the question is whether North Korean policies constituted faminogenesis. Practically, the question is how North Korea could be persuaded to ameliorate its policies and what, if anything, could be done under international law to punish perpetrators of faminogenesis and assist both those North Koreans who stayed in the country and those who fled. These latter questions will be addressed in Part III, Chapters 8 and 9.

Historical Background

A state severely isolated from the international community, North Korea is a creation of the Cold War. From 1910 to 1945, the Korean Peninsula was colonized by the Japanese. At the end of WWII, the defeated Japanese withdrew from their colony and the Americans and Soviets agreed that Korea would be split at the 38th parallel, a line arbitrarily chosen as it roughly divided the ancient kingdom into two equal parts. Kim Il Sung, purportedly a former guerilla leader against the Japanese in Manchuria (Hwang 2010, 185), was chosen by the Soviet Union to lead the North. In 1950 he attacked the South, anticipating an easy victory. The United States and other countries came to the South's defense, with United Nations approval, leading newly Communist China to enter the war on the side of the North. An extremely brutal three-year war ensued in which hundreds of thousands died, many in the North from American bombs and napalm (Hwang 2010, 210): North Korea is estimated to have suffered 300,000 military and 400,000 civilian deaths during the war (Bluth 2008, 22). In 1953 the two parties signed a truce and retreated to their respective sides of the 38th parallel. There was no peace treaty, and as of 2015 the two Koreas were still technically at war, maintaining a heavily defended demilitarized zone between the two countries.

The official organ controlling the North Korean state was the Korean Workers' Party (Bluth 2008, 25), supplemented by an extremely large military of approximately 1.1 million people out of an estimated population of 22.7 million in 2011 (International Institute for Strategic Studies 2011, 412), but in practice the North Korean regime was a hereditary dictatorship. Introduced in 1970, North Korea's official ideology was called *Juche*, comprising "self-control, independence, and self-sufficiency" (Rigoulot 1999, 548); in a word, self-reliance or extreme autarky (Cumings 2005, 429). This alleged self-reliance consisted of a combination of a command economy, collectivization of agriculture, and heavy dependence on imports of cheap goods, fuel, and food from North Korea's allies, especially the former Soviet Union and China. However, no one except the extremely corrupt elite was legally permitted access to foreign goods, thought, or media. In practice, *Juche* meant that North Koreans relied completely on the whims of the state for fulfillment of their basic needs. The government was characterized by deep paranoia, massive corruption, and fascistic racism, as well as by almost complete control over a devastated and severely inefficient economy. The regime also perpetuated a mythology that its hereditary rulers represented "the will of both heaven and earth" (Rigoulot 1999, 559). Kim Il Sung died in 1994 and was succeeded by his son, Kim Jong Il, who ruled North Korea until his own death in December 2011; in turn, he was succeeded by his son, Kim Jong Un, thought at the time of his succession to be only 29 or 30 years old.

In the 1950s and 60s North Korea was more prosperous than its Southern counterpart (Bluth 2008, 34). In part, this was because it had inherited most of the country's industrial capacity and infrastructure (Hassig and Oh 2009, 69); in part it was because the Soviet Union heavily subsidized its economy (French 2007, 76). When the Soviet Union de-Stalinized in the 1950s, North Korea turned to China for infrastructure, energy, and food support. Food shortages occurred in 1945–46 (just after WWII), 1954–55 (just after the Korean War), and 1970–73 (Haggard and Noland 2007, 9); food rations began to decline steadily from about 1970 (Feffer 2006, 5). Moreover, industry and infrastructure quickly deteriorated as a result of inadequate maintenance, poor management, lack of spare parts, and lack of an external market for the shoddy goods that factories produced (French 2007, 73–114).

Food production problems were caused in large part by highly inefficient collectivized agriculture. Immediately after WWII the government seized all land belonging to Japanese colonialists and Korean landlords and redistributed it to peasants. The initial redistribution of land was unsuccessful and food production fell. The government then collectivized all land in the 1950s (French 2007, 117). Above a certain minimum left for their own consumption, farmers were obliged to turn over the entire harvest to the state, which distributed food to citizens through the Public Distribution System (PDS), adopted in 1950. Outside the collectivized farms, only very tiny "micro-farms" on which citizens could cultivate fruits and vegetables and keep small animals, poultry, and bees for their personal consumption or for periodic legal farmers' markets were allowed (French 2007, 119).

About 62 percent of the people, mainly urban, were dependent on the PDS for all their food. Even with the PDS in place, however, the country relied on food aid from the Soviet Union and China as early as the 1980s, as its own production of food declined (Natsios 2001, 10). Thus, North Korea's collectivized system of food production, its refusal to allow almost any private production of food, its prohibition of food markets, and its reliance on food rationing all set the stage for the famine of the 1990s and severe malnutrition in the 2000s.

Famine

In order to understand the extent of famine and malnutrition in North Korea, it is first necessary to absorb the shocking statistics about hunger and malnutrition presented by the Food and Agriculture Organization (FAO). In 1990 25.4 percent of the population was undernourished: that figure rose to 34.8 percent in 1995, 36.9 percent in 2000, and 38.3 percent in 2005, before dropping slightly to 32 percent in 2010 (Food and Agriculture Organization 2013, indicator V12). The percent of the population suffering from food inadequacy was 36.4 in 1990, rising to 47.4 in 1995 and 51.8 in 2000, before dropping slightly to 50.6 in 2005 and 49 in 2010 (Food and Agriculture Organization 2013, indicator V15). The depth of the food deficit (the number of calories below the minimum needed per person) was 183 in 1990, 261 in 1995, 282 in 2000, 295 in 2005, and 249 in 2010 (Food and Agriculture Organization 2013, indicator V14).

Figures on children are available only for 2000 and after, but present the effects of famine even more vividly than figures on nutritional inadequacy for the North Korean population as a whole. In 2000 51 percent of children were stunted (too short for their age), dropping to 43.1 percent in 2004 and 32.4 percent in 2010 (Food and Agriculture Organization 2013, indicator V16). 24.7 percent of children were underweight in 2000, dropping to 20.6 percent in 2004 and 18.8 percent in 2009 (Food and Agriculture Organization 2013, indicator V18). Wasting (being severely underweight) is the most severe indicator of malnutrition among children: In 2000 12.2 percent of children were wasted, dropping to 8.5 percent in 2004 and 5.2 percent in 2009 (Food and Agriculture Organization 2013, indicator V17).

These figures cover the period of famine in the 1990s; its long-term consequences, especially for children; and the continued severe malnutrition in North Korea in the first two decades of the twenty-first century. In the early 1990s, the World Food Programme (WFP) described the food situation in North Korea as a "famine in slow motion" (Natsios 2001, 21). By the mid-1990s, there was a major famine. While many reports cited figures of up to three million out of a then population of 22 million having died from 1994 to 2000 (e.g., Becker 2005, 211), scholarly accounts present a lower figure of about 600,000 to one million dead (Haggard and Noland 2007, 1; Goodkind and West 2001, 220). A South Korean scholar using several types of demographic and statistical data concluded that between 580,000 and 1.1 million people lost their lives, or between 2.6 and 5 percent of the population (Lee 2005, 47). The 2014 United Nations Committee of Inquiry into Human Rights in North Korea cited estimates of from 490,000 to 2.1 million dead, (the latter figure for the period of 1995 to 1998 only) (COI: United Nations General Assembly 2014, February 7, par.668, pp. 203–24), or 2.2 to 9.5 percent of the then population of 22 million.

North Korea attributed the famine of the 1990s to natural disasters, citing poor harvests and flooding in 1995. But these "natural" disasters were in large part a consequence of poor decisions by the central government in the 1980s about agricultural policies, which exacerbated the earlier food shortages caused by collectivized food production and distribution. During the 1980s, the government ordered continuous cropping and overuse of chemical fertilizers, which eroded soil quality; there was also much soil erosion and deforestation as hills were denuded of trees to provide more land for cultivation (Noland 2007, 201). When the floods came, terraced hillsides simply collapsed. By this point there was very little agricultural machinery or fuel; much cultivation was by hand.

Both Russia and China cut their food and fuel aid to North Korea in the early 1990s, exacerbating the extremely poor agricultural policy (Goodkind and West 2001, 220–21). Russia, the successor state to the Soviet Union, had no interest in subsidizing Communist states abroad. Chinese exports of maize to North Korea declined by 80 percent from 1993 to 1994, in part because of a poor harvest in China itself and in part because China was punishing North Korea for opening up diplomatic relations with Taiwan (Lee 2005, 35–36). Both countries informed North Korea that it would have to start paying for their exports in hard currency (Bluth 2008, 38).

The regime responded by describing the famine as an "Arduous March" (Natsios 2001, 5). Adopting a disingenuous approach to its causes, Kim Jong Il first urged on his subjects the virtues of eating only two meals a day (COI: United Nations General Assembly 2014, February 7, par. 511, p. 149), then one, meantime attributing the famine to an imperialist blockade (Myers 2010, 118). At the same time, the regime reduced farm families' grain rations by 35 percent, far below subsistence level (Marcus 2003, 260). Nevertheless, privileged groups, especially members of the government, the military, and the Korean Workers' Party continued to receive rations (Noland et al. 2001, 747).

Reports on the famine, many by refugees, were heart-breaking. A refugee doctor described wasted children whose desperate mothers fed them weeds and wild grasses. Unable to digest this food, children appeared in the doctor's under-equipped North Korean hospital with severe medical complications, or simply with a vague malaise that preceded their deaths. Babies died from lack of mothers' milk, and often parents and grandparents denied themselves food so that children could eat (Demick 2009, 113, 167); sometimes entire families killed themselves (Becker 2005, 29). Women prostituted themselves to buy food for their children, while homeless children were reputed to be cannibalized (Demick 2009, 153, 168). One refugee reported witnessing the public execution of a 28-year-old man accused of eating a four-year-old child (Kim 2008, 50), and the WFP requested the right to inspect farmers' markets where it was reported that "special meat" on offer was actually human flesh (French 2007, 130). Ironically, in this devastated land, the very children dying of starvation were taught a song about how they had "nothing to envy" from the rest of the world (Demick 2009, 195).

In 1998, a survey by the WFP, the FAO, and the European Union (EU) found that 60 percent of North Korean children were stunted and

50 percent malnourished (Lee 2005, 13). Indeed, the height requirement for entry into the military was reduced because so many military-age men were stunted (Demick 2009, 188). Once the actual famine ended around 2000 as a result of better weather, international food aid, and some policy reforms, a "chronic food emergency" ensued, well into the twenty-first century (Haggard and Noland 2007, 2).

After the worst of the famine in the 1990s, the government introduced some reforms in food production and distribution. As early as 1987 it had decided to permit industrial workers to cultivate small plots of land at their under-producing factories and farmers to expand their personal plots and trade in illegal – though tolerated – farmers' markets (Lee 2005, 6). The factories were given some autonomy from state control and permitted to trade manufactured products among themselves and in international markets (Bluth 2008, 41). The state de-regulated cooperative farms and permitted farmers to keep a portion of the surplus food they produced (Lee 2005, 13). The state turned a blind eye to private markets that sprang up in urban areas, indeed legalizing them in 2002 (Caryl 2008, 26). The government also decided to change the pricing structure to reflect real market conditions, aligning official prices more closely with black-market prices, but not increasing wages proportionately (Lankov 2013, 119–20). Men were sometimes obliged to spend time at factories even if there was neither work nor wages for them, while women, who were less likely to be obliged to spend time at factories, began to engage in petty trade, selling home-cooked food or handicrafts (Park 2011).

Unfortunately, the reforms also had their own detrimental consequences. Although wages were increased, prices also rose; after the 2002 reforms, the price of rice rose by a multiple of 550 (Lankov 2013, 120). Moreover, the reforms did not appear to cause a substantial increase in production (Hassig and Oh 2009, 103), as farms and factories still lacked necessary inputs and fuel (Economist 2008, September 27, 14). As a result, North Korea faced the classic inflationary scenario of too much money chasing too few goods – especially too little food.

By 2005, a new system of stratification between rich and poor had developed. Some people had access to hard currency (Hassig and Oh 2009, 130) either through remittances (mostly from Japan or China); smuggling across the border with China; or crime, such as exporting arms or narcotics (French 2007, 99). These individuals could buy what little food was in the market, while those dependent on meager state wages could not. Thus, this incomplete, regulated "socialist" marketization resulted in high rates of post-famine malnutrition for those who could not earn hard currency. Moreover, after its effective collapse in the late 1990s (Lankov 2013, 78–79), the government abolished the PDS in 2002, except for the top one or two million people in the country (Hassig and Oh 2009, 114). Those many other North Koreans who had relied on the PDS were suddenly forced to either cultivate their own food or buy it in markets; many lacked the resources to do either. About 50 percent of formerly PDS-dependent households were unable to meet their caloric requirements (French 2007, 143).

Complicating matters even further, in 2005 the state overturned some of its reforms. It once again banned the private buying and selling of grain (Feffer 2006, 17) and reintroduced the PDS (Human Rights Watch 2006a, 2–3; Lankov 2013, 121), although rations were tied to attendance at and performance in the workplace (Gause 2011, 81). Age and gender restrictions were imposed on those still allowed to sell (non-food) items, permitting only older women to trade (Lankov 2013, 123), and price controls were imposed on marketed goods (Gause 2011, 81). As of 2008 markets were again closed, and women under forty were no longer allowed to trade, even though women were the mainstays of their families (Economist 2010, January 16). Nevertheless, by 2009 North Koreans relied on private economic activities for about 70 to 80 percent of their actual family income (Lankov 2009, 99), eking it out in the interstices of the supposedly socialized economy. Realizing it could not control the informal markets, in 2010 the government reversed its policies and issued orders not to intervene with them (Lankov 2013, 130). By 2011 it appeared that some official markets were permitted, but they could not sell staple cereals (FAO/WFP 2011, November 25, 25).

Finally, a currency reform in late 2009 effectively wiped out the savings of those North Koreans who were managing to make money in private markets, which they could use to purchase food: Citizens were obliged to turn in their banknotes, to be replaced at a rate of 1 per 100 wons (COI: United Nations General Assembly 2014, February 7, par. 531). This was one of the few times that some parts of the population showed their displeasure, demonstrating against the government. In response, the regime reportedly executed Pak Nam Gi – the official in charge of the reform – and sent three dozen of his relatives to prison (China Post 2010, July 7), although the government never confirmed the execution (Lankov 2013, 131).

Partly as a consequence of these incomplete and erratic reforms, severe food shortages causing malnutrition and death returned by the end of the decade. This food shortage was a result in part of lack of seeds, fertilizer, fuel, storage capacity, and advanced agricultural technology (Human Rights Watch 2010b, 326). By 2008, the country was "once again on the brink of mass starvation," (Economist 2008, May 10, 50) with families eating grass, tree bark, and poisonous mushrooms that could cause death by diarrhea in young children (Amnesty International 2010, July 15). Matters were made worse by periodic campaigns to boost industrial production, which removed farmers from their fields: "we are being led to our deaths," said one such farmer (Economist 2009, October 24). These campaigns continued in 2010–11 as preparations were made to celebrate the 100th anniversary of the birth of Kim Il Sung in April 2012.

Rations in 2010 met less than half the daily food needs of the 68 percent of the population dependent upon them (World Food Programme 2010). In March 2011, estimates were that 6.1 million people, about a quarter of the population, were food insecure, especially in the northern and eastern provinces (World Food Programme et al. 2011, 29). "Feral children" ate dead dogs and rotted food in the markets (Economist 2011, September 17). In October 2011, the PDS rations were only one-third of the daily requirement (COI: United Nations General Assembly 2014, February 7, par. 536, p. 161), and a WFP mission in November 2011 found signs of edema, a symptom of extreme malnutrition: Only about 6 percent of households had acceptable diets. Households were reducing the numbers and sizes of their meals and adding water to their food to increase its volume: Many also foraged for wild foods. By November 2011, about a third of the children under five were at risk of long-term effects of malnutrition (FAO/WFP 2011, November 25, 26, 28).

Drought followed by severe flooding exacerbated the threat to North Korea's food supply in 2012. By May 2012 there were reports that workers were dying at three major steel works because their rations had been stopped (Good Friends: Research Institute for North Korean Society 2012, May 23), and 10,000 people were believed dead of starvation in two provinces (COI: United Nations General Assembly 2014, February 7, par. 538, p. 162). Although the WFP reported in August 2012 that North Korea was not facing a famine (Blanchard 2012, August 9), starving children reappeared on the streets, and even members of the military were malnourished, with parents sending food to their sons in the army (Demick 2012, October 14). Ordinary soldiers were expected to find food through foraging or theft from civilians (COI: United Nations General Assembly 2014, February 7, par. 565, p. 170).

By March 2013 over two-thirds of the population were judged to be food insecure, while 2.8 million needed regular food aid: 28 percent of children under five suffered from chronic malnutrition and 4 percent were acutely malnourished (United Nations News Centre 2013, March 15). In April 2013 North Korea went so far as to ask Mongolia for food aid (Kwaak 2013, April 22), and in August Kim Jong Un ordered the military to release its stores of rice to the general population (Yoo 2013, August 26). One estimate was that North Koreans were obtaining 50 percent of their calories from the informal, "underground" market, as the formal distribution system could not provide enough food (Hanke 2013, June 22). While the food situation appeared to improve in 2014 and 2015, partly as a result of private food markets springing up, it was still bad enough that members of the military began raiding nearby villages in China for food (Zhai and Kim 2015, January 13), and the weight of military backpacks was reduced because it was too heavy for malnourished soldiers (Moon 2015, January 14).

One strong indication of the depth of a food crisis is cannibalism. Reports of cannibalism resurfaced in 2006 (COI: United Nations General Assembly 2014, February 7, par. 528, p. 157) and 2012 (Wallace 2012, December 19). An official North Korean document leaked in mid-2011 reported five cases of cannibalism, including one in which a guard killed one of his colleagues, ate some of his flesh and sold the rest on the market disguised as mutton (Lodish 2011, June 24), although the date of these cannibalistic acts is unclear.

Some of the starvation and malnutrition after 2005 might have been avoided if the regime had continued its path of reform, however erratic, rather than retrenching. The reasons for the post-2005 rollback of reform (Gause 2011, 77–86) are unknown, but it appeared that the regime feared development of a social class that might challenge its power. The political advantage of a public rationing system in a non-democratic state is that the population is completely dependent on the government for its subsistence. If governments can respond to unrest by withdrawing or drastically cutting the food supply, then rebellion is unlikely. The currency reform wiped out the incipient class of wealthy people who were beginning to extricate themselves from the state's totalitarian control. Severe curtailment of private trade in food, limiting it to older women – probably the least likely demographic category to rebel – meant that young men were less likely to remove themselves from the state's grip.

This short description of North Korean economic policy cannot explain all the various decisions that caused famine in the 1990s and mass hunger, if not famine, in the twenty-first century (for a detailed description of North Korean economic policies, see French 2007, 73–182). In brief, until 2000 North Korea was a dogmatic, totalitarian state that refused to institute even the mildest reforms. In the twenty-first century, reform was erratic and internally contradictory; in a word, incompetent at best. Regime security took precedence over food security. It was not communist ideology that impelled Kim Jong Il to reinstate almost complete control over production and distribution of food as of 2005: It was a cold-blooded calculation of how to retain his personal power and pass it on to his son.

As explained in Chapter 1, I use the term "right to food" as shorthand for the rights to adequate food and freedom from hunger, protected in the 1976 International Covenant on Economic, Social and Cultural Rights (ICESCR) by Article 11, 1 and 2. Freedom from hunger is more urgent than the right to adequate food: This minimalist approach is what concerns us in this chapter. North Korea ratified both the ICESCR and the ICCPR on September 14, 1981, although it withdrew from the latter Covenant on August 23, 1997.

As noted in Chapter 1, Article 2, 1 of the ICESCR mandates that each state party to the Covenant should take steps "to the maximum of its available resources, with a view to achieving progressively the full realization of the rights recognized." This clause is usually interpreted to mean that developing states are not expected to provide all human rights immediately but should so do progressively as the resources become available. However, North Korea was not a developing state that could not provide enough food because it did not have enough resources. Rather, the government deprived its citizens of food as a matter of policy. Collectivization of agriculture, prohibition of private production of food, and abolition of the market were all policy decisions that prevented citizens from feeding themselves. Complete prohibition of civil and political rights, as discussed below, meant that citizens could not protest these measures, nor could they take part in government or elect leaders who might change food policies.

In 2012 even the United Nations General Assembly (UNGA) urged reform in North Korea, in a notable departure from the principle of state sovereignty over internal economic matters. The UNGA noted the "serious deterioration in the availability of and access to food... partly as a result of frequent natural disasters, compounded by structural weaknesses in agricultural production resulting in significant shortages of food, and the increasing State restrictions on the cultivation and trade in foodstuffs." Going even further, the UNGA recommended that North Korea "implement more effective food security policies, including through sustainable agriculture, sound food production [and] distribution measures and by allocating more funds to the food sector" (United Nations General Assembly 2012, March 29, pars. 3 and 5 (h)). The UNGA's resolution indicated the seriousness of the ongoing food crisis in North Korea. In 2014 the UNGA voted to establish a Commission of Inquiry into human rights abuses in North Korea, as discussed in Chapter 12.

The Crime of Faminogenesis

Were there such an international crime as faminogenesis, the North Korean regime would surely be guilty of it. As discussed in Chapter 1, Marcus defined four categories of faminogenesis: intentional, reckless, indifferent, and incompetent. Famine is intentional if the state deliberately uses it as a means of extermination and is reckless if the state continues its food policies despite evidence of famine.

Marcus argues that some of the North Korean government's actions during the 1990s famine constituted the first degree crime of intentional faminogenesis. He accuses the government of "knowingly manipulating the famine to target certain populations that threaten its political survival," denying them food rations (Marcus 2003, 260). Supporting Marcus' viewpoint, Suk Lee noted that during the 1990s famine "It was persistently reported that PDS rations were delayed or temporarily suspended in the northern parts of the country" (Lee 2005, 6–7); rations under the PDS appeared to have been completely cut off to the northeast in 1994 (Natsios 2001, 109). However, Haggard and Noland state that they "find no evidence that particular segments of the population were deliberately starved" (Haggard and Noland 2007, 10). They consider the evidence that the regime cut off rations to four northern provinces (COI: United Nations General Assembly 2014, February 7, par. 512, p. 150) to be circumstantial, although they note that there is evidence that the government focused food aid on the western coast, despite knowing that the [north] east coast was facing particularly severe food shortages (Haggard and Noland 2007, 64–65).

Haggard and Noland's view is that "informational failures and the lack of accountability characteristic of authoritarian regimes played a crucial role" in the famine (Haggard and Noland 2007, 10). This suggests that the government was guilty of Marcus' second-degree crime of reckless faminogenesis, continuing policies that caused famine even when their consequences were known (Marcus 2003, 260). Not permitting citizens to farm small plots of land was reckless, as such farms could have produced food to supplement official rations. Prohibition of trade was also reckless. The same might be said of the food shortage of 2010–14, which was caused in part by the regime's 2005 decision to rescind the earlier reforms that had helped create a market economy.

Incompetence, Marcus' fourth degree of faminogenesis, is the most generous description of a regime that followed policy prescriptions from the Soviet Union and China, which by 1990 had been abandoned by both countries. On the other hand, the fact that North Korea did accept some food aid, as discussed in Chapter 9, suggests that it was not indifferent to the famine, thus not guilty of the third degree of faminogenesis. However, there was some suspicion that the food aid was not disbursed to the most needy citizens: rather, it seemed, the military was well-fed while others starved (Rigoulot 1999, 563).

Feffer argues that the famine was not intentional but rather was a result of "atrocious policy" (Feffer 2006, 6). Haggard and Noland also argue that "the famine was a classic case of state failure" (Haggard and Noland 2009, 1), rather than having been deliberately created. However, these arguments seem to inadvertently imply that the policies were made by honest bureaucrats who accidentally made poor decisions; an alternative view is that the regime made decisions in its own interests regardless of the deleterious effects on some sectors of the population. As long as members of the Korean Workers' Party and the military – along with the relatively privileged inhabitants of the capital, Pyongyang – were fed, the regime could ignore other people. The deliberate denial of civil and political rights also suggests intentionality.

Civil and Political Rights

Lack of civil and political rights meant that North Koreans could not protest their government's policies nor bring to its attention the fact that they were starving. Systematic denial of human rights during severe food shortages suggests at minimum reckless faminogenesis. The state deliberately denies itself a key resource – the voices of its own people – that could help to rectify its faminogenic policies. North Koreans enjoyed no freedom of speech, assembly, or press; no political right to vote; and no protection from torture or arbitrary execution. Citizens could not protest the policies causing starvation, nor could they vote their leaders out of office; if they did protest, they risked imprisonment, torture, or death. Nor could citizens fulfill their need for food when they were not permitted freedom of movement to leave the country or travel within it.

Article 12 of the Universal Declaration of Human Rights (UDHR) states that "No one shall be subjected to arbitrary interference with his privacy, family, home or correspondence ... " Violation of the right to privacy is characteristic of totalitarian states. North Koreans enjoyed no right to privacy whatsoever. Neighbors were encouraged to spy on neighbors, and all citizens had to attend self-criticism sessions where they were obliged to confess and repent for even the tiniest acts that might be considered disloyal to the regime. Thus, independent thought and conversation were blocked by a system in which neighbors could and did report each other for "crimes" against the state such as foraging for, producing, and selling food, or even complaining about food shortages. Radios and televisions were wired so that they could receive only state channels (Human Rights Watch 2006a, 6), which broadcast propaganda into every household (Caryl 2010, 30), thus prohibiting the spread of information that might cause unrest about food shortages.

North Korea also prohibited private property. The right to own property is protected by Article 17 of the UDHR. This right helps individuals to be self-sufficient, rather than relying on the state to provide everything they need. Aside from the micro-farms described earlier, no personal cultivation of land was permitted in North Korea until the 1990s, and as of 2015 there was still no private ownership of land. Even in the brief period of flowering markets in the early 2000s, no reforms were introduced to enable individuals to own the land they farmed. Yet individual land rights have been shown to result in "higher productivity, cultivation and yields, as well as the retention of surpluses against the risk of climatic disaster" (French 2007, 136).

The denial of citizens' human rights in North Korea was a consequence of deliberate policy decisions. A government concerned with the welfare of its citizens would not continue policies that cause its citizens to starve. Thus, the regime was recklessly faminogenic, prohibiting human rights that could avert or modify famine. It is not quite as easy to make a case for intentional faminogenesis, especially given the inconsistent and erratic policy changes that the state introduced as of the mid-1990s. In either case, though, denial of citizens' civil and political rights was a key cause of the starvation. Not enjoying any of these rights, North Koreans resorted to occasional protests, strikes, uprisings, sabotage, and even murders of local officials (Becker 2005, 36). There were also reports of attempted assassinations and coups d'état, suggesting dissent within the ruling clique and/or the military (Bluth 2008, 31).

The complete denial of civil and political rights meant that North Korea violated the United Nations Committee on Economic, Social and Cultural Rights General Comment 12 on the right to food, as discussed in Chapter 1, which prohibited the use of food as a political weapon. North Korea prohibited all the civil and political rights mentioned in the Guidelines, used food as a tool of political and economic pressure, and did not protect individuals' rights to the assets that could provide them with food. It also violated the voluntary guidelines on food security adopted by the FAO, as discussed in Chapter 1, which noted the importance of civil and political rights to the economic human right to food, and specifically mentioned the human rights to freedom of opinion and expression, information, press, and assembly/association (Food and Agriculture Organization 2005, Guideline 1.2, p. 9). The North Korean regime never had the political will to protect the right to food; quite the opposite, as shown most clearly in its abominable treatment of its prisoners.

Penal Starvation

The North Korean government was responsible not only for famine but also for a deliberate policy of subjecting its prisoners to starvation rations. The government maintained a large system of repressive slave labor camps – in effect, a gulag – in which prisoners were even more likely than the general population to starve. Rations were far below what was needed to maintain health and were so even before the food shortages and famine of the 1990s: Prisoners were "provided only enough food to be kept perpetually on the verge of starvation" (Hawk 2003, 25). Food was allocated on the basis of productivity; the less a prisoner produced, the less he ate, resulting in a spiral downward as those deprived of even more food produced less and less. Many in the camps died because of lack of food, while some were executed for foraging; in one case a prisoner was executed for collecting ripe chestnuts that had fallen at the entrance of a slave-labor mine (Hawk 2003, 37). There were no health facilities to speak of, and prisoners often died of malnutrition-related diseases.

I use the term "penal starvation" to describe this phenomenon. Penal starvation attacked a significant percentage of prisoners who could not live on rations constantly below subsistence level, or whose food rations were even lower than the prescribed level because they did not work hard enough or had angered the authorities in some way. Estimates vary of how many people were in the prison camps at any time. Some sources suggest about 200,000 every year (Human Rights Watch 2011, 345), although a more conservative estimate by the United Nations Commission of Inquiry estimated that there were 80,000 to 120,000 prisoners (COI: United Nations General Assembly 2014, February 7, par. 61, p. 12). However, there is some suspicion that the lower figure might be a consequence of recent mass executions of prisoners (Bellamy 2015, 231). Published originally in 1997, Rigoulot estimated that 1.5 million people had died in the camps since the creation of North Korea (Rigoulot 1999, 564).

Inhabitants in these camps fell into two major groups. The first was people imprisoned for political reasons. Party purges began in 1953 to rid North Korea of any former guerillas not content with Kim Il Sung's rule and continued until at least 1997 (Rigoulot 1999, 550–2). About 15,000 "anti-revolutionaries," along with 70,000 family members, were sent to camps in purges from 1966 to 1970 (Hassig and Oh 2009, 208). The state also classified every citizen on the basis of perceived loyalty, or lack thereof, to the regime: the three classes were the core, or loyal, class; the wavering class; and the hostile class. South Korea estimated that these categories constituted 30, 50, and 20 percent of the population respectively (Hassig and Oh 2009, 198). Membership in the three classes was hereditary; for example, an individual might be deemed a member of the hostile class because his great-grandfather had been a landlord. Members of the hostile class were most likely to be sent to the gulag; they were also the first to have their rations cut during the 1990s famine (Hassig and Oh 2009, 203).

Several other categories of people were so despised that they were frequently sent to prison camps. North Korea imprisoned Koreans who had lived in Japan when Korea was under Japanese colonial rule but had been badly treated there. Some of the estimated 93,000 returnees from Japan were incarcerated (Hassig and Oh 2009, 208). Christians were also imprisoned or executed (Goedde 2010, 554; Hawk 2003, 67); the earliest massacre of Christians appears to have taken place in November 1945 (Hwang 2010, 216), and it is believed that the government executed about 400,000 religious practitioners (not necessarily all Christians) during the 1970s (Human Rights Watch 2007, March, 7).

North Korea was also explicitly racist. Basing his analysis on the regime's propaganda, Myers argues that far from being a Communist state, North Korea was actually a fascist, racist state along the lines of Hitler's Germany, and that it derived what little legitimacy it had in part by convincing the populace that it was a superior race (Myers 2010, 14–15). Thus people who were of mixed "racial" background were likely to be incarcerated. Some women refugees repatriated from China (as discussed in Chapter 8) were imprisoned, many after severe torture, because in addition to fleeing they had committed the crime of racial pollution by having had sexual relations with Chinese men. Some of these women had voluntarily married Korean-Chinese or ethnic Chinese men. Some were trafficked to Chinese husbands, as China's one-child policy has caused a surplus of men over women and many men therefore resorted to purchasing wives. Others became sex workers, usually through coercion (Muico 2005). Women who were pregnant when they were returned to North Korea were forcibly aborted. If they were in the late stages of pregnancy, delivery was induced and the infants then murdered or tossed alive into garbage cans before their mothers' eyes (Hawk 2003, 61–62; Haggard and Noland 2011, 97).

The regime's racist ideology stressed the perfection, as well as the purity, of the Korean people. Until the 1980s if not later, people with disabilities were sent to special concentration camps in accordance with the Kims' belief that North Koreans ought to be physically perfect. The Kims had a particular aversion to "dwarfs," who were put in special prison camps and subjected to forced sterilization (Natsios 2001, 37). It appears, however, that as of the 1990s people with disabilities were somewhat better treated and less likely to be imprisoned; indeed, in 2003 the regime passed a law for their protection, although discrimination against the disabled was still very common (Young-ho et al. 2010, 64, 249–60).

The second group of prisoners was people whose actions in search of food were considered illegal. Their crimes consisted of engaging in petty trade, cultivating small plots of land, hoarding food (French 2007, 144), foraging for food, travelling within the country in search of food (Moon 2009, 112), stealing food, smuggling and other black market activities, and cannibalism (COI: United Nations General Assembly 2014, February 7, pars. 610–22, pp. 185–88). In addition, it is estimated that about 200–300,000 people fled to China during the 1990s famine (Hawk 2003, 56); China returned refugees to North Korea where most were then imprisoned, as discussed in Chapter 8. In effect, these individuals were "re-starved." Having committed what the state considered to be crimes in order to survive famine, they were incarcerated and deliberately subjected to starvation rations. However, during the food shortages of 2010–15 officials appeared to be somewhat more lenient regarding travel within the country and may even have encouraged foraging. In exchange for bribes, they were also willing to turn a blind eye to smuggling or migrant work abroad (Lankov 2009, 99); thus, by 2010 the estimated number of refugees in China was only 20–40,000 (Lankov 2013, 123).

Not only those convicted of crimes but also their families, including their parents, spouses, siblings, and children, were imprisoned in the gulag. This was in accordance with Kim Il Sung's 1958 directive that "[Prison] inmates are class enemies and must be actively exterminated to three generations" (Becker 2005, 90), which was apparently repeated in 1972: "Factionalists or enemies of class, whoever they are: their seed must be eliminated through three generations" (Park 2011, 11). Thus, for example, Kang Chol-Hwan, the author of a rare memoir of the camps, was incarcerated at the age of nine because his grandfather was suspected of a crime (Kang , 2006, 684). This form of collective punishment was one reason why the gulag contained so many prisoners.

Referring again to Marcus' four categories of faminogenesis, it is clear that penal starvation was intentional. The state decided whom to imprison, it decided on food rations for prisoners, and it decided that prisoners could be deprived of food for further transgressions while in prison, such as not working hard enough. Thus, as a subset of faminogenesis, penal starvation is a first-degree famine crime, to which I return in Chapter 8.

Conclusion

As of the time of writing in early 2015, the regime had remained stable under the leadership of Kim Jong Un, who appeared to have consolidated his position as head of the military, the Korean Workers' Party, and the government. When he first succeeded his father, it was thought that his uncle by marriage, Jang Sung Taek, would effectively act as regent. Jang showed signs of being interested in Chinese-style economic reforms, which would have introduced a more productive market economy while retaining authoritarian rule (Nathan 2013, December 4; Economist 2013, December 14). However, in December 2013 Kim ordered that his uncle be executed, possibly in a dispute over who would profit from North Korea's exports (Choe and Sanger 2013, December 23).

Although it seemed that for the time being market-style reforms were thwarted, there were still signs of interest in reforms, such as setting up Chinese-style economic development zones (Economist 2014, March 8). There were reports that farmers were to be permitted to sell produce in excess of government quotas at market prices (Lankov 2013, 141), which would encourage production. There were also reports that state collective farms were to be replaced by smaller, family-based units (Sullivan 2012, September 12), and that small private factories were being set up. By 2015 it seemed that some of these reforms were taking place (Economist 2015, February 28). Moreover, managers of state enterprises were being encouraged to run them like profit-making private corporations (Evans 2015, January 14).

These small signs, however, did not thwart the hunger still stalking the country in 2015. Under Kim Jong Un, hunger and starvation continued to be policy choices, as they were under his grandfather and father. They were the result of the regime's unwillingness to reform its economic policies, which were designed to produce massive food insecurity not by accident or incompetence but as a means of keeping the population under complete totalitarian control. That it was a policy choice is evidenced by the regime's complete denial of civil and political rights to its subjects. The government knew of the detrimental consequences of its policies, but preferred regime stability to any attempts to protect the human rights to freedom from hunger and adequate nutrition of ordinary North Koreans.

5   Zimbabwe

The period 2000–2008 in Zimbabwe is known as the "Zimbabwe crisis." Unlike North Koreans in the 1990s, Zimbabweans during this period did not suffer widespread famine. However, they did endure widespread food shortages and severe malnutrition, and some people may have starved to death. Although independent Zimbabwe had always suffered from chronic infrastructural problems and periodic drought (Jayne et al. 2006, 533) during the twenty-first century food shortages were principally the result of deliberate government actions and reckless incompetence. The government deliberately manipulated food supplies and international aid to favor its supporters and suppress the opposition. It also instituted a recklessly incompetent and politically motivated system of land reform that undermined national productive capacity. Even if there was no actual famine, the food crime conformed to all four of Marcus' (Marcus 2003, 46–47) categories of faminogenesis, showing signs of intentionality, recklessness, incompetence, and indifference. Moreover, although the worst of the crisis was over after 2008, similar policies continued through early 2015.

North Korea, one of Zimbabwe's political allies, illustrates what can happen to food production and distribution when a totalitarian dictatorship institutes irrational food policies, combined with complete denial of civil and political rights. Zimbabwe illustrates what can happen when a formal democracy descends into authoritarian dictatorship, progressively undermining civil and political rights and the property laws that had previously facilitated the efficient production, distribution, and acquisition of food.

Historical Background

Formerly a British colony, Zimbabwe became independent in 1980. Its population consisted of two major ethnic groups, the Shona, about 80 percent of the population, and the Ndebele, about 10 percent. About 5 percent of the population was white at independence, reduced to less than 1 percent by 2000 and 0.5 percent by 2007 (Bourdillon 2008, 333–34).

In 1889 the British South Africa Company, a private corporation controlled by Cecil Rhodes, took power over Southern Rhodesia, now Zimbabwe. With good arable land and a climate conducive to European settlement, Southern Rhodesia became a settler colony. In 1923 the British government took control, but rather than administering Southern Rhodesia as a formal colony with a Governor responsible to the Colonial Office in London, it granted the settlers a form of political autonomy that excluded the much larger African population from political affairs. In 1930, the government passed a Land Apportionment Act that allocated the best farmland to the colony's tiny white minority, expelling Africans without compensation from their land and setting the seeds for conflict over land after independence. One million blacks were allocated 29 million acres, while 48,000 whites were allocated 49 million acres (Rukini 2006, 34).

After WWII, the government violently expropriated another 100,000 black farmers to make way for white British war veterans who were enticed with free land to settle in Southern Rhodesia (Hanlon et al. 2013, 35–36). This fairly recent loss of land remained within the living memory of those who fought for independence and who later supported the violent takeover of land from whites (Meredith 2007, 118; Lamb 2006). By 1980, white commercial farm owners owned 27 million acres of land, or 33 percent of prime farmland, while 800,000 peasant households lived on 39.5 million acres (Dashwood 2004, 223). White-owned farms accounted for three-quarters of agricultural output and employed about one-third of the wage-earning labor force (Meredith 2005, 618).

When in the late 1950s Britain began to grant independence to other African colonies, whites formed the Rhodesian Front Party, and in 1965 issued a Unilateral Declaration of Independence to prevent Britain from giving independence to black Southern Rhodesians. A war of liberation against white minority rule ensued from 1972 to 1980. In this war Robert Mugabe led the Zimbabwe African National Union (ZANU), roughly representing the majority Shona, and Joshua Nkomo led the Zimbabwe African Peoples' Union (ZAPU), roughly representing the minority Ndebele. The two parties united in 1976, becoming the Zimbabwe African National Union-Patriotic Front (ZANU-PF).

A peace treaty known as the Lancaster House Agreement was negotiated in 1979, and Zimbabwe attained independence under black majority rule in 1980. Under the Agreement property rights were protected, although the government was permitted to acquire under-utilized land for agricultural settlement as long as adequate compensation was promptly paid (Southern Rhodesia Constitutional Conference 1979, Annex C, C, V.1). This implied that any land transferred from white settlers to the government for purposes of redistribution to black Zimbabweans was to be sold on a willing seller-willing buyer basis. Yet there was no provision for compensation to the Africans who had lost so much of their land to Europeans, many after WWII.

Robert Mugabe became Prime Minister of Zimbabwe in 1980 after competitive elections, and President in 1987 after signing a Unity Agreement with Nkomo (Dashwood and Pratt 1999, 232). He was still President in 2015. Although initially Zimbabwe was by African standards a prosperous country, in the 1990s it was hit by economic crisis, caused in part by the adoption of an Economic Structural Adjustment Programme meant to solve Zimbabwe's growing indebtedness (Human Rights Watch 2002, 8). Rising unemployment increased resentment against white commercial farmers, many of whom were by now Zimbabwean citizens. Aside from agriculture, the Zimbabwean economy was based on mining – especially of gold and platinum – and some industry.

Mugabe and his ZANU-PF party were re-elected in parliamentary and presidential elections throughout the 1980s and 90s; however, political violence marred even these very early elections (Kriger 2005). Mugabe began to build a coterie of supporters who enriched themselves at the country's expense. Many came not merely from his larger ethnic group, the Shona, but from his smaller clan, the Zezuru (International Crisis Group 2005, 11).

Mugabe was re-elected President in 2002 and 2008. The 2008 election was marred by severe violence and intimidation of voters by ZANU-PF activists, worried about the rising popularity of the opposition Movement for Democratic Change (MDC), led by Morgan Tsvangirai. In order to forestall more violence after 2008, Tsvangirai agreed to a "unity" government and became Prime Minister, serving under Mugabe, who continued as President. The MDC took over portfolios such as health and finance, leaving the crucial military and security sectors in ZANU-PF hands. Mugabe again triumphed over Tsvangirai in a 2013 snap election, but with notably less violence than 2008. This time, however, there were allegations of severe electoral irregularities, including votes by one million dead or absent Zimbabweans (Byom 2013, July 24, 2), repeat-voting, and child voting (Economist 2013, August 10, 41).

Famishment and Malnutrition

From 2000 to 2014 Zimbabwe experienced an extremely severe food crisis: only the World Food Programme (WFP) and its sister agencies, along with many non-governmental organizations (NGOs), prevented an actual famine. If, as suggested in Chapter 1, one views famine as a process comprised of three stages of dearth, famishment, and morbidity (Rangasami 1985, 1749) rather than a state of mass starvation, then Zimbabwe was well into that process in the early 2000s. Zimbabweans suffered for several years from a politically induced dearth of food that resulted in famishment for hundreds of thousands, if not millions, even if the country was not experiencing widespread starvation.

In October 2003, half of Zimbabwe's population was considered "food-insecure, living in a household that is unable to obtain enough food to meet basic needs" (Human Rights Watch 2003b, 1). These problems continued through later years. Many Zimbabweans in 2008 were living on one meal a day or even one meal every second day, yet the WFP, lacking resources, had had to reduce its rations to a level below the minimum needed for survival. Many were eating seeds meant for planting in 2009; some of these seeds had already been treated with pesticide. People were also eating cattle suspected of infection by anthrax (The Elders 2008, November, 3, 5). Others foraged for wild foods, even eating tree bark and soil, as well as selling all their household assets to buy food (World Food Programme 2009, February 24). By early 2009, approximately 75 percent of the estimated nine million people left in the country (many others having fled, mostly to elsewhere in Africa) relied on the WFP and other agencies to keep them alive; this was the highest percentage of population needing food aid of any country (USAID: United States Agency for International Development 2009, February 13).

In 2010 Zimbabwe was listed as one of the ten countries most at risk for food supplies (Sibanda 2010, August 26). A 2011 survey in Gwanda, Matebeleland South, discovered that only 17 percent of families were eating three meals a day, and almost half had gone an entire day without food in the previous two months (Solidarity Peace Trust 2011, November 2). In 2012 food shortages were so severe in some parts of Zimbabwe that in classic signs of famine, farmers were starting to sell off their cattle at reduced prices (Dube 2012, May 8), children were being sent into the forest to forage for wild fruits (Mhofu 2012, August 13), and the government did not have enough funds even to feed all of the military (Chinaka 2012, June 14). The WFP estimated that 2.2 million people would need food in 2014 (World Food Programme 2013, October).

These widespread food shortages, combined with declining health services and a high rate of HIV/AIDS in the 2000s, resulted in severely declining living conditions. The under-five mortality rate rose from 76 per thousand in 1990 to 132 in 2006, and the percent of the population living below $US 1.00 per day rose from 25.8 in 1990 to 56 in 2006

(Besada and Moyo 2008a, 9). The maternal mortality rate rose from 168 per 100,000 live births in 1990 to 1,100 in 2005, the increase caused both by HIV/AIDS and a significant decline in maternal health services (Physicians for Human Rights 2009, viii). By 2007 1.3 million children were orphans (UNICEF 2008) and 23 percent of children under five were malnourished (World Bank 2009). In 2006, 35.8 percent of children under five were stunted, as compared to 28.9 percent in 1994 (Food and Agriculture Organization 2013, indicator V16)). Wasting affected 7.3 percent of children under five in 2006, as compared to 6.3 percent in 1994 (Food and Agriculture Organization 2013, indicator V17), and 14 percent of children were underweight in 2006, as compared to 11.7 per cent in 1994 (Food and Agriculture Organization 2013, indicator V18).

These indicators suggest that Zimbabweans' right to adequate nutrition and freedom from hunger was indeed undermined in the first few years of the twenty-first century. However, the prevalence of food inadequacy decreased from 52.9 percent of the population in 2000, a peak year for under-production of food as a result of the land invasions (to be discussed below), to 42.4 percent in 2010, and the overall prevalence of undernourishment decreased from 44.1 percent in 1990 to 32.8 percent in 2010 (Food and Agriculture Organization 2013, indicators V15 and V12). The percentage of children under five who were wasted declined from 8.5 in 1999 to 3.1 in 2010, while the percentage of children under five who were stunted declined from 33.7 in 1999 to 32.3 in 2010, and the percentage of children under five who were underweight declined from 11.5 in 1999 to 10.1 in 2010 (World Bank, Zimbabwe, indicators 16, 17, 7 and 8). These later figures reflect some improvements that occurred after the height of the crisis.

Exacerbating the food shortages, extremely high rates of HIV/AIDS caused poor health among many Zimbabweans. Indeed, Zimbabwe could be considered to have endured a "new variant famine," in which HIV/AIDS is a core aspect of overall famine conditions (De Waal and Whiteside 2003). The HIV/AIDS rate in 2008 in Zimbabwe for individuals aged 15–49 was 15.3 percent (UNAIDS 2008). This catastrophe was further exacerbated by severe erosion of health services, incapacity to import necessary drugs, poor sanitation, lack of access to clean water, and high rates of emigration of medical personnel (Chikanda 2010). In late 2008, cholera broke out as a result of the almost complete breakdown of Zimbabwe's sanitary systems and clean water supplies; there were over 98,000 cholera cases between August 2008 and mid-July 2009 (Office for the Coordination of Humanitarian Affairs 2009, July 15, 1).

Despite the plethora of statistics presented above, however, I could find no reliable estimates of how many Zimbabweans actually died from starvation or diseases related to malnutrition after 2000; thus, we do not know how much, if at all, dearth and famishment contributed to morbidity. We do know that government policies to expropriate large farms from white owners after 2000 caused massive, unnecessary disruptions in food production and distribution. Assaults on livelihoods also made it very difficult for Zimbabweans to buy food. These policies were facilitated by widespread denial of civil and political rights.

Land Redistributions

The violent redistribution of large-scale commercial farms, mostly owned by whites (both Zimbabwean citizens and foreigners) was the chief cause of food shortages during the Zimbabwe crisis. After independence, the government had encouraged white farm owners to stay and continue to produce for the domestic and external markets, with their property rights protected and land transferred only on a willing seller-willing buyer basis. From 1980 to 1996 the government engaged in a legal land purchase and resettlement process that gave land to about 75,000 black families (Hanlon et al. 2013, 54). Black Zimbabweans also bought about 500 large-scale commercial farms (Wright 2008, 331).

Many Zimbabweans criticized Britain for using the Lancaster House Agreement's protection of property rights to favor white commercial farmers instead of the black Zimbabwean peasantry. In fact, however, following the Agreement Britain had promised to help finance purchases of white-owned land (Dashwood 2004, 226), although in the event it apparently spent only about £44 million before cutting off further financial support for land transfers in 1994 because of corruption (Meredith 2005, 631; Cliffe et al. 2011, 912, fn. 4). Many of the transferred farms had been given to Mugabe's cronies, and many resettled black farmers had been obliged to join ZANU-PF (Karimakwenda 2012, October 4). Nevertheless, Britain offered a further £36 million in 2000 to fund land reform but imposed conditions such as fair pricing, a guarantee that the rural poor would benefit from the land reform, and conformity to the rule of law: Zimbabwe refused to accept these conditions (Taylor and Williams 2002, 554).

In 2000, Mugabe began a more violent path to land reform. He encouraged land invasions of white-owned farms by persons alleged to be veterans of the 1972–80 war of independence (Sithole 2008, 78), although many of the invaders were too young to have fought in it. An Amendment to the Constitution in 2000 absolved the government of any responsibility to pay compensation for expropriated land (Nading 2002, 773). Commercial farmland was officially nationalized by another Amendment in 2005, which specifically prohibited any appeal to the courts to challenge the government's acquisition of land, although it permitted appeals to challenge the amount of compensation, if any (President and Parliament of Zimbabwe 2005, Article 2, 2) a and b; and 3), a and b).

A new constitution was passed in 2013: It stipulated that no one could go to court to claim compensation or challenge any land acquisition on grounds that it was discriminatory (Government of Zimbabwe 2013, Article 72, 3, c). This new clause was to prevent more court actions such as had resulted in 2008 in an aborted ruling by the Tribunal of the Southern African Development Community that white farmers should be compensated as they had been victims of racial discrimination, discussed in Chapter 10. The 2013 Constitution also insisted that Britain was responsible to pay compensation to former landowners and that if it did not do so, Zimbabwe had no such responsibility (Government of Zimbabwe 2013, Article 72, 7, C, i and ii).

A draft of the 2013 Constitution had been published in 2010, and had resulted in a further round of land invasions, including black invasions of land owned by blacks – for example a ZANU-PF militia invasion of a farm owned by an MDC official – as it became clear that the Constitution would prohibit any former owners from using the courts to retain their land (Karimakwenda 2012, August 23; Share 2012, November 6). The government redistributed land through the legal fiction of simply publishing the names of farms to be taken over, while making offers of occupancy to those Zimbabweans it favored (Mutenga 2012, August 10). Despite these procedures and their lack of access to the courts, by the end of 2012 an estimated 210 remaining white farmers were under prosecution for refusing to vacate their land (Maodza 2012, December 7). Land requisitioning continued through early 2015.

The earliest land requisitions dispossessed not only members of the white minority but also about 150,000 to 200,000 black farm workers. Including their families, these workers constituted about a million and a half to two million people (Human Rights Watch 2003b, 18). Many were MDC supporters, and the invasions of the farms on which they worked were intended to intimidate them (Meredith 2007, 177; Hill 2005, 78). Many farm workers, however, had been badly treated by their white employers before the expulsions (Moyo 2006, 155) and thus may have supported land reform. But by 2004 only 1 percent of "resettled" black farmers (those who took over expropriated land) were estimated to have formerly been farm workers (Hellum and Derman 2004, 1795). Some farm workers were immigrants from other African countries, thus not eligible for the land that was, in principle, earmarked for redistribution to black Zimbabwean citizens (Human Rights Watch 2003b, 18).

The ostensible reason for land invasions was that whites had taken over land while Zimbabwe was under colonial rule; however, over 80 percent of white-owned land had changed hands since independence (Blaire 2002, 177). These farms had by law to be first offered to the government, which had refused the offers (Lessing 2003, 8). One reason for this refusal may have been lack of funds despite the British loans, especially as the price of commercial farmland increased (Dashwood 2004, 224). Moreover, there was pressure on the government to pay white farmers in foreign currency, as the Lancaster House Agreement had specified that landowners were to be permitted to remit their compensation to any country outside Zimbabwe without paying tax on it (Southern Rhodesia Constitutional Conference 1979, Annex C, C, V.3).

Many of the farms taken over after 2000 were distributed to single black owners, not to landless peasants. One scholar estimated that middle-class and urban "new farmers" received about 40 percent of the land, among whom at least 10 percent were members of Zimbabwean elites (Makadho 2006, 181). Much of the redistributed land went to Mugabe's relatives and allies, or to ZANU-PF supporters. For example, the Minister of Home Affairs received five farms, and Mugabe's wife received two (Power 2003, 4). Some of these individuals did not cultivate the land they received, instead using it and the former owners' houses as country estates. By mid-2008, many farms remained empty, not yet allocated to new settlers of any kind (Besada and Moyo 2008b 11). Subsistence peasants and urban poor who did receive land were often unable to produce for the market.

The land expropriations caused a severe downward spiral in the Zimbabwean economy. Food was no longer available at reasonable prices to urban and other Zimbabweans who did not produce their own food. An unprecedented need to import food caused a drain on foreign currency. This caused severe inflation, which the government tried to ameliorate by imposing price controls on food, resulting in even more severe shortages as producers refused to sell at prices below the cost of production, forcing even more of them to revert to subsistence production. In October 2008 the official inflation rate was estimated at 231 million percent per year (Dugger 2008, October 12, 10): By mid-November, it took only 24.7 hours for prices to double (Hanke 2009). In early 2009 prices finally stabilized after the new unity government decided to make US dollars legal tender and pay government employees in dollars, leaving other Zimbabweans to rely on barter (Hammer 2009b, October 25, 48–49), smuggling, or illegal importation of foreign currency.

During this period more and more Zimbabweans relied on remittances from relatives abroad, especially emigrants to South Africa, to support themselves. Emigrants were estimated to have sent $US 680–905 million in cash and goods to Zimbabwe in 2011 alone (von Burgsdorff 2012, April 11, 3). To evade price controls, many Zimbabweans resorted to smuggling goods into and out of the country (Besada and Moyo 2008a, 16). Finally, the general economic chaos meant that even after the currency was stabilized and inflation controlled the government did not have funds to pay reasonable wages to its civil servants, including teachers and medical personnel (Dube 2011, June 2), who in consequence had difficulty buying food.

At the same time, lost taxation revenue from displaced large-scale farmers meant that the government no longer subsidized inputs such as fertilizer and seed needed by peasants living in the "communal" areas set aside for them under colonial rule, as well as by the newly resettled farmers on formerly white-owned land. These losses should not be overestimated, however, as many of the large-scale farmers had been proficient at evading taxes (Makasure 2014, December 7). There were also accusations that distribution of inputs was politically biased, with MDC supporters denied fertilizer and seed (Gonda and Zulu 2012, February 8), causing a downward spiral in the amount of crops communal and peasant farmers could produce. The severe inflation also eroded farmers' capacity to buy seeds and fertilizers at market prices (Zimbabwe Independent 2009, August 20).

Moreover, many people who were genuinely attempting to farm expropriated land were undermined by a government policy that ostensibly gave them 99-year leases but stipulated that the leases could be cancelled at 30-days' notice; the actual guaranteed lease of one month was insufficient to use the land as collateral for bank loans (Internal Displacement Monitoring Centre 2008, August, 38, fn. 158). Land that had previously produced food surpluses sufficient not only to feed the entire country but also to export reverted at best to subsistence production, while many communal farmers also reverted to subsistence from commercial agriculture (Richardson 2005, 531).

Mugabe encouraged invasions even of farms owned by foreigners whose property rights were supposedly guaranteed by bilateral Zimbabwean agreements with governments such as Germany and South Africa (Shaw 2010, July 2). Even farms that the Zimbabwean High Court had protected were invaded, in defiance of the rule of law (Bell 2010, July 2). Meanwhile, there were reports that senior military and political figures were evicting black small-holders, the very people the land reforms had ostensibly been designed to help (Mashiri 2010, October 15), and that ZANU-PF was encouraging illegal takeovers of urban land from MDC supporters (Corcoran 2012, February 2). While this did not appear to disturb Mugabe, he objected when he heard that some new owners were leasing their land back to former white owners (Bhebhe 2011, September 8).

Ironically, in 2010 Zimbabwe began to import maize from Zambia, to which it had previously exported food. Even more ironically, some of Zambia's new surplus food was produced by white Zimbabwean immigrant farmers (Lessing 2003, 10; Whande 2010, July 8; Newsdze Zimbabwe 2012, June 11). Whereas in 1996 Zimbabwe had produced 263,000 tons of wheat and 3,131,000 tons of cereal, by 2011 the respective figures were 44,000 and 1,768,000 tons. Wheat exports declined from 54,900 tons in 1996 to only 100 pounds in 2011, while cereal exports declined from 317,900 to 1,300 tons (FAOSTAT). Thus, resettled farmers were producing far less food for themselves, the urban market, and export than the expropriated commercial farms. Resettled farmers seemed most successful in producing tobacco for export (Smith 2013, September 4; Hanlon et al. 2013, 180–81), thereby contributing to their own personal capacity to buy food but not increasing the country's overall food stocks.

Despite these problems, two reports after the crisis period suggested that land reform was somewhat successful. Among the million people settled on land expropriated from white farmers, some managed to cultivate both subsistence and market crops (Scoones et al. 2010, 233). This suggested some hope for economic progress after the land seizures ended, assuming that the government adopted sensible farm support policies such as making sure that the new occupiers received secure land tenure, either in ownership or genuine 99-year leases (Mangudhla 2013, May 24) that could be used for collateral, and supplying inputs such as fertilizers and seeds (Scoones et al. 2010, 243; for a critique of Scoones et al., see Dore 2012, November 13). Another imperative was to institute a land audit to reduce multiple farm ownership, especially among Mugabe's family members, members of his entourage, and politicians and military men who had received land that they did not farm and in which they did not invest (Chivara 2013, May 3). Given that the land expropriations were a *fait accompli*, it seemed best to focus on ways to assist resettled farmers. "Repeasantization" (Cliffe et al. 2011, 909) of Zimbabwe's agriculture, supported by appropriate land tenure arrangements and agricultural inputs, could result in widespread household production of nutritious food, as long as centralization of land ownership in the hands of the black elite could be controlled.

In 2013 a new book by Joseph Hanlon, Jeannette Manjengwa (herself the recipient of a farm under the fast-track land reform (Hanlon et al. 2013, 233)), and Teresa Smart caused a media stir and was used as propaganda by the government. Hanlon et al. argued that there were now more resettled farmers (with their families and their workers) on formerly white-owned land than there had been expelled farm workers and their families; thus, in an end-justifies-the-means approach, they argued that the land reform was successful (Hanlon et al. 2013, 193). Tony Hawkins, a University of Zimbabwe economist, disputed their claim that more people were resettled than had been employed on large farms before 2000, arguing that the actual net employment creation was only about 6,000 persons per year (Hawkins 2013, June 5).

Hanlon et al. estimated that fewer than 5 percent of new farms, covering less than 10 percent of the land taken over by settlers, had been given to Mugabe's family or entourage (Hanlon et al. 2013, 91), although another scholar, Sam Moyo, estimated that by 2009, 30 percent of the redistributed land had gone to 15,500 members of parliament, civil servants, judges, ministers, and security and army officials (Economist 2009, March 7). Hanlon et al. also argued that production on these farms was increasing, but Hawkins replied with statistics showing that food and livestock output in 2012 was less than half the output in 2000, with cereal output down by 55 percent. Hawkins also criticized Hanlon et al. for not taking into account other ways the Zimbabwean economy had deteriorated since 2000, and for not acknowledging how corruption and the undermining of human rights and the rule of law had harmed it (Hawkins 2013, June 5).

The violent and illegal expropriation of land from white owners raised the question, discussed in Chapter 10, of what it meant to be a citizen in Zimbabwe. Some of the whites who lost their land were indeed descendants of European settlers who had been given large grants of land stolen from indigenous Africans. These Africans were never compensated for their stolen land. Thus it was easy for Mugabe to stir up a politics of vengeance against whites as a group, regardless of their citizenship, their ties to Zimbabwe, or the date of purchase of their farms. As early as 1996 he said "We are going to take the land and we are not going to pay for the soil. Our land was never bought by the colonists and there is no way we can buy back the land" (The Herald 2011, December 27). In 2014, still denying the citizenship and equality rights of white Zimbabweans, he said "The British who are here should all go back to England" (Majaji 2014, September 11).

Resentment of these perceived wealthy "outsiders" masked the corrupt allocation of many farms to the new black elite, which left many properties poorly managed or completely uncultivated, while many farm workers were unemployed. Orderly land redistribution in conformity with the rule of law, by which the state could have purchased land from white owners, might have had the same redistributive outcome at a much lower price of political violence, malnutrition, and disease. Hanlon and his colleagues argued that it was not their role to discuss the rights and wrongs of either the colonial or the contemporary Zimbabwean government (Hanlon et al. 2013, 13). But aside from the ethical implications of ignoring them, this approach assumes that human rights violations have no effect on the right to food.

The takeovers of large, white-owned farms were not the only reason for food shortages in Zimbabwe, especially after 2008. Zimbabweans were vulnerable to the international food price hikes that began in that year (Howard-Hassmann 2010, 76–82); they were also vulnerable to climate change. Food shortages also tended to be seasonal, as Zimbabweans waited for the next year's harvest. However, the poor harvests after 2000 were in large part a consequence of redistribution of the land, much of which was never cultivated by rich new owners. In other cases, new smallholders either did not know how to cultivate the land they received or lacked the necessary inputs to do so.

It seemed by 2015 that there was no turning back from the expulsions of white farmers: the most that they might hope for, someday, was modest financial compensation. One may still question, however, whether the possible positive long-run outcome of the forced land redistribution justified the years of intense national suffering that coincided with it. Aside from violations of the right to food during the actual period of redistribution, the consequences for the children who suffered from wasting and stunting were life-long, and would affect not only their health but also their capacity to learn. Thus, state-induced malnutrition undermined Zimbabwe's future human capital.

Assaults on Livelihoods

Aside from land invasions, the Zimbabwean government instituted other policies that deprived citizens of their capacities to buy food. In 2005, it instigated Operation Murambatsvina (loosely translatable as "Operation Drive Out Trash"), a cruel name for a decision to destroy the homes and small businesses of approximately 700,000 urban Zimbabweans, ostensibly human "trash" with no right to live in urban areas, severely compromising their housing, nutrition, and health (UN-Habitat 2005, July 27). This affected a total population of 2.4 million (Potts 2006, 276). One motive for this attack on urban dwellers was to punish supporters of the opposition MDC (Bratton and Masunungure 2006, 26), including displaced farm workers who had drifted to the cities hoping to find housing and work (Romero 2007, 277), although many of those affected were ZANU-PF supporters. The government also wanted to gain control of the foreign currency that circulated in the informal economy (Bratton and Masunungure 2006, 25). No food was provided for those driven out of urban areas.

In November 2006 the government expelled tens of thousands of gold panners and their families from gold-producing areas. Some of these people had already been displaced by the land reforms (Maguwu 2008, 37) or by Operation Murambatsvina and were trying to eke out a living looking for gold. The government argued that the panners were depriving the Zimbabwe Reserve Bank of gold it should be able to sell on the international market (Internal Displacement Monitoring Centre 2008, August, 39). As new gold deposits were found, Mugabe and/or ZANU-PF took control of them too; the biggest gold trader in Zimbabwe in 2012 was rumored to be a very powerful ZANU-PF cabinet minister (Smith 2012, January 9).

In 2006 enormous diamond deposits were discovered in the Marange region and immediately populated by small diamond diggers. These deposits could have been a boon to Zimbabwe's economy, had they been properly managed and the revenues gone to the state rather than private individuals. But in October 2008 the military overran the diamond deposits, killing at least 200 small diamond diggers and displacing over 4,000 families (Human Rights Watch 2010a, 1). Mugabe and his coterie used the diamond wealth to buy votes in the 2013 election (Economist 2013, February 23, 45). Thus, deprived of income, the small diamond-diggers, like the gold panners, were at risk of malnutrition and starvation.

In March 2008 the government passed the Indigenization and Economic Empowerment Act, intended to intensify a long-standing indigenization program by transferring 51 percent of corporate ownership to indigenous Zimbabweans (Besada and Moyo 2008b, 16), although later it decided to vary the percentage of a company that a foreign investor could control, depending on the economic sector (Bhebhe 2010, August 28). Indigenous Zimbabweans were defined as "any person who, before 18 April, 1980, was disadvantaged by unfair discrimination on the grounds of his or her race, and any descendant of such person," as well as any business firm in which indigenous Zimbabweans held the controlling interest (Government of Zimbabwe 2007, Part IV, 12). Thus, white Zimbabweans were not considered indigenous.

Indigenization further eroded the fragile Zimbabwean economy, as investor trust was undermined by the threat of indigenization and the capricious ways in which it proceeded. It seemed the government was also targeting British and European-owned companies in retaliation against the European Union's travel ban against Mugabe and about 200 senior officials, discussed in Chapter 9 (Mashiri 2010, October 15). Some commentators viewed indigenization as a vehicle for corruption, in which shares in foreign companies would be handed out liberally to Mugabe's family and allies (Dore 2012, May 4, 2).

It seemed the government was particularly interested in indigenizing the diamond and platinum mines; Zimbabwe had the world's second-largest platinum mines after South Africa (Lourens 2011, September 1). Foreign owners argued that indigenization failed to take account of the need for capital investment (Banya and Dzirutwe 2011, September 14), which they supplied but to which new Zimbabwean co-owners would not be able to contribute. This would be especially so if the Zimbabwean co-owners obtained their shares via corruption, not through an open market mechanism (Vigil 2011, October 5). It appeared likely that if the government enforced its indigenization policy, some mining companies would leave the country, thus reducing employment opportunities as well as tax revenues. Reduced employment meant less opportunity for Zimbabwean workers to acquire food, while reduced tax revenue meant that the government would have lessened capacity to provide food to the poor. In any event, it appeared that the real meaning of "indigenization" was accumulation of gold and diamonds by members of the political and military elite (Mtondoro et al. 2013). Indeed, it seemed that none of the revenue from gold and diamonds was flowing into government coffers, although one estimate was that they should have generated about $US 2 billion per year (Hawkins 2009, vii).

Urban expulsions, expulsions of small-scale gold-panners and diamond miners, indigenization, and economic chaos all undermined Zimbabweans' capacities to earn their own living and feed themselves and their families; it was estimated that in 2009 the unemployment rate was 95 percent (Central Intelligence Agency 2015). Yet displaced and unemployed Zimbabweans had to pay very high prices for such food as they could obtain. Even taking into account climate change and lack of rainfall, as well as rising international food prices after 2008, the major reason for lack of food was incompetence at best, and corrupt and racist at worst, government policies. Nor could Zimbabweans protest against these measures, rely on the courts for relief, or vote against them without fear of immediate and violent reprisals, as they were increasingly denied civil and political rights.

Civil and Political Rights

Civil and political rights were already fragile in Zimbabwe before 2000, but after 2000 became increasingly so. In order to successfully promote land invasions, the government had first to ensure that it had no political opposition and would not be subject to the rule of law.

Although it had seemed that elections in the 1980s and 1990s were free and fair, in fact Mugabe had intimidated, threatened, and imprisoned members of the opposition (Kriger 2005), and undermined the rule of law, freedom of the press, and free speech. As early as 1982 Mugabe said of the opposition, "An eye for an eye and an ear for an ear may not be adequate in our circumstances. We may very well demand two ears for one ear and two eyes for one eye" (AIDS-Free World 2009, 8). In 1993, anticipating the land invasions, Mugabe challenged the courts, saying, "We will not brook any decision by any court [preventing us] from acquiring any land" (Meredith 2005, 631). In 2001 the Supreme Court ruled against land invasions on the grounds of procedural flaws and political discrimination, as the government had announced that only ZANU-PF supporters would receive redistributed land (Meredith 2007, 197–98). The government retaliated by harassing judges. In 2000 a mob invaded the Supreme Court shouting "Kill the judges" (Meredith 2005, 641), and the next year Chief Justice Anthony Gubbay, whom Mugabe himself had appointed, resigned after Mugabe accused him of aiding and abetting racism (Martin 2006, 251).

In 2002 the government passed the Public Order and Security Act and the Orwellian-named Access to Information and Protection of Privacy Act, both laws that "stifled almost all public criticism of Mugabe" (Hammer 2008a, June 26, 27). Independent media were also harassed. In 2002 the government closed and burned offices of independent newspapers. In 2010, it issued an arrest warrant for the editor of *The Zimbabwean*, an opposition newspaper edited from Britain (Greenslade Blog 2010, November 22). In 2012, the government barred unregistered foreign newspapers, many of them opposition newspapers published by exiles (Banya 2012, February 3).

Mugabe and his inner circle also encouraged violent attacks against the opposition, especially in 2008 when it seemed likely that the MDC might win a free and fair presidential election. As the election approached, murder, torture, sexual violence, and intimidation of members of the opposition and their families were common (for many horrific stories of torture see Godwin 2010). Despite the violence, Tsvangirai won a plurality of 47.9 percent of the votes (Pan-African Parliament 2008, June 27, 10), but was too intimidated to stand against Mugabe in the run-off election required when no candidate received over 50 percent. After pressure from the international community, Mugabe agreed to share power with his opponent; nevertheless, for several months after the 2008 election, Tsvangirai stayed in South Africa, refusing to return to Zimbabwe for fear of his life. At least 163 MDC supporters had been killed between March and June 2008 (Human Rights Watch 2009b, 8).

Despite agreeing to share power with Tsvangirai, Mugabe and ZANU-PF retained control of key aspects of the government, including the military and police (Dugger 2008, October 12, 10), defense, justice, and national security. ZANU-PF also retained control of the courts and jails, as well as the Ministry of Information, responsible for regulating the press (Hammer 2009b, October 25, 49). Opposition members and human rights activists continued to be subject to arbitrary arrest, imprisonment, and torture (Amnesty International 2012a): ZANU-PF militants plundered the private granaries and killed the livestock of MDC supporters (Human Rights Watch 2009a, 13). In 2011 ZANU-PF youth were reported to be mobilizing again, attacking, for example, citizens' meetings (Madongo 2011, June 27).

These violations of civil and political rights reinforced the economic policies that devastated the Zimbabwean economy and contributed to malnutrition, if not outright deaths from famine and disease. Mugabe and his cronies progressively implemented a dictatorship that merged political repression and violation of the rule of law with violation of property rights and the right to work.

Penal Starvation

Amongst the many Zimbabweans suffering food shortages, perhaps prisoners suffered the worst. In 2008 prison rations were cut from three meals to one a day (Godwin 2010, 308). By 2009, prisoners were "moving skeletons, moving graves," dying of starvation and often left as maggot-infested corpses because there was no place to bury them. Prisoners fought over food, traded sex for food, and ate food waste (Alexander 2009, March 21, 995). In 2014, an estimated 19,000 prisoners faced starvation because of lack of food; at least one hundred prisoners had died of starvation in 2013 (Mathuthu 2014, January 16).

It is difficult to determine whether the mistreatment of prisoners was deliberate penal starvation, a matter of policy as in North Korea, or a consequence of incompetence and lack of resources combined with indifference. Prisoners have no influence in dictatorial societies, and when economic crisis means resources are almost non-existent many other people take precedence over them. On the other hand, starvation in Zimbabwean prisons may have been a result of corruption. Top military personnel had taken over prison administrative positions, while members of ZANU-PF militias had replaced trained, experienced guards

(Alexander 2009, March 21, 996). Moreover, the regime imprisoned many of its political opponents – including Morgan Tsvangirai himself before the 2009 Unity Government – and might have deliberately imposed starvation rations to punish them. The mere awareness of malnutrition and starvation in Zimbabwean prisons functioned as a warning to political opponents of what awaited them, should they be incarcerated (Gavaghan 2009, April 2).

A Faminogenic State

The government of Zimbabwe was at best indifferent to and at worst intentionally disregarded the food crisis after 2000. It maintained a Grain Marketing Board, but distributed state-owned grain only to ZANU-PF's political supporters and withheld it from those thought to be its opponents (Human Rights Watch 2003a, 2008b). It also denied international food aid to its perceived opponents, requiring recipients to produce ZANU-PF party cards (International Crisis Group 2004, 103). Moreover, the maize it distributed was often too expensive, partly because of corrupt dealings between government officials and private businessmen, and partly to accumulate funds that would support ZANU-PF while undercutting the private market in grain (Human Rights Watch 2009a, 16). Mugabe prevented NGOs from distributing food (Oborne 2003, 9–10), while food-for-work programs were confined to ZANU-PF supporters. The government relied on ZANU-PF militias, the armed forces, traditional leaders, and indeed even school principals to control food distribution. Indicating a complete breakdown of community and solidarity, teachers denied food to students and neighbors denied it to children, if the children were thought to come from MDC families (Physicians for Human Rights Denmark 2002, May 21, 15).

All of the actions enumerated above violated the International Covenant on Economic, Social and Cultural Rights, whose Article 2 prohibits discrimination on political grounds: Zimbabwe ratified this treaty in 1991. The policies of the Zimbabwean government after 2000 thus confirm Marcus' view that state-induced famine, or faminogenesis, should be considered a distinct crime. Working upward from Marcus' least criminal fourth degree of faminogenesis, one cannot argue that famine in Zimbabwe was simply caused by incompetence. Rather, at minimum, Mugabe and his colleagues were guilty of the third degree of faminogenesis, indifference. In 2002, faced with accusations that people were starving, Didymus Mutasa, then minister of national security and head of the secret police, said "We would be better off with only 6 million people, with our own people who support the liberation struggle.

We don't want all those extra people" (Grundy 2006, October 2; Lamb 2006, xxvii).

Moreover, the government was not simply indifferent to hunger that was the result of natural causes or inadvertent political or economic incompetence. Rather, it recklessly pursued its policies even when there was clear evidence of their detrimental consequences, thus engaging in second-degree faminogenic behavior. In fact, the government pursued first-degree faminogenic policies: Mugabe and his cronies intentionally implemented policies that would enrich themselves, even when they knew the results would be a decreased food supply. The core cause of the food deficit situation was the interests and ambitions of Mugabe and his inner circle.

Mugabe's intent to induce starvation, if not famine, can be shown by his deliberate decisions at various times after 2000 to stop the WFP from importing grain or distributing it to regions where there were many MDC supporters, as discussed in Chapter 9. His deliberate policies to distribute government relief grain only to his political supporters also show his intent to induce starvation. Politicized distribution of food aid – often presented as a "gift" from Mugabe (The Herald 2013, July 10) – was especially pronounced in the months before the 2013 election (Laing 2013, May 6), perhaps meant both to buy votes and to warn MDC voters about what would happen after the election.

The almost-famine in Zimbabwe after 2000, then, was not a result of natural disasters; nor was it a result, as polite commentators suggested, of policy "failure" (The Elders 2008, November 3). It was the result of policy success; the policy was to maintain Mugabe and his inner circle in power. Nor was the situation in Zimbabwe merely a "complex emergency," a result of "poor governance" (USAID January 5, 2009). The emergency was a consequence of the decisions of active political agents engaged in successful governance strategies advancing their own interests; while its consequences were complex, its causes were not. Land theft; attacks on livelihoods; corruption; denial of civil and political rights; and torture, violence, and murder were all policies whose intent was to assist Mugabe and his inner circle to stay in power, and whose consequence was severe malnutrition.

6   Venezuela

In contrast to the horrific food policies in Zimbabwe and North Korea, Venezuela from 1999 to 2013 under the rule of President Hugo Chávez seems at first glance to have been a case of food insecurity via incompetence, Marcus' fourth category of faminogenesis (Marcus 2003, 246). Chávez's policies were originally intended to improve the access of the poor to food. He used Venezuela's oil wealth to establish food "missions" (*misiones*) that distributed free food to the poor, and opened state-owned markets (*Mercals*) that sold food in poverty-stricken areas at subsidized prices (Gott 2011, 256–59; Jones 2007, 395). Chávez also imposed price controls on food. Thus, in the very short term he improved fulfillment of Venezuelans' right to food.

However, food shortages became common during the later years of Chávez's presidency, yet he recklessly continued his policies. He also intentionally imposed controls on civil and political rights, thus depriving himself of the chance to respond to criticisms and rectify his policies, as the North Korea and Zimbabwean governments had also done.

Historical Background

From 1958 to 1998 Venezuela was ruled by a "pact" (Kornblith 2006, 290) that allowed the major political parties to alternate power while also accommodating the interests of minor parties. While it was based particularly in the middle classes, the pact also accommodated the interests of other social groups including organized labor, the church, businesspeople, and the armed forces. The pact's economic basis lay in "clientelistic distribution of the petroleum income" (Duarte Villa 2007, 154).

The pact encountered trouble in the 1980s and 90s. In 1983 currency devaluation ushered in a period of social and economic decline during which poverty rates rose (Kornblith 2006, 291). That same year witnessed an end to the "petro-bonanza," or high price of oil, that had started in 1973 and had permitted government to dispense benefits to its supporters (Myers 2008, 290). The period 1987–98 was characterized by a drop in income per capita, rising inflation, depreciation of the currency, and a boom-and-bust economy that followed fluctuations in oil prices (Kelly and Palma 2004, 206–18). In 1989 shortages of basic foodstuffs along with an increase in the price of gasoline caused riots in Caracas, in which from 300 to 1,000 people were killed (Kornblith 2006, 291; Duarte Villa 2007, 157).

During the 1990s, economic decline, increased unemployment, and high rates of poverty continued (Kornblith 2006, 298). By 1998 between two thirds and three quarters of Venezuelans lived below the poverty line (Myers 2008, 288; Shifter 2006, 47). In 1999 the purchasing power of the average Venezuelan salary was only about 33 percent of what it had been in 1978 (Kelly and Palma 2004, 207). Thus, if Chávez mismanaged the economy, undermining long-term food security, he was certainly not the first Venezuelan president to do so. Nor was Chávez the first president to rely on oil rents to subsidize government expenditures, rather than trying to encourage a more efficient economy (Briceno-Leon 2005, 3–4).

In 1992 Chávez, then a member of the military, attempted a coup d'état. The coup failed and he was jailed for two years; on his release, he established a mass political movement, the Movement of the Fifth Republic (Duarte Villa 2007, 159). In 1998 he successfully ran for president, receiving 58 percent of the vote (Duarte Villa 2007, 160).

In 2002 Chávez overcame an attempted coup by middle-class and military elements (Duarte Villa 2007, 163; Marcano and Barrera Tyszka 2006, 169). He remained in power through a combination of genuine support from some of the poor, some policies such as cheap gas and expanded state employment that benefited the middle classes as well as the poor (Lupu 2010; Corrales 2013, 32), and a good dose of electoral chicanery (Corrales 2011), winning every election in which he ran from 1998 to 2012. He also won a recall referendum in 2004, although he lost a 2007 referendum on constitutional amendments. However, only in 1998 were the poor more likely to vote for Chávez than other income groups, though throughout his tenure the rich were disproportionately unlikely to vote for him (Lupu 2010, 23). By the end of his tenure many among the poor were fed up not only with food shortages but also with the corruption and nepotism that characterized his rule. Chávez died of cancer on March 5, 2013, to be succeeded by Nicolás Maduro, who continued and intensified his policies.

Many commentators consider Chávez to have been a populist leader (e.g., Castaneda 2006, 38–42). Populist political leaders appeal to the underprivileged masses; often this appeal relies on a perceived personal relationship between a charismatic leader and his followers rather than on an explicit policy platform (Sandbrook et al. 2007, 28). This appears to have been the case in Venezuela, where Chávez relied on his identification with the poor and his self-portrayal as a man of the masses of non-European descent, as opposed to the white elite. Chávez also exemplified economic populism, relying on "the creation of a material base for the public's support and the distribution of favors to constituents," while ignoring resource constraints (Cordova Cazar and Lopez-Bermudez 2009, 401). But Chávez also relied for support on the military, from which he himself had emerged (Kornblith 2006, 311): Members or former members of the military occupied many positions in government and the nationalized sectors of the economy (Briceno-Leon 2005, 19).

The Right to Food

Scholarly evaluations of Chávez's record as President are mixed; some focus on the good he did for Venezuela's poor while others emphasize the economic harm he caused. Those who praise him mention in particular his food policies. Chávez established the *Mercals,* special people's markets, where a large range of subsidized goods could be purchased. By 2006 almost 16,000 stores throughout Venezuela offered subsidized food at about 30 percent less than private market prices (Weisbrot and Sandoval 2007, 2): By 2007, a little over nine million people (of a total population of about 28 million) shopped for food at the *Mercals* (Penfold-Becerra 2007, 74). Moreover, as of 2008 3.9 million children benefited from a school food program (Weisbrot 2008, 6), as against only 252,000 children in 1999 (Weisbrot and Sandoval 2007, 8). The missions also distributed free food to the very poor (Duarte Villa 2007, 166).

However, "shortages of foods such as beef, sugar, corn oil, milk, chicken and eggs" (Weisbrot and Sandoval 2007, 16) began as early as 2007. By late 2007 other basic foodstuffs such as sardines and black beans were also scarce (Rodriguez 2008, 4). Price controls were a major cause of these shortages. Producers lacked incentives to produce and sell food at control prices that were less than the costs of production and distribution. By 2008, a "steep drop in food production and widening food scarcity" resulted from price and exchange controls and Chávez's threats to expropriate property, policies discussed below (Rodriguez 2008, 57). Prices of non-controlled goods rose as producers tried to compensate for their losses on controlled goods; for example, some dairy producers substituted non-controlled cheese for controlled milk (Daniel 2008, April 30), and one rice-processing plant started to sell non-controlled flavored rice (Economist 2009, March 12). Demand for these non-controlled goods rose as a reaction against shortages in the controlled sector.

The sale of food at control prices also opened up opportunities to exploit the dual price system, as entrepreneurs bought food at *Mercals* and then resold it, illegally, at higher prices; managers of *Mercals* stole food from inventory and sold it at home or abroad (Corrales 2013, March 14). This method of exploiting the dual price system was especially lucrative because of the food shortages. Prices of non-subsidized and non-controlled foods also rose drastically as a consequence of inflation, which averaged about 22 percent annually from 2003 to 2011 (Weisbrot and Johnston 2012, 21). In order to combat inflation, Chávez ordered controls on more and more items, so that by 2012 the prices of hundreds of foods were controlled (Devereux 2012, September 4).

The more controlled goods, the higher the prices on the black market became when goods could not be found at *Mercals*. Thus in a vicious spiral, price controls encouraged higher black market prices, which in turn resulted in more controlled prices and more shortages. In January 2013 the Venezuelan Central Bank reported that 78 percent of retail establishments it had surveyed did not have enough sugar, while the figures for other staples were 67 percent shortage for vegetable oil, 57 percent for corn oil, 86 percent for sunflower oil, 77 percent for wheat flour, and 43 percent for precooked corn (DVA Group and Selinger Group 2013, January 18). Over one year, from January 2011 to January 2012, the price of a kilogram of sugar rose from 87 cents to $2.56, while the street price of a bottle of corn oil was over $4.50, three times the control price of $1.40 (Sanchez 2012, January 3). 2.2 monthly salaries at minimum wage were required in January 2013 to buy the monthly food basket (DVA Group and Selinger Group 2013, January 15).

Nor was food necessarily distributed equitably; rather, it was distributed on a clientelistic basis either to neighborhoods that already supported Chávez politically (Penfold-Becerra 2007, 78–79), or whose support Chávez hoped to obtain (Hidalgo 2009, 81). Indeed, the Inter-American Commission on Human Rights tactfully warned in 2009 that since mission policies were "determined at the discretion of the executive branch" the impression might be garnered that "some persons are not eligible for these benefits as a result of their political position vis-a-vis the government" (Inter-American Commission on Human Rights 2009, December 30, 267).

The food missions were used as political tools to persuade people to vote for Chávez in the 2004 recall referendum and the 2006 and 2012 elections: for example, during the 2006 election the missions allocated resources to "groups whose votes President Chávez sought"

(Myers 2008, 313). In the run-up to the 2012 election, Chávez imposed controls on a far wider range of goods in an attempt to ensure that the poor could buy them. Despite the shortages, the *Mercals* remained extremely popular, and Chávez's opponents promised to keep funding them even if he lost office (Daguerre 2011, 843). Yet at least in the early years the missions were not subject to auditing; spending on them was entirely a matter of Chávez's discretion (Marcano and Barrera Tyszka 2006, 269–70). Nor was it possible to ascertain whether, later on, more accountable budgeting procedures were instituted. The government was "reluctant" to release information specifically on mission programs, including the food mission (Penfold-Becerra 2007, 75).

Despite the food shortages, statistics on the right to food in Venezuela showed marked progress from 1999 to 2012. The number of undernourished people fell from an estimated four million in 2000 to one million in 2010 (Food and Agriculture Organization 2013, indicator V01). In 2000, 27.1 percent of the population was estimated to be without enough food for normal physical activity, but by 2010 that figure had declined to 6.4 percent (Food and Agriculture Organization 2013, indicator V15). The depth of the food deficit (the number of calories per day per person needed to end malnourishment) fell from 108 in 2000 to 16 in 2010 (Food and Agriculture Organization 2013, indicator V14). The prevalence of stunting, or child malnutrition under five as measured by height per age, was 17.4 percent in 2000 but 15.6 in 2007 (Food and Agriculture Organization 2013, indicator V16). The infant mortality rate declined from 19.6 per 1,000 in 1999 to 12.9 per 1,000 in 2011, while the under-five mortality rate declined from 23.1 per thousand in 1999 to 15 in 2011 (World Bank 2013a).

During the first few years of Chávez's tenure the poverty rate rose as a result of a temporary drop in the price of oil and destabilizing political events, including the 2002 attempted coup and a protracted strike by oil workers in 2002–03. The percentage of people living below $1.25 per day rose from 11.4 in 1999 to 19 in 2003, and the percentage of people living below the national poverty line rose from 48.7 in 1999 to 62 in 2003. Later statistics, however, show a significant drop in poverty, reflecting Chávez's consolidation of power, recovery in the price of oil, and creation of the social welfare missions. By 2006, the percentage of people living below $1.25 per day had fallen to 6.6, while the percentage living under the national poverty rate had fallen to 36. By 2012, the national poverty rate had dropped further, to 25.4 percent (all statistics in this paragraph from World Bank).

These statistics suggest that Chávez's policies did indeed assist Venezuelans to realize their right to food in the short run. In the longer run, though, when food shortages began, citizens were increasingly unable to criticize Chávez's policies or vote against them.

Civil and Political Rights

Populist claims to represent "the people" do not extend to standard liberal forms of democratic rule. Rather, populist rulers tend to assume that once they win democratic elections they have license to act as they wish, abjuring legislative checks and balances, undermining the rule of law, and violating those civil and political rights such as freedom of speech and press that might allow their opponents to garner support. This was the pattern in Venezuela under Chávez, who attempted to implement "twenty-first century socialism" to reign in the excesses of "savage capitalism" (Myers 2008, 285, 319). Yet without the protections of civil and political rights, citizens opposed to or adversely affected by government policies cannot make their concerns known. This occurred in Venezuela, as Chávez became increasingly dictatorial.

Chávez interpreted his electoral victories as mandates to institute whatever policies he preferred, often ruling by emergency decree. He was determined to impose his policies even in the face of evidence that they were depriving the very people he wished to help of food. Although he conducted periodic elections, he otherwise became increasingly autocratic. He intimidated or restricted the media, the judiciary, and ordinary voters: thus, elections could not be considered free or fair.

Chávez's many assaults on civil and political rights are too numerous to detail; here I discuss only some of the most egregious (for details up to 2010 see Brewer-Carias 2010). After the recall referendum in 2004 the government published a list of 2.5 million people who had signed the petition to recall him, thus making known his opponents' names (Hidalgo 2009, 83); some citizens were denied state benefits because they were known to have signed the petition (Marcano and Barrera Tyszka 2006, 283). During the 2006 election, Chávez used public assets for his campaign and the head of national oil company, Petróleos de Venezuela (PDVSA), threatened that workers who did not support Chávez would lose their jobs (Naim 2006, xvii).

On December 2, 2007, a proposal for constitutional amendments which would have given Chávez the right to be elected president in perpetuity was barely defeated in a referendum (Myers 2008, 286). Chávez was reputed to have expedited citizenship for between two and three million new voters so that they could vote for him (Gott 2011, 261). In 2009 Chávez won a second referendum to abolish term limits – allowing him to run for a third term as president in 2012 – in part by threatening people who voted against government candidates with loss of benefits (Kornblith 2013, 53), and also threatening that civil war might result if he were no longer president (Economist 2009, February 21). By law Chávez could requisition television time whenever he wanted in order to give long, rambling speeches, yet his opponents were limited to three minutes of television time per day during the 2012 election (Economist 2012, September 29, 16). Chávez again illegally used state resources to finance his campaign and threatened a civil war if he did not win (Cawthorne 2012, September 10).

In 1999, the legislature passed an Enabling Act that enabled Chávez to rule by decree; by the end of 2000 he had issued 49 decrees (Duarte Villa 2007, 162). Chávez also undermined the rule of law and independence of the judiciary. In December 2004 the Supreme Court was expanded from twenty to thirty-two members, ostensibly to reduce judges' workload; this tipped the partisan balance in favor of the government as all the new judges were Chávez's political allies (Human Rights Watch 2008a, 3–4).

Chávez instituted measures to undermine any interest group perceived to oppose his policies. Although he appointed many members or former members of the military to his Cabinet and various other positions, he also attempted to replace or supplement the military, whom he did not entirely trust after the attempted coup of 2002, with a private militia that would be personally loyal to him (Shifter 2006, 49). By 2012 there were 125,000 members of this militia, providing an armed counterweight to the ostensibly neutral military (Economist 2012, August 11). Chávez discharged 17,000 people belonging to the oil workers' union after the strike in 2002–03 (Myers 2008, 306), fostering pro-government workers' councils in their place (Human Rights Watch 2008a, 6–7). Scores of trade unionists were reported murdered and dozens arrested (Economist 2009, May 9). Chávez also passed a law prohibiting foreign funding of Venezuelan non-governmental organizations (Economist 2011, January 1).

In general, Chávez engaged in political discrimination against his real or perceived enemies, denying citizens he perceived to oppose him access to social programs, and/or blacklisting and firing opponents from the PDVSA and other state-run organizations (Human Rights Watch 2008a, 2). Human rights defenders were intimidated, threatened, and assaulted (International Bar Association Human Rights Institute 2007, 3). By 2012 there were reports of torture, death threats, and assassinations, as well as politically motivated charges brought against Chávez's opponents (Amnesty International 2012b, 2).

Chávez also undermined freedom of the press. He cancelled licenses of opposition radio stations (Inter-American Commission on Human

Rights 2009, December 30, par. 20, p. xii), increased penalties for so-called defamation, and expanded laws of contempt, thus pressuring the media to censor itself (Vivanco and Wilkinson 2008, November 6, 68). He passed laws permitting the state to supervise the content of the media and permitting imprisonment of any citizen showing "disrespect" to or supposedly insulting government officials (Human Rights Watch 2008a, 4). Judges supportive of Chávez refused to accept decisions critical of the government rendered by the Inter-American Court of Human Rights (Brewer-Carias 2010, 140) and in 2012 Venezuela withdrew from all human rights organs of the Organization of American States (Sanchez 2012, July 26).

Often, violations of civil and political rights signal concomitant violations of economic, social, and cultural rights, as they did in North Korea and Zimbabwe. Venezuela, however, shows that authoritarian populism is capable of fulfilling some citizens' economic human rights at least in the short term, as long as the economy will support the leader's intentions to distribute economic goods. After 2003 Chávez benefitted from very high prices for Venezuela's oil, yet he did not manage the economy in such a way as to ensure Venezuelans' long-run food security. In particular, his attitude to property rights and his mismanagement of overall economic policy caused severe food shortages. Yet he closed off avenues that might have been able to show him how his policies adversely affected Venezuelans' right to food. They might also have shown him how his undermining of the right to own property had adverse effects on the production and distribution of food.

Property Rights

From 2000 on, Chávez issued various decrees that "raised doubts about the protection of private property" in Venezuela (Kelly and Palma 2004, 225), despite a guarantee of the right to property in Article 115 of the 1999 Venezuelan Constitution (Bolivarian Republic of Venezuela 1999). The 2001 Land Law permitted expropriation with compensation of idle land from estates that owned a minimum of 5,000 hectares (12,355 acres) of such land; in 2005 the amount was reduced to 3,000 hectares (7,413 acres) (Wilpert 2006, 254). The law also permitted the government to regulate what was produced on private farms; for example, it could decide that a cattle ranch should produce sorghum (Marcano and Barrera Tyszka 2006, 146–47). Chávez had some justification in redistributing land: in 1997 the bottom 75 percent of Venezuelan landowners possessed only 6 percent of the land, while the top 5 percent possessed 75 percent (Wilpert 2006, 252).

Awash as he was in oil money, Chávez did promise to compensate former landowners at market rates (Wilpert 2006, 254); thus, this program was not originally analogous to Zimbabwe's arbitrary expropriations without compensation. Later, however, he reneged on his promises of compensation or offered it only in the local currency, *bolivares* (Associated Press 2011, October 30). Some landowners wanted compensation in dollars, as consistently high inflation rates devalued the *bolivar* (Corrales 2013, March 7, 3, online version). Nor did landowners want compensation in government bonds, which by 2011 some analysts believed would soon become worthless (Economist 2011, February 26). There were also concerns because the Land Law stated that the government was not obliged to compensate landowners for investments they had made (Wilpert 2006, 256).

Moreover, officials began to question the legality of ownership of productive large estates so that they could expropriate them even if they were not idle (Wilpert 2006, 259; Jones 2007, 438): They also claimed privately owned properties were actually state-owned (Corrales 2006, 37). Chávez instituted by decree many of the proposed constitutional reforms of 2007 undermining the right to own property, even though the reforms had been defeated in a referendum. The result was many takeovers of property, including large estates previously protected from takeovers as long as their land was not idle (Brewer-Carias 2010, 318). Thus, it appears that many "rescued" lands were not paid for, as they were considered to have been left idle or not legally acquired in the first place (Paullier 2012, January 2).

Chávez encouraged landless Venezuelans to invade large landholdings even before the legality of expropriation had been determined. By 2007 180,000 families had received almost 8.9 million acres of expropriated land. Any Venezuelan head of household or young person could apply for land, regardless of whether he or she was an experienced farmer; however, new peasants often had difficulty obtaining credit to buy seed (Wilpert 2006, 255–62). Thus the land resettlement policy did not seem to increase food production, as had been its intent.

The frequent extra-legal expropriations caused chaos in farming and ranching. As early as 2001 the Venezuelan cattle ranchers' federation reported that 139 farms had been invaded, although the government claimed the figure was an exaggeration (Economist 2001, April 26). By 2010, the government had reportedly seized between five million (James 2010, August 31) and 7.5 million acres of farmland (PROVEA [National Program of Human Rights Education and Action] 2012, trans. Antulio Rosales), out of a total of about 67 million acres considered suitable for cultivation, or 7.5–11 percent of Venezuela's cultivable land. In late

2011, the Venezuelan Supreme Court ruled that it would not enforce laws against occupation of private land, arguing that "above private rights are those rights for the common good destined to the production of food or other products for human consumption" (MercoPress 2011, December 17).

There is some debate as to whether land redistribution increased the food supply. Carlos Machado, an agricultural expert, calculated that from 2004 to 2012 rice production fell by 34 percent, cattle production by 27 percent, and maize production by 25 percent (Munoz 2013, April 10). Reliance on imports rose from 64 percent of food in 1998 (Gott 2011, 164) to 75 percent in 2005 (Wilpert 2006, 262). Another agricultural expert, Alejandro Gutierrez, noted that during the period 2003–11 Venezuela imported agricultural products in which it had previously been self-sufficient, while its food exports declined by 93 percent from 1998 to 2011. Insecurity of land tenure and fear of expropriation; lack of investment in infrastructure; scarcity of inputs; and lower prices paid to producers caused this decline in productivity and food exports (Gutierrez 2013a, 26–28, 32–34, trans. Antulio Rosales).

Yet statistics from the Food and Agriculture Organization for 1999 and 2011 show increased production in such staples as milk, rice, maize, and chicken (Food and Agriculture Organization). These FAO statistics, however, might have been drawn from unreliable figures produced by the Venezuelan government, figures that might have been deliberately rigged, especially by over-calculating production from expropriated land (Gutierrez 2013b). Alternatively, the problem of food shortages might have resulted not from decreased production but from decreased processing and retailing of food.

Chávez not only attacked landowners and other food producers; he also attacked wholesalers and retailers. When oil earnings declined and he was not able to subsidize Venezuelan consumers as much as he wished, Chávez blamed the market economy, claiming that price-gougers and hoarders were responsible for the high price of food. Increasingly, he used the slogan "exprópiese!" ("expropriate it!") (Grant 2010, November 15), proposing that expropriations would release food supplies and lower their prices.

By 2010 Chávez had nationalized almost 400 businesses, although these were not only in food (Corrales 2011, 125); many of these nationalized industries underutilized their capacity, went into debt, and produced less than they had under private owners (El Universal 2013, November 18, trans. Antulio Rosales). Although he had promised to pay market prices for nationalized industries, Chávez reneged when his expenditures on other parts of the economy outstripped his revenues from oil. Faced with price controls and threats to imprison those who violated them (Romero 2007, February 17), private businesspeople withdrew from food production and distribution, as they could not afford to produce or sell at the prices Chávez decreed. In early 2010 Chávez closed down hundreds of stores for "speculation," and seized a French supermarket chain (Economist 2010, January 30, 46). In May 2010 forty butchers were detained and strip-searched on the grounds that they were driving up prices; consequently many butchers stopped selling beef entirely (Sanchez 2010, May 7). High inflation rates also raised the costs of inputs for food producers, yet price controls meant that they could not raise prices, driving some producers out of business (Corrales 2013, March 7, 3, online version).

Unsurprisingly, the government had to spend more money on food imports as the local supply shrank (Ellsworth 2009, March 7). Nor did the state properly manage these imports: In June 2010 the government admitted that 30,000 tons of food were rotting on the docks, although opposition media claimed the figure was 75,000 tons (Economist 2010, June 12, 43). In January 2013 it was reported that imported goods were delayed for an average of 45 days at the docks: This might have been in part because many port managers were members of the military, some of whom demanded bribes before they would release food (DVA Group and Selinger Group 2013, January 22). Delays, wastage, and sale of controlled food on the black market explain why food imports from other countries rose; from 2006 to 2012, grain imports from neighboring Latin American countries increased by 375 percent (El Universal 2012, November 1).

Reports from 2010 to 2015 of mismanagement of food production, distribution, and imports, as well as of threatened and actual takeovers of farms, ranches, and factories were numerous. Productivity in nationalized industries was low: for example, the government owned half the productive capacity of pre-cooked maize flour but supplied only a fifth of the market (Economist 2013, February 9); this flour was the central ingredient of Venezuela's staple food, the *arepa*. The government's response to shortages was often to blame private producers for hoarding (which some may have done) rather than to rectify inefficiencies in production, storage, and transportation of food.

Macro-Economic Policies: Undermining Food Security

The statistical data above on reduced rates of malnutrition and undernourishment suggest improved distribution of food to the poor during the first few years of Chávez's rule, despite his undermining of the property rights of those who produced and sold it. Thus, Chávez's populist policies were successful in fulfilling Venezuelans' right to food. This also suggests that violations of civil and political rights do not necessarily mean concomitant violation of economic human rights, at least in the short term. Redistributive (quasi) socialist policies can be implemented without civil and political liberties.

However, such short-term improvements in the human right to food undermined Venezuelans' longer-term food security, as Chávez mismanaged temporary oil profits. Chávez used profits from the state-owned oil company, PDVSA, nationalized in 1976 by an earlier government (Duarte Villa 2007, 156), to finance food imports as well as his health, education, and food missions. As of 2002 the PDVSA was required to release at least 10 percent of its annual investments for social spending (Gott 2011, 312); for example, in 2006, it was responsible for $13.3 billion in social spending, or 7.3 percent of GDP (Weisbrot and Sandoval 2007, 8). In 2012 it donated $15.5 billion directly to the National Development Fund (Fondo de desarollo nacional: FONDEN) and spent another $28 billion on social development, or about a quarter of its reported earnings (Petroleos de Venezuela 2012, trans. Antulio Rosales). Money that might have been used to pay PDVSA employees, to maintain its equipment, and for reinvestment was instead diverted to social projects.

The state takeover of the PDVSA resulted in inefficiency and mismanagement, as Chávez frequently put military officers, his own family members, and political supporters in charge of PDVSA and of other important economic assets, regardless of whether they were qualified. The PDVSA suffered from loss of technical capacity and the problem of having to satisfy a "growing web of political patronage" (Rodriguez 2008, 6). By 2013 PDVSA had cut its production from a planned 5.8 million barrels per day to between 2.8 and three million barrels (Economist 2013, February 9). An explosion at an important refinery in August 2012, killing at least forty-two people, showed how the PDVSA was deteriorating (Economist 2012, September 1).

Chávez used Venezuelan oil as a personal asset to promote his political agenda. He sent 90,000 barrels of oil per day to Cuba in return for 30,000 doctors (Azieri 2009, 100). Jamaica, the Dominican Republic, and ten other Caribbean states signed an accord with Venezuela in 2005, allowing them to pay 40 percent of their oil debts over twenty-five years in either cash or food such as bananas, sugar, or rice (Ellner 2007, 16). Oil from Venezuela also supported Nicaragua, one of the poorest countries in the Americas, where the business and investment communities were still treated with suspicion (Kinzer 2008, June 12, 60). Indeed, through the

PDVSA-owned American retailer, CITGO, Chávez even supplied cheap fuel to several poverty-stricken areas in the United States, undoubtedly to emphasize the poverty in his imperialist enemy (Marcano and Barrera Tyszka 2006, 311, n. 17): This generous subsidy to Americans ended in 2009 when the Venezuelan economy began to unravel (Economist 2009, June 6).

Subsidizing foreigners was not a sound economic decision, as Chávez could have sold subsidized oil at higher prices on the international market and invested the profits in Venezuela. Nor was it a sound economic decision to subsidize oil for Venezuelans. In 2012 Venezuelans paid as little as 1.6 cents a liter for oil (Associated Press 2012, February 2), yet this was partly a subsidy to wealthier Venezuelans, who were far more likely to own cars than the poor. Combined with reduced production at PDVSA, these subsidies meant that by 2013 Venezuela faced a hard currency shortage and could not import enough food (Naim 2013, January 3).

Much of the money that Chávez requisitioned from PDVSA was invested in FONDEN, the agency he used to finance his missions. By 2013, FONDEN had received $56.9 billion from the PDVSA and another $45.3 billion from the Central Bank (DVA Group and Selinger Group 2013, January 25, 2). At least during the early years of his rule, Chávez personally controlled FONDEN, rather than allocating its funds to ministries in charge of social services. Neither professional bureaucrats nor anyone else knew how Chávez spent its assets; FONDEN was unaudited and disbursal of its funds not subject to normal oversight or decision-making (Corrales and Penfold 2011, 57–59).

The "off the balance-sheet spending" (Penfold-Becerra 2007, 75) enabled Chávez to distribute food and other goods to his supporters and withhold it from his opponents. Indeed, Chávez had dismantled previously existent social programs established by earlier governments before he set up FONDEN (Penfold-Becerra 2007, 64–65). Yet neither criteria for citizens' access to benefits nor rules for allocation of resources were clear (Inter-American Commission on Human Rights 2009, December 30, 266–67). Moreover, despite his control of FONDEN, Chávez still did not have enough money to finance the missions, and he began to look for new sources of funds in the later years of his presidency. Starting around 2008, he borrowed from China in exchange for cheap oil. By 2013, these loans were in the range of $46.5 billion over the preceding four years (DVA Group and Selinger Group 2013, January 18).

Chávez also increased the number of people employed by the state, thus removing some people from poverty while ensuring his own popular support. By 2009, public sector employment had doubled to two million people (Economist 2009, January 3). This is a standard populist measure that can become economically unsustainable in the longer term and was only sustainable in Venezuela because of the country's oil wealth. Some of these new jobs were given to people who were not competent, as in the case of political and/or patronage appointments to the PDVSA.

Whatever Chávez's attempts to improve access to food were, they were undermined by extremely high inflation during the second half of his rule. This inflation was caused in part by devaluation of the *bolivar*. During the first few years of Chávez's tenure, the *bolivar* was overvalued relative to foreign currencies; this encouraged food imports that would have been more expensive if it had not been over-valued: Indeed, it was often cheaper to import food than to produce it locally (Corrales 2011, 126). Thus over-valued currency permitted imports of protein-rich foods such as chicken, improving Venezuelans' overall diet during this period (Rodriguez Rojas 2009, 49, trans. Antulio Rosales). From 2003 on, however, the government devalued the *bolivar* a minimum of five times (Corrales 2013, March 7, 2). Imported food was now more expensive, so less was brought in; this new shortage was exacerbated by the requirement that importers apply for allocations of foreign exchange from the government (DVA Group and Selinger Group 2013, January 25). Company managers would queue for days hoping to receive a foreign exchange allocation, then give up and reduce imports (Rodriguez Pons and Cancel 2011, February 21).

At the same time, the changes in property relations discussed above meant that less food was being distributed internally. The result was the classic definition of inflation, "too much money chasing too few goods"; in this case, the scarce goods included food. The food price level index, an index of the price of food relative to the price of a generic consumption basket in the US in 2011, rose from 2.15 in 2000 to 4.06 in 2013 (Food and Agriculture Organization 2013). Chávez tried to encourage more food imports by introducing dual exchange rates for essential (food) and non-essential goods; for example, to buy essential goods in May 2010 one dollar cost 2.6 bolivars, whereas for non-essential goods a dollar cost 4.3 bolivars (Daniel 2010, May 16). The official rate later rose to 6.3 bolivars per dollar (Gupta 2014, January 23) for essential goods, and a higher rate for non-essential transactions (Economist 2014, February 1, 28). However, dual exchange rates increased the likelihood of currency manipulation, as businesses and individuals could buy dollars at the official rate and then sell them at the much higher black market rate.

In an attempt to counteract inflation during the run-up to the 2012 elections, Chávez announced controls on almost one hundred new food and other essential products. However, because both food imports and internal distribution had been reduced, the one because of devaluation and the other because of price controls, the sporadic food shortages that had been occurring since 2007 became quite severe. While the cost in money of controlled foods might have been very low, the cost in time to obtain food was very high as consumers spent long hours in line searching for food at different *Mercals* in their neighborhoods.

Finally, corruption contributed to economic mismanagement. Chávez appointed family members, friends from his days in the military, and political allies not only to senior positions in government but also to senior management jobs in nationalized industries. Corruption and nepotism resulted in mismanagement and underproduction, resulting in fewer exports and fewer dollar earnings that could be used to buy food: Underproduction at food-producing and processing facilities also resulted in less food both for the *Mercals* and the open market. Even if individual appointees were not corrupt, their incompetence adversely affected the food supply. As an example of nepotism, one banker originally close to Chávez was granted a monopoly to supply staple foods to the *Mercals*, thus presumably charging more than would have been the price had there been some competition among suppliers (Economist 2009, December 12). In 2014 Transparency International ranked Venezuela 161st out of 175 countries: in this corruption perception index, the higher the number, the more corrupt the country is perceived to be (Transparency International 2014).

Chávez: An Incompetent Steward of the Right to Food

If one looks at the three aspects of the right to food, to respect, protect, and fulfill it (Eide 2006), then Chávez's record is mixed. He did respect the right to food, instituting *Mercals*, free food distribution, school feeding programs, and price controls. Moreover, whatever their defects, his policies may have two positive long-run effects. Economically, his food policies may have improved Venezuela's human capital, as Venezuela's Ambassador to the US noted in 2006: "Although some critics have called these programs [the missions] clientelistic, they are simply responding to long-ignored needs and building much-needed human capital in Venezuela" (Alvarez Herrera 2006, 198). For example, programs providing school meals meant that children would be better able to learn: this may have long-run positive effects. Politically, Chávez made it difficult for future leaders to ignore the poor.

Despite these programs, Chávez's short-term fulfillment of nutritional needs undermined citizens' longer-term food security; in effect, he did not protect the right to food. In a 2004 speech at the United Nations,

Chávez spoke of his goal of food security (Gibbs 2006, 270), yet far from increasing the amount of food available, nationalizations and price controls undermined food distribution. The inflationary pressures caused by economic mismanagement priced much food out of reach of ordinary Venezuelans, while mismanagement at the ports meant imported food was delayed and sometimes rotted. Expropriation and redistribution of land may also have decreased food production. Under-pricing and bartering of oil rather than selling it on the world market undermined Venezuela's long-term capacity to protect the right to food because fewer funds were available for imports. And the clientelistic distribution of food to supporters over opponents meant that individual food security became a relatively scarce political good.

Nevertheless, these conditions do not suggest that Chávez was engaged in faminogenesis, nor was he committing what I call a state food crime. Marcus' fourth, and least blameworthy, category of faminogenesis is by incompetence. Chávez was indeed an incompetent steward of his country's economic future, wasting oil resources, expropriating food producers without planning how to replace them, and driving food distributors out of business via unrealistic price controls. Venezuela would have been better off had Chávez respected property rights and the market while subsidizing food for those who needed it. But statistics do not indicate that in the short run Venezuelans suffered severely from food shortages; certainly, there were no reports of starvation or of high malnutrition rates. Moreover, many of Chávez's planning, management, and distribution errors had also been made by preceding regimes that relied heavily on oil revenue, endured high inflation rates, and instituted price controls (Daguerre 2011). Chávez is distinguished mainly by his focus on the poor (albeit more on his perceived supporters among the poor) and by his attack on private property. The former is laudable: the latter economically unwise.

Nor could one reasonably argue that Chávez was responsible for state food crimes as I defined them in Chapter 1; that is, crimes by states that deny their own citizens and others for whom they are directly responsible the right to food. Chávez's populist platform was to provide for the poor the food to which they had previously had no access. The support he received in the 2012 elections, despite food shortages, was in part because many people believed that he cared about them in a way his predecessors had not. The fact that before that election the opposition had to assure voters that they would continue the missions – albeit with more efficiency and accountability – may indicate that politics in Venezuela had changed for the better for the long run (Reuters 2011, November 7; Economist 2012, February 11).

On the other hand, Venezuelans continued to face food shortages after Chávez's death as his successor, Nicolás Maduro, continued his policies, imposing price controls on many more items (Corrales 2013, March 7, online edition). The twelve-month inflation rate was close to 70 percent in 2014 (Economist 2015, April 4). The price of food rose by 210 percent between August 2012 and August 2014 (Salmeron 2014, September 11), partly as a result of continued devaluation of the *bolívar* but also as a result of food scarcities. Rice, coffee, and beef, previously produced in Venezuela, now arrived from other countries (Anderson 2103, April 10).

As the price of oil plummeted in 2014–15, Maduro spent much of his time making deals with other Latin American countries to import food from them, but it often rotted as ships could not unload at congested, inefficiently run ports (El Universal 2013, September 19). He encouraged more land invasions – with some retaliatory murders of peasants by landlords – (Robertson 2014, January 13); expropriated more privately owned food chains; and arrested more food producers for profiteering (Cawthorne 2014, April 26). By 2015 the government had introduced de facto rationing, for example by fingerprinting food shoppers (Wyss 2014, March 31), while citizens were arrested for tweeting photographs of empty shelves in government-owned food stores (Investor's Business Daily 2015, January 16).

Information technologists developed mobile apps and websites to provide information about what goods were available where (Associated Press 2013, June 9), and about the real (black-market) as opposed to the official exchange rate: Maduro responded by ordering arrests of the individuals maintaining the exchange-rate website (Delgado 2013, March 27). When not blaming the shortages on an imperialist, CIA-led conspiracy, Maduro explained them away as a consequence of "overconsumption" by Venezuelans (El Universal 2013, June 12). He also blamed shortages on a deliberate campaign of sabotage by food producers and distributors, ordering government agents to raid private companies' warehouses for allegedly hoarded food. The private producers responded that much of the "hoarded" food was simply what was needed to produce finished goods. Meantime, smugglers were selling price-controlled food over the border in Colombia, exacerbating the food shortages (Rueda and Bajak 2013, June 4; Kurmanaev and Willis 2014, January 8).

Ironically, as food shortages worsened Maduro accepted an award from the FAO for Venezuela's success in reducing malnutrition (El Universal 2013, June 12). While this success was real, it was due in large part to Venezuela's high oil revenues and to general and unsustainable mismanagement of the economy. Indeed, in August 2013 forecasters predicted a

7.5 percent decline in food consumption by 2017 (The Small Business Newswire 2013, August 12).

Statistics reported in 2014 by the Economic Commission for Latin American and the Caribbean showed an increase in poverty in Venezuela from 25.4 percent of the population in 2012 to 32.1 percent in 2013, and an increase in "indigence" from 7.1 percent to 9.8 percent (CEPAL 2014, 17). In April 2015 forty-three of the fifty-eight products in the Venezuelan basic shopping basket were no longer available; in any event, the cost of this shopping basket was six times the monthly wage (Martin 2015, April 24). In 2014 an independent study conducted by scholars at three Venezuelan universities concluded that although the government claimed that 95 percent of Venezuelans ate at least three meals a day, in fact 13 percent of Venezuelans did not; independent observers reported in mid-2015 that malnourished children were arriving in hospitals, some dying from starvation (Economist 2015, June 20).

In early 2014, there were large anti-Maduro demonstrations in the streets of Caracas and elsewhere protesting food shortages, during which about forty-four people (both opposition and government supporters) were killed, according to official figures (Economist 2014, May 17). Detainees accused the government of torture and death threats (Economist 2014, February 22, 31) as well as of encouraging pro-government private militias to quell the protestors (Associated Press 2014, March 11). In 2015 the Ministry of Defense authorized the armed forces to use "potentially lethal force" to control public protests (Government of Venezuela 2015, January 27). Maduro's insistent continuation of Chávez's economic policies did not bode well for Venezuelans' future human right to food.

7   The West Bank and Gaza

Unlike North Korea, Zimbabwe, and Venezuela, Israel was a democratic state. However, it was also a *de facto* colonial power. After it was attacked by Egypt, Jordan, Syria, and Lebanon in 1967, Israel conquered the territories of the West Bank (so-called because it is on the west side of the Jordan River) and Gaza. These two areas are generally known internationally as the Occupied Palestinian Territories (OPT), but after 2005 Gaza was not technically occupied, as Israel had withdrawn its settlements from the territory. As will be shown below, however, Israel did maintain effective control of Gaza, not least via the blockade it imposed in 2007. Israel also disputed that the West Bank was occupied, although the consensus of international legal opinion was that its rule did indeed constitute an occupation. Therefore, in order to focus on Palestinians' right to food, I will refer to these territories throughout as simply the West Bank and Gaza (WBG).

This chapter cannot document all Israeli laws and policies that had the effect of denying Palestinians their right to adequate nutrition: I merely indicate some major factors in the WBG. Nor do I suggest that Palestinians' own leaders bore no responsibility for these problems. Yasser Arafat, who was Chairman of the Palestine Liberation Organization and the leader in the WBG until his death in 2004 was notorious for his corruption, channeling funds meant for all Palestinians to his supporters (Allen 2006, 15). 84 percent of Palestinians responding to a 2003 survey thought there was corruption in the institutions of the Palestinian Authority (PA), a semi-autonomous body established in 1993 to govern the West Bank (Dowty 2012, 179). The PA was known to be dysfunctional and to rely on patronage and cronyism as well as outright corruption: such corruption may well have contributed to malnutrition in the WBG. Somewhat offsetting this may have been the activities of Islamic charities that provided food aid as well as other services to Gazans (Gordon and Filc 2005, 553; Masters 2012, November 27, 1, 5).

Egypt also contributed to the high rate of malnutrition in Gaza. Fearing terrorist infiltration into the Sinai Peninsula by Hamas, the

114

Islamist political movement that ruled Gaza as of 2007, Egypt sealed its border with Gaza. As a result, Gazans could not buy food and other goods they needed in Egypt. Some of the Palestinians' food problems were also caused by international increases in the price of food after 2008, over which neither Egypt, Israel nor Hamas or the PA had control. It is impossible to quantify how much of the malnutrition in the WBG was caused by Israel and how much by Palestinian authorities, by Egypt, or indeed by the international food market. Nevertheless, as the occupier of the West Bank and with *de facto* control over Gaza, Israel bore the legal responsibility to respect, protect, and fulfill the right to food in the WBG.

Historical Background

It is extremely difficult to summarize the complex history of the relations between Israel and Palestinians. Moreover, much discussion of this history is permeated by anti-Semitism and sometimes Islamophobia. The purpose of my intervention in this discussion is solely to analyze violations of Palestinians' right to food. My personal position on Israeli-Palestinian relations is that like any other state, Israel has an absolute right to exist. Like any other state, it also has an absolute right to live in peace, not subjected to terrorist attacks. Since its establishment, Israel has had major security concerns, not least of which are threats to completely delegitimize its right to exist as an independent state. But, like any other state, Israel is also obliged to respect international law, including laws that protect the right to food of the people for whom it is responsible. Conversely, Palestinians, like all other people, are entitled to protection of their human rights.

On November 29, 1947 the United Nations General Assembly in Resolution 181 called for partition of the former British mandate of Palestine into two separate states, one Jewish and one Arab; on May 15, 1948 Israel declared its independence (Dowty 2012, 270). The Arab League, however, rejected the partition plan and immediately declared war, which Israel won.

What Jewish Israelis celebrate as the day of independence is marked by Palestinians as the *Nakba*, or catastrophe (Manna' 2013). An estimated 600,000 to 760,000 (Morris 2004, 604) Palestinians either fled or were expelled from Israeli territory before, during, and after the independence struggle (for a detailed account of the expulsion of one Palestinian village, see Shavit 2013, 99–132). Some went to Gaza, a small strip of territory on Israel's southern border then administered by Egypt, while others went to Jordan (which controlled the West Bank until 1967), Syria, or Lebanon. By 1949 only about 156,000 non-Jews remained in Israel (Morris 2004,

589). By 2012 there were 1,167, 572 registered refugees living in Gaza and 727,471 in the West Bank; however, these included both the original refugees and their descendants (UNRWA 2013a; UNRWA 2013b). The total populations of these areas were 1,763,387 and 2,676,740 respectively in 2013 (Central Intelligence Agency 2013a, 2013b), including inhabitants who were not originally refugees from Israel. Israel's population in 2013 was 7,707,042 people, of whom 23.6 percent were non-Jewish, mostly Arab (Central Intelligence Agency 2013c).

Israel fought several wars against some or all of its Arab neighbors, of which the most relevant to this background section is the war of 1967. After Egypt closed the Straits of Tiran to Israeli ships, Israel attacked and occupied Egypt's Sinai Peninsula (including Gaza), the West Bank, East Jerusalem, and the Golan Heights (formally Syrian territory) (Dowty 2012, 271). The war also reflected ongoing tensions between Israel and Iraq, Syria and Jordan, all of whose militaries Israel quickly defeated (Bickerton 2012, 132). During this war 200,000 to 250,000 Palestinians fled the West Bank for Jordan, of whom only about 17,000 were ultimately permitted to return (Gordon 2008, 6).

Palestinians in the WBG were relatively quiescent until 1987, when the first *intifada,* or mass uprising against Israel, commenced. In 1993 Israeli and Palestinian representatives signed the Oslo Accords, which ostensibly laid out the responsibilities of each group to govern the WBG, allowing the Palestinian political party, Fatah, semi-autonomous authority in some but not all of the West Bank, which was divided into Areas A, B, and C. Area A, where most Palestinians lived, was under full Palestinian control; Area B was under Palestinian municipal and Israeli military control; Area C, where most Israeli settlers (see below) lived, was under full Israeli military control. A second *intifada* began in 2000. Israel withdrew its military and twenty-one settler communities from Gaza in 2005 (Gordon 2014, April 21) but retained control of land access to Gaza from its border as well as sea and air access to all of that territory. Meantime, Egypt controlled access to Gaza from its border.

The Islamist political party, Hamas, was democratically elected ruler of Gaza in 2006 and used Gaza as a base for rocket attacks against Israel. This convinced many Israelis that if they withdrew from the West Bank, Palestinians would also attack Israel from that territory. In 2007 Hamas further consolidated its power through repression of members of the more moderate Palestinian party, Fatah, murdering some Fatah members and exiling others to the West Bank (Helfont 2010, 428), while Fatah used similar tactics to rid itself of Hamas supporters. Gaza remained under Hamas rule and the West Bank under Fatah rule, although many aspects of Palestinians' day-to-day lives in the West Bank were controlled by

Israeli military rule, as discussed below. Israel defended its progressive occupation of the West Bank on security grounds, a defense that had some justification but did not preclude its obligations to protect the human rights of Palestinians.

Hamas periodically attacked Israel with home-made rockets, resulting in around thirty-two deaths inside Israel between 2004 and 2014 (B'Tselem 2014, July 24). Israel retaliated in several short battles and two very serious attacks on Gaza, from December 27, 2008 to January 18, 2009, and from July 8 to August 26, 2014. Known as Operation Cast Lead, the 2008–09 attack resulted in between 1,385 (B'Tselem 2009) and 1,419 (Palestinian Center for Human Rights 2011, December 27) Palestinian deaths, as opposed to 13 Israeli deaths. The number of Palestinian deaths in the 2014 war was estimated at a minimum of 1,473 by the United Nations (Office for the Coordination of Humanitarian Affairs: Occupied Palestinian Territory 2014, September 4), and 2,191 by the Palestinian Center for Human Rights (Palestinian Center for Human Rights 2015, March 4).

This chapter does not propose a solution to the Israeli-Palestinian conflict. My concern is solely with the right to food. Some of the complexities of the Israeli-Arab conflict will be referred to in Part III, where I consider Israel's obligations under international law to protect Palestinians' right to food, and what might have been done by the international community to ensure that right.

Malnutrition

Before the outbreak of the first *intifada* in 1987, Israel tried to justify its control of the WBG in part by maintaining that it had improved inhabitants' standard of living, boasting that Palestinians' per capita food consumption had increased from 2,460 calories per person per day in 1966 (before Israeli conquest) to 2,719 calories in 1973 (Gordon 2008, 165). But as Israel tightened border controls after 1987, simultaneously expropriating more land and water in the WBG, nutritional standards began to decline. Official figures from the Food and Agriculture Organization (FAO) reveal disquieting trends of malnourishment. Some of this malnourishment might be a result of factors that also affect other Middle Eastern countries, such as lack of arable land or poor weather conditions. For example, in 2012 the rate of malnourishment in the Arab world as a whole was about 10 percent; the rates in Jordan, Lebanon, and Syria were 5, 5, and 6 percent respectively (World Bank 2013a: no figures available for Israel). Nevertheless, the standard must be comparison with Israel, which had legal responsibility for the WBG.

In 2014, it was reported that about 894,000 Israelis suffered from hunger (not an exact comparison to malnutrition) or 11.6 percent of the population, among whom were many Arabs (YNet news.com 2014, August 8).

The percentage of people in the WBG who were undernourished (that is, suffered from hunger) increased from 17.9 in 1990 to 31 in 2012; the percentage of people who suffered from food inadequacy (a measurement of food deficiency for normal physical activity) increased from 26.6 in 1990 to 42.4 in 2012. The food deficit – that is, the difference between average dietary energy consumption and average dietary energy requirements – increased from 104 calories in 1990 to 204 in 2012 (Food and Agriculture Organization 2013, indicators V12, V15, and V14). Access to food appears to have varied in part according to the political conditions of the time. For example, in 1996, 10.6 percent of children under five were stunted, or too short for their age: in 2002 this figure had increased to 16.1 percent, but it decreased to 11.8 percent in 2007. The 2002 figure is two years after the beginning of the second *intifada*, when Israel was particularly exigent in controlling borders. Similarly, the percentage of children under five who were wasted, or underweight, increased from 3.6 in 1996 to 9.4 in 2002, but declined to 1.8 in 2007 (Food and Agriculture Organization 2013, indicators V16, V17).

A 2002 nutritional assessment of 1,000 Palestinian households in the WBG found that 2.5 percent of children suffered from acute malnutrition and 9.0 percent from chronic malnutrition (Qouta and Odeh 2005, 76). A 2003 study of 102 children in the Gaza Strip found that 34 percent were wasted and 31 percent stunted, while 73 percent were anemic (Radi et al. 2009, 163). A 2007 study of the village of Beit Haroun in Gaza found that more than half the population went without fruit, vegetables, fish, and meat on most days (Massad et al. 2011, 12). About 80 percent of Gazans relied on food aid by the 2010s (UNRWA 2013a), and the World Food Program estimated that in 2012 34 percent of Palestinians were food insecure, an increase of 7 percent over 2011 (World Food Programme 2013, June 21).

Some of the specific mechanisms by which Israel violated the right to food are discussed below.

Civil and Political Rights

Palestinians suffered, in the first instance, because they were stateless. Article 15 of the Universal Declaration of Human Rights (UDHR) states that: "1. Everyone has the right to a nationality. 2. No one shall be arbitrarily deprived of his nationality nor denied the right to change his nationality." Thus, in principle all human beings have the right to be citizens of one country or another, yet residents of the WBG endured a citizenship limbo. They had no state to represent them or to which to turn to have their concerns addressed. They were not citizens of Israel, the state that controlled them.

The United Nations Resolution that created the state of Israel mandated that everyone residing in the territory at the time of independence become a citizen. However, Israel passed a law in 1952 that defined residency as continuous presence in Israel since 1948, especially presence during a registration survey in 1952. Thus, it effectively denied citizenship to Palestinians who had been expelled or fled and had not returned (Baer 2015, 56). Palestinians who had always lived in the WBG – that is, who were not expellees or refugees – also lacked citizenship rights. Before Israeli occupation Gaza was administered by Egypt while the West Bank was controlled by Jordan, but after 1967 Palestinians in Gaza and the West Bank – whether refugees or indigenous residents – were not citizens of Egypt, Jordan, or Israel.

Palestinians in the West Bank enjoyed no civil and political rights in their interactions with Israel. They lived under pervasive and arbitrary military rule, obliged to obtain permits for many aspects of their daily existence, however miniscule (Gordon 2008). These permits made it difficult for Palestinians to establish and run businesses, farm their own land, or even graze sheep or grow vegetables (Ron 2003, 132). The Israeli military detained Palestinians without trial and tortured them; even minors were sometimes tortured (Amnesty International 2011, 4). Israel also violated other civil and political rights, for example the right to freedom of assembly, and arbitrarily closed civil society groups. Press freedom was also undermined: Israel censored Palestinian newspapers (Nossek and Rinnawi 2003, 190), and was particularly careful to censor discussion of settlers' seizures of land and water (Gordon 2008, 37), as discussed below. These violations of civil and political rights also contributed to violations of Palestinians' economic human rights; Palestinians could not speak out to defend their right to food.

However, Israel was not responsible for all violations of civil and political rights: indeed, the principal violators in the WBG after 2006 were the PA in the West Bank and Hamas in Gaza (Bazian 2009, 177). In Gaza these violations included political assassinations of (alleged or known) supporters either of Israel (Human Rights Watch 2012, October 3; Human Rights Watch 2013, April 4) or of Fatah, and severe repression of freedom of expression (Human Rights Watch 2013, July 28). Fatah responded with political repression of its own, including torture of suspected Hamas supporters in the West Bank (Blecher 2009, 68) and beatings of protestors (Human Rights Watch 2013, July 30). The PA also co-operated with Israel, for example by detaining without charge people whom Israel suspected of violence against Israel or Israelis (Bazian 2009, 175). Nor was there an independent judiciary or rule of law in the WBG (Bazian 2009, 177; Frisch and Hofnung 2007). The PA also censored newspapers critical of its rule (Nossek and Rinnawi 2003, 198–200). Thus Palestinians were caught among three separate authorities, none of which protected their human rights.

One illegal aspect of Israeli rule was collective punishment in the form of house demolitions to punish real or perceived crimes against Israel or Israelis. The Israeli human rights organization B'Tselem estimated that for every individual accused of attacking Israel, twelve innocent Palestinians lost their homes (B'Tselem 2005, February 17). One can assume that the homelessness caused by these demolitions was one cause of malnutrition: it is difficult for people without access to cooking facilities to prepare nutritious food for their families. Israel frequently demolished buildings for security reasons; for example, if it assumed a building was an entrance to a tunnel to Egypt from Gaza, as discussed below. From 2000 to 2007, almost 45,000 buildings in the West Bank and 29,000 in Gaza were damaged (Bazian 2009, 178).

Israel also undermined Palestinians' capacity to work. From 1967 to 1987, Palestinians were encouraged to work in Israel; their earnings made up for losses in agricultural production as the government of Israel and Jewish settlers took over land in the West Bank. However, access to work in Israel became increasingly restricted after the first *intifada* began, and about 100,000 people lost their jobs (Ziegler et al. 2011, 179). Once the second *intifada* started in 2000, borders were closed and restrictions on access became even tighter (Gordon 2008, 83). Earlier, Palestinians simply had to be hired by an Israeli employer to work in Israel; now, their right to work there was regulated by the military and the state. Without work, Palestinians found it difficult to buy food for themselves and their families. Restrictions on access to Israel proper were justified as a security measure, to counter frequent suicide bombings and other attacks within Israel after 2000.

Finally, Palestinians suffered particular hardships because Israel violated their right to freedom of movement (Kretzmer 2009, 318), protected by the International Covenant on Civil and Political Rights (ICCPR) in its Article 12, which mandates that people should enjoy freedom of movement within their own state. Article 4, 1 of the ICCPR mandates that states can derogate from its provisions only "to the extent strictly required by the exigencies of the situation." Yet it is not at all clear that restrictions on Palestinians' freedom of movement within the

West Bank were necessary for Israel's security. Along with frequent road closures and checkpoints, curfews prevented people from going to their own farms and from shopping for food (Ziegler et al. 2011, 178). Palestinian access to many areas of the West Bank, including Jewish settlements and military bases, was prohibited. Palestinians were forbidden to enter protective zones around Jewish settlements, nor could they enter areas where settlements' sewage, electricity, and water facilities were located (Gordon 2008, 132–36).

Moreover, Israel built roads on which cars with Israeli license plates – including the cars of Jewish settlers – could travel among settlements and between the settlements and Israel, but on which West Bank Palestinians were not permitted to drive. Indeed, by 2008 West Bank Palestinians were divided up into more than 200 enclaves, kept from each other by Jewish settlements, restricted roads, military bases, and roadblocks (Gordon 2008, 179). In July 2004, for example, there were 700 checkpoints and other physical boundaries to freedom of movement in the West Bank (Gordon and Filc 2005, 550). All these policies deprived Palestinians of the freedom of movement necessary to get to their farms or paid work. Economic development was hindered as businesspersons within the West Bank could not easily trade with one another or between the West Bank and Israel (Middle East Monitor 2011, February 24, 2).

Restriction on movement between the WBG and Israel was a matter lawfully within Israel's control, as there is no right under international law for individuals to enter states of which they are not citizens. Border controls with Israel meant that Palestinians from the West Bank could not shop there for foods available only in Israel. These border controls – and the frequent closings of the few crossings that existed – also limited the movement of people and food into and out of Gaza.

The rest of this chapter considers the West Bank and Gaza separately, to pinpoint distinct factors that contributed to malnutrition in each territory.

The West Bank

Denial of property rights and water rights particularly affected residents of the West Bank. The creation of a "seam zone" behind the wall that purportedly separated Israel from the West Bank but was actually built in the West Bank proper meant that some Palestinians were denied access to their own agricultural land.

A major cause of malnutrition in the West Bank was landlessness, caused by takeovers of Palestinian land by both the Israeli state and "private" (though state-supported) individuals. Some of the land was taken by Jewish settlers, who settled in it because of their beliefs in political Zionism, because they believed that the West Bank was actually Jewish holy land (Judea and Samaria), or simply because state-subsidized housing was cheaper in the West Bank than in Israel proper (Dowty 2012, 139, 231; Sasley and Sucharov 2011, 1005–06). By 2011, 325,000 settlers lived in the West Bank (Dowty 2012, 120). Israel actively encouraged these settlements, offering tax exemptions (Sasley and Sucharov 2011, 1006), grants and loans to settlers (Zartal and Eldar 2007) as well as providing schools for Jewish – but not Palestinian – children (Human Rights Watch 2010, December 19, 2), thus indicating that settlement was actual government policy. Many of these settlers felt it their right to destroy Palestinians' land and crops. For example, a Palestinian group claimed that between September 29, 2000 and May 21, 2003 hundreds of thousands of citrus, olive, and other trees were uprooted (Ziegler et al. 2011, 187). Settlers also stole Palestinians' olive harvests (B'Tselem 2012, October 11; B'Tselem 2013, December 25).

Israel expropriated land for nature reserves and military firing ranges, although the latter were so numerous and extensive that it is difficult to believe that they were all necessary for their stated purpose. In 2011, 46 percent of the land Israel had expropriated in the Jordan valley and Northern Dead Sea areas was for firing zones and another 20 percent for nature reserves (B'Tselem 2011, May). Israel also expropriated land on which to build its restricted roads. It used a variety of legal ruses to justify these expropriations, including a rather specious resort to the Jordanian law that had ruled the West Bank until 1967; Jordan had relied in part on Ottoman customary law, which permitted the state to expropriate "unused" land (Carter 2006, 124). By 2010 Israel occupied 42 percent of the West Bank (B'Tselem 2010, July), including settlements, nature reserves, military zones, and transportation corridors.

In effect, these settlements and expropriations meant that West Bank Palestinians enjoyed no property rights (Kretzmer 2009, 317); their farms, grazing lands, citrus and olive groves were routinely expropriated without compensation by the government, the military, and settler communities, undermining subsistence cultivation. Palestinians also lost their homes; in the first four months of 2013, Israel dismantled over 200 Palestinian homes in the West Bank (Economist 2013, May 4, 51). Israel also demolished water cisterns and animal shelters, so that it was difficult for Palestinians to keep cattle, sheep, and goats (Amnesty International 2012c, 2).

Land seizures affected Palestinians who practiced commercial agriculture, exporting food and using their profits to feed their families. Israel also imposed many measures to protect its own agricultural producers from competition with Palestinian producers (Benvenisti 2004, 125); for example, frequently Palestinian farmers were not permitted to replace dead trees in their orchards (Carter 2006, 121). Some Palestinians cultivated olive trees instead of other crops because the trees were present on the land all year round; thus, Israel could not claim their groves were "uncultivated" land eligible for takeover by the state, according to Israeli interpretations of Ottoman law (Butterfield et al. 2000, 6).

Palestinians lost not only land but also water. Clean water is a prerequisite to the right to food; without it, food cannot be cultivated, cleaned, or cooked. Access to clean water was a major problem for West Bank Palestinians. While Israelis in 2009 consumed about 300 liters of water per person per day, Palestinians consumed 70 (Amnesty International 2009, 3). The percentage of people with access to improved water in the WBG as a whole declined from 97 in 1995 to 85 in 2010 (Food and Agriculture Organization 2013, indicator V10). While Jewish settler farmers had plentiful water to irrigate their crops, Palestinians had to neglect previously cultivated land because of lack of water (B'Tselem 2011, May 2). Yet the right to water includes the right to be free from discrimination in its allocation (Committee on Economic Social and Cultural Rights 2002, Par. 12, c, iii). Israel expropriated much of the water in the West Bank for its own use or use by settlers. The main source of water was the Mountain Aquifer, but Palestinians had access to only 20 percent of the water it produced, while Israel used the rest (Amnesty International 2009, 9–10). Land expropriations and the creation of the seam zone between Israel proper and the Separation Wall also limited Palestinians' access to water (Amnesty International 2009, 36, 46).

The right to water includes protection from arbitrary interference in the water supply (Committee on Economic Social and Cultural Rights 2002, Par. 10), yet Israeli authorities frequently cut off Palestinians' water. The Israeli army destroyed private water cisterns (Amnesty International 2009, 1, 29, 35) and other traditional means by which Palestinians collected and conserved water, violating the rule that "Access to traditional water sources in rural areas should be protected" (Committee on Economic Social and Cultural Rights 2002, Par 16, c). The Israeli military required Palestinians to obtain permits to build new cisterns yet often did not grant them (Amnesty International 2009, 5). Israel destroyed some Palestinian wells and denied permits for new ones; between 1967 and 1996 it granted only thirteen permits to build new wells in the WBG (Amnesty International 2009, 12).

States are also obliged to "prevent third parties from interfering in any way with the enjoyment of the right to water" (Committee on Economic Social and Cultural Rights 2002, par. 23), yet Israel permitted

Jewish settlers in the West Bank to draw on water supplies traditionally used by Palestinians, even permitting Jewish families to have swimming pools while nearby Palestinians endured severe water shortages; this also violated the principle of equitable distribution of water. Without access to clean water, many Palestinians relied on water brought in by tankers, which could be contaminated (Stefanini and Ziv 2004, 168); segregated roadways often rendered it difficult for tankers to reach Palestinian villages (Amnesty International 2009, 53). Palestinians also sometimes endured deliberate contamination of their water supply by settlers who, for example, threw garbage or even dirty baby diapers into Palestinians' water containers (Amnesty International 2009, 39).

Lack of water also constrained Palestinian export agriculture (Butterfield et al. 2000, 17). By 2009 the shortage of irrigation water had undermined the West Bank Gross Domestic Product by as much as 10 percent, and had cost perhaps 110,000 jobs (Amnesty International 2009, 15). Lack of water for agriculture obliged Palestinian farmers to rely on purchased food, as one farmer told Amnesty International: "We can't keep more goats because we can't afford the water, and we can't grow food for us and fodder for the animals, so we have to buy it" (Amnesty International 2009, 23). Many families sold their livestock because they could not afford water for the animals (Amnesty International 2009, 38).

In general, "Water should never be used as an instrument of political and economic pressure" (Committee on Economic Social and Cultural Rights 2002, Par. 32), yet Israel controlled the West Bank water supply in its own economic and political interests. While in the early years after 1967 Israel used West Bank water to make up for its own water shortages, in later years it constructed desalinization plants, which supplied much of its water, reducing, if not eliminating, its reliance on West Bank water (Elizur 2014, January 24; Associated Press 2014, May 31). Thus, while settlers continued to use disproportionate amounts of West Bank water, Israel proper no longer needed it. In the light of Israel's ability to use desalinization to provide for its own needs, it was all the more troubling that Palestinians continued to be plagued by water shortages.

Meantime, Palestinians lost even more land after 2002, when Israel began to build an 800-kilometer "Separation Wall," actually a combination of a wall, fencing, and sensors (Thein 2004; Ben-Eliezer and Feinstein 2007, 178), in order to separate Israel proper from the West Bank for security reasons. This attempt was successful: suicide attacks on Israel in the first six months of 2004 declined 75 percent compared to the first six months of 2003 (Thein 2004, 6). However, approximately 85 percent of the Wall was actually built within the West Bank (B'Tselem 2012, October 1) in order to separate Palestinians from Jewish settlements (Cohen 2006, 684). By 2012, 8.5 percent of the West Bank was confined between Israel proper and the Wall (B'Tselem 2012, July 16). This seam zone also hemmed in about a half million Palestinians who lived there (Goldstone 2009, 48, par. 185).

Palestinian residents in the seam zone could move freely neither into Israel nor through the wall into other parts of the West Bank, including their own farms (Cohen 2006). Some lived on the east side of the Wall, but their land was on the west side; the Wall also cut off farmers from their wells and irrigation networks (Trottier 2007, 115, 120). Israel opened gates in the wall through which farmers could go to their land only for short periods every day (Stefanini and Ziv 2004, 165). Yet the seam zone contained some of the West Bank's most productive farmland: there was a 65 percent decline in agricultural productivity in this breadbasket region after the Wall was constructed (Bazian 2009, 180), in part because an estimated 86 percent of the land confiscated in order to build the Wall was agricultural (Turner 2006, 746). The Wall also made it much more difficult to work in Israel or export commercial crops, both sources of livelihood necessary to buy food.

The combined effect of land confiscations for the Wall, for military use, for restricted roads, and for Jewish settlements was "a slow dispossession of the Palestinian people, depriving them of their means of subsistence" (Ziegler et al. 2011, 180). On the other hand, the number of attacks on Israel declined after the Wall was built, thus justifying its construction from the point of view of Israel's security. I will discuss the legality of the Wall and other aspects of Israel's rule in the West Bank in Chapter 8.

The Gaza Strip

Israel withdrew from the Gaza Strip in 2005; before its withdrawal, 8,000 Jewish settlers had controlled 40 percent of the arable land, 25 percent of the territory, and most of the water in Gaza (Shlaim 2009, January 7, 2). Thus, Gazans no longer suffered the same problems of illegal land acquisitions as Palestinians in the West Bank, nor were there restricted roads or Israeli military installations to prevent Gazans from reaching their farms. Nevertheless, Israel controlled all access to Gaza by air and sea, as well as over the Israeli border (B'Tselem 2013, January 1). Israel also declared about 29 percent of Gaza along its eastern and northern borders to be a "no-go" buffer zone closed to Gazan farmers and herders (Food and Agriculture Organization and Office for the Coordination of Humanitarian Affairs 2010, May, 2), yet almost a third of Gaza's arable land lay in that zone (Roy 2012, 81).

In 2009 Israel imposed a three nautical mile limit on Gazan fishermen, even though Gazan fishing waters were supposed to extend for twenty nautical miles (Goldstone 2009, 84, par. 321); 85 percent of Gaza fishing water was blocked by Israeli warships (Hogan 2012, 109). In negotiations after the 2014 war, the limit was changed to just over five nautical miles (Economist 2014, August 30).

Gazans also suffered two other problems; namely, an Israeli blockade and the destructive effects of attacks on Gaza, the latter justified as retaliation for rocket attacks by Hamas on Israel. From 2001 to 2009 Palestinian groups fired about 8000 mortars and rockets into Israel (Goldstone 2009, 31, par.103). In September 2007, after Hamas took power, Israel blockaded Gaza, declaring it hostile territory (Goldstone 2009, 51, par. 192). It cut food supplies to Gaza by half in November 2007 and announced a total blockade on fuel – used to transport and cook food – in January 2008 (Pelham 2012, 8). According to some critics, the purpose of this blockade was to completely disable the economy (Roy 2012, 85). Indeed, one commentator referred to the blockade as "thoroughly planned impoverishment" that actually began before 2007 with, for example, a 2000 Israeli ban on imports into Gaza of cooking fuel and gas (Usher 2001, 3).

Before the blockade, Israel's Ministry of Defense had calculated the minimum number of calories that Palestinians would need to stay healthy and had then translated that figure into the minimum number of truckloads of food and other humanitarian goods it would permit into Gaza every day. Whereas before 2007 about 400 truckloads per day had entered Gaza (Gisha 2012, October 17), the permitted number was proposed to be 106, including seventy-seven truckloads of food and twenty-nine of other humanitarian goods (Ministry of Defence 2008, January 27, slides 2, 4). The military proposed prohibiting supplies of food to Gaza that were not "of a humanitarian character" or that were "in quantities exceeding... [those] required for humanitarian needs" (Gisha 2008, December, 6–7, n. 27).

This cynical calculation of necessary truckloads of foodstuffs did not take into account that agricultural production in Gaza had fallen as a result of shortages of seeds and chickens caused by the blockade (Cook 2012, October 24). Nor did it take into account possible inequities in distribution of food within Gaza (Ministry of Defence 2008, January 27, slide 2) and the possibility that some individuals would not receive the minimum they needed. Food was often wasted as truckers waited at the border for clearance: much food spoiled because it had to be removed from Israeli trucks, driven through the border by "neutral" trucks, and then re-loaded on the other side into Gazan trucks (Cook 2012, October 24). In Israel's defense, however, the average number of calories it calculated Palestinians needed was 2,100 per day, conforming to guidelines from the World Health Organization (Ministry of Defence

2008, January 27, slide 9); moreover, the military claimed it had never actually implemented the policy of permitting only the minimum number of truckloads of food into Gaza (Ministry of Defence 2008, January 27, cover message to Gisha).

The blockade affected not only food but also water. In early 2009 only 20 percent of Gaza's water was drinkable, as a result of Israeli restrictions on fuel and chlorine necessary for water treatment plants. 70 percent of agricultural land was un-irrigated, while 80 percent of Gaza's wells were only partly functional (Anonymous 2009, 170). Many children suffered from disease caused by polluted water, especially as Gaza lacked electricity to treat sewage facilities and run desalinization plants that could produce drinkable water. By 2014 only one-tenth of the water available to Gazans was fit for drinking, and only 6.5 percent of Gaza's wells provided water meeting WHO standards (B'Tselem 2014, February 9). However, in acknowledgment of this problem Israel announced in 2015 that it would double the supply of water it provided to Gaza (Khoury 2015, March 4).

Food shortages in Gaza during the blockade were not a consequence only of Israeli policy. Egypt also closed its border with Gaza after Hamas took over (Helfont 2010, 428), presumably because the then Mubarak regime feared the influence in Egypt of Islamist radicals supported by Hamas. In practice, however, the border with Egypt was very porous, and Gazans dug hundreds of sophisticated tunnels under it through which they imported all manner of goods, including weapons and drugs (Almog 2004, 2) as well as food and other consumer items (Helfont 2010, 430). Many tunnels were dug from the basements of houses on the Gaza side, causing Israel to demolish the homes (Verini 2012, 2).

The tunnels became the largest source of non-governmental employment in Gaza (Pelham 2012, 19) after employment within Israel was cut off, and the tunnel economy helped Gazans to rebuild rapidly after the 2008–09 war. Hamas also taxed the goods brought in via tunnels: these taxes were an important source of its revenue (Verini 2012, 3). In 2010, thirty tunnels brought in livestock to Gaza; farmers also imported seeds, pesticides, and tools prohibited by Israel, while a food-processing plant resumed business after the 2008–09 invasion and received supplies from Switzerland brought in via the tunnels (Pelham 2012, 15, 16). According to Gazan wholesalers, about 60 percent of the food in Gaza entered through the tunnels, although after the blockade was eased in 2010 many retailers resumed importing food from Israel (Pelham 2012, 17, 28 notes 41 and 48).

Nevertheless, the harmful effect of the Egyptian blockade can be understood in the breach: in late January 2008 explosions set off by Hamas broke down the frontier wall, and some 200,000 (Sharp 2008, 9) to 350,000 people immediately entered Egypt to buy goods, including food (McGirk 2008). As a result of this security breach, Egypt started to construct an underground steel wall to block smuggling, especially of arms (Helfont 2010, 426): Egypt had a peace treaty with Israel and did not want Hamas to undermine it. Egypt also worried that Hamas might attack its own territory, such as tourist sites in the Sinai Peninsula frequented by Israelis (Helfont 2010, 432–33), or that Hamas might export arms to militants in Sinai opposed to the central government (El Amrani 2013, February 20). Egypt was also concerned that weapons acquired by Hamas from its Islamist ally, Hezbollah, might be used against it, perhaps in alliance with Egypt's Muslim Brotherhood. Finally, Egypt feared loss of US aid if it did not try to control smuggling into Gaza (Helfont 2010, 432–34). Tunnels were blocked in 2013 when the Egyptian military regained power after overthrowing President Mohamed Morsi, a representative of the Muslim Brotherhood who had been democratically elected in 2012 after the dictator Hosni Mubarak was removed from power (Yaari 2013, 2).

For its part, Israel feared Hamas' smuggled weapons and during the 2008–09 war it bombarded the tunnels, continuing to destroy them after the war by other means, such as flooding them with sewage (Pelham 2012, 13–14). During the 2014 war Israel again tried to destroy all the tunnels, while Egypt also reinstated its blockade of Gaza after the war (Economist 2014, October 4). Certainly if Gazans had had easier access to Egypt, they could have alleviated some of their food shortages.

All of these problems were exacerbated by periodic wars between Israel and Hamas. At the time of writing, no official report existed on the 2014 war, but there was a report on the 2008–09 war. From December 27, 2008, to January 18, 2009, Israel invaded Gaza, a response in large part to Hamas' continuous attacks on Israeli civilians. This attack was the subject of an investigation led by Justice Richard Goldstone of South Africa and commissioned by the United Nations Human Rights Council. As had been the case in its predecessor United Nations Commission on Human Rights, this Council was composed of official representatives of states, some of which were themselves guilty of gross human rights abuses. It devoted a disproportionate amount of its attention to Israel (Navoth 2014, April 6; Landes 2009b, 4), perhaps because Israel was seen as a colonial state or as an ally of the United States (Lebovic and Voeten 2006, 864, 879). Anti-Semitism may also have influenced the inordinate amount of attention the Human Rights Council paid to Israel.

Goldstone and his colleagues discovered deliberate destruction of and damage to greenhouses, wells, and agricultural land in Gaza during the 2008–09 war. They concluded that this destruction indicated "the specific purpose of denying their use for the sustenance of the civilian population of the Gaza Strip" (Goldstone 2009, 280, par. 1320). The Goldstone Report also considered "unlawful and wanton destruction" of a flour mill and a chicken farm that reportedly supplied over 10 percent of Gaza's eggs to be potential war crimes (Goldstone 2009, 21–22, pars. 50 and 51). By one estimate, 60 percent of all agricultural land in Gaza was destroyed (Goldstone 2009, 261, par. 1230), as also were markets, slaughterhouses, and some food businesses (Goldstone 2009, 93, par. 365; 215, par. 1010). Israel also inflicted massive damage on housing during the war (Goldstone 2009, 210–14, pars. 990–1007). Without housing and the means with which to prepare their own food, Palestinian families were left dependent on charity and food aid. Finally, Israel damaged the water supply.

The Goldstone Report did acknowledge that Israel attempted to fulfill its obligations to make sure that residents of Gaza had enough food during the war. Israel imposed a unilateral ceasefire for three hours each day to send in food (Dershowitz 2010, 22, 25), but the overall level of supplies was still insufficient. Thus the Report concluded that "Israel violated its duty to respect the right of the Gaza population to . . . adequate food [and] water," stating that at the time of its investigation, "most people [were] destitute" (Goldstone 2009, 26, pars. 72 and 73; 259, par. 1219). At the same time, unemployment increased as Gazans who worked in Israel or in other Arab countries found their mobility blocked (Goldstone 2009, 260, par. 1225). The only reason why starvation was not imminent in Gaza in 2009, the Report added, was humanitarian assistance (Goldstone 2009, par. 935). By 2011, half of all Gaza's households were still food insecure (Qarmout and Beland 2012, 42).

Some critics argued that Goldstone and his colleagues were too credulous in accepting Gazans' accounts of the 2008–09 war, especially as some Gazan witnesses might have been intimidated by Hamas. Goldstone decided to make all testimony public, possibly intimidating individuals who feared Hamas' retaliation if they did not criticize Israel's invasion (Landes 2009a, 4; Dershowitz 2010, 32). Moreover, critics noted that the Commissioners did not hear Israel's account of the war, without which it was difficult to know why soldiers bulldozed a chicken farm or bombed a flour mill (Halbertal 2009, November 6, 17). Israel, however, had refused to co-operate with the Goldstone Commission, although it did reply to some charges against it, for example saying that it did not deliberately target the flour mill but accidentally hit it during a firefight with Hamas militia. If this were the case, then the destruction of the flour mill would not have been a war crime (Dershowitz 2010, 20–21).

Conclusion

Gordon suggests that Israel's occupation of the West Bank changed from colonialism to separation (Gordon 2008). In the early years after 1967, he contends, Israel presented itself as a benevolent conqueror, under whose rule the lives of Palestinians had improved; nevertheless, it began expropriating land and encouraging settlements in the 1970s. After the 1987 *intifada*, however, Israel's goal was to separate Palestinians from Israel for security reasons. This was the change that resulted in increased malnutrition. Whereas in the early period Palestinian laborers had been encouraged to work in Israel, thus providing incomes for their families, in the later period migration was discouraged as all Palestinians were perceived as security threats. Thus, migrant labor income no longer replaced income lost from dispossession of land.

Israel prided itself on being the only democratic country in the Middle East and on extending that democracy to its non-Jewish citizens. Yet its actions in the West Bank resembled settler colonialism. Like nineteenth-century Britain and Canada, it did not seem to perceive any contradiction between colonialism and democracy. Israel's severe shortage of land and water (in the early period) made Jewish settlement in the West Bank very attractive, whether or not settlers also believed that Israel was religiously or historically justified in taking over Palestinians' property.

To return to Sen's view that there are no famines in democracies (Sen 1999), Israel shows that democracies can be cavalier about nutritional standards in conquered areas. Its careful calculation of the amount of food Gazans needed in order to consume exactly 2,100 calories per person per day suggests a formal concern with the right to food, but the impediments it imposed on production and importation of food in Gaza put the lie to that concern. Nor could Israel claim a formal concern for the right to food when it deprived West Bank Palestinians of farmland, water, and indeed the very homes in which they should have been able to prepare nutritious meals.

At minimum, then, in Marcus' terms (Marcus 2003, 246) Israel was guilty of indifference to the right to food in the WBG. Its actions cannot be excused on the grounds of incompetence: it had the capacity to organize and implement plans to make sure the inhabitants of the WBG did not suffer malnutrition. Security needs do not explain theft of water and land by the Israeli government, military, and settlers, or restrictions on freedom of movement and all other civil and political rights within the West Bank. On the other hand, Israel did not seem to be intentionally starving Palestinians or causing their malnourishment, although it did indirectly, and sometimes directly as through the blockade of Gaza, deprive them of food. Its concerns were security and protection of settlements.

It seems most likely that Israel was guilty of recklessness (Marcus 2003, 247); it persisted in policies that deprived Palestinians of food and increased malnutrition among them, even when it was aware of their consequences. Israel appeared to be carefully following international law to make sure that Palestinians did not starve, yet policies guaranteeing only minimal caloric intake, controlling Gaza's borders, depriving the occupants of the West Bank of land and water, and denying civil and political rights contributed to Palestinians' malnutrition. Israel had the right to take measures to protect its own security, but it was also obliged under international law to protect the human rights – including the right to food – of all those under its control. Most of the measures described in this chapter went far beyond what was necessary to protect Israel's security; rather, they suggest an illegitimate colonial policy in the West Bank and a policy of extreme containment in Gaza.

Nevertheless, Israel was not the only perpetrator of human rights abuses in the WBG. During the periods that Egypt blockaded its border, it was very difficult for Gazans to obtain food. And the Palestinian Authority and Hamas violated the civil and political rights of the people for whom they were responsible; Palestinians in the WBG also endured massive corruption among their leaders. The degrees of responsibility for malnutrition of these various actors cannot be quantified, but Egypt, the Palestinian Authority, and Hamas also treated Palestinians with reckless indifference.

Part III

Implications for the International Human Right to Food

8   International Law and the Right to Food

Changes in international law and practice might help protect people from state-induced famine and malnutrition. International laws prohibiting genocide and crimes against humanity, the international law of occupation, and refugee law could all be used to remedy such crimes. This chapter will first discuss these four types of law, and will end with brief discussions of international law regarding penal starvation, and evolving soft law. North Korea, Zimbabwe, Venezuela, and Israel/Palestine raise different questions regarding international law; not all types of law apply to each case.

The International Law of Genocide

The state food crimes described in Part II fall most precisely into the legal category of crimes against humanity. However, critics sometimes claim that North Korea, Zimbabwe, and Israel have committed or are committing genocide. It is necessary to dispose of these arguments before proceeding to discuss crimes against humanity.

The 1948 United Nations Convention on the Prevention and Punishment of the Crime of Genocide (UNGC) contains no specific mention of state-induced famine, although some consequences of intentional and reckless faminogenesis could be described as aspects of genocide. The definition of genocide in Article 2 of the UNGC is:

any of the following acts committed with intent to destroy, in whole or in part, a national, ethnical [sic], racial or religious group, as such:
(a) Killing members of the group;
(b) Causing serious bodily or mental harm to members of the group;
(c) Deliberately inflicting on the group conditions of life calculated to bring about its physical destruction in whole or in part;
(d) Imposing measures intended to prevent births within the group;
(e) Forcibly transferring children of the group to another group (United Nations General Assembly 1948a, Article 2)

Intentional state-induced famine kills people, the first aspect of genocide (Article 2, a of the UNGC). It causes serious bodily harm to members of groups (Article 2, b of the UNGC) and also deliberately inflicts "conditions of life calculated to bring about [a group's] . . . physical destruction in whole or in part" (Article 2, c of the UNGC.). State-induced famine also prevents births within a group (Article 2, d of the UNGC) as starving women cannot conceive.

However, the UNGC refers only to victims who are members of specific national, ethnic, religious, or racial groups. According to this definition, most of the famine victims in the three cases discussed in Chapter 2 were not victims of genocide. Starvation in Ukraine and other parts of the Soviet Union occurred before the UNGC was drafted, but scholars dispute, in any case, whether the famine in Ukraine was directed against Ukrainians as such or whether they were victims of a national policy of collectivization not directed at any particular ethnic group. Chinese famine victims died as a result of collectivization and other draconian agricultural policies but were not singled out because of their ethnicity. Only in Cambodia did some victims fit the UNGC definition: the Muslim Cham and ethnic Vietnamese and Chinese were condemned to death on the basis of their religious/and or ethnic identities.

The Ukrainian and Cambodian famines did contain elements of politicide, a type of genocide in which "victim groups are defined in terms of their political status or opposition to the state" (Harff and Gurr 1988, 359). The term, "politicide," however, is not recognized in law. During the debate in the late 1940s on the definition of genocide, the Soviet Union, Poland, and some non-communist countries that were worried that their conflicts with insurgent groups could be characterized as genocide opposed attempts to describe people oppressed for political reasons as victims of genocide (Naimark 2010, 21–22; Alsheh 2011).

Yet the politicides in Ukraine and Cambodia were precursors of the manner in which the Zimbabwean government targeted groups of people who opposed or were thought to oppose its rule, regardless of their ethnicity, race, religion, or nationality. They were also precursors of the large-scale murder by famine in North Korea. In this sense they fit the sociological definition of genocide proposed in 1990 by Frank Chalk and Kurt Jonassohn, "Genocide is a form of one-sided mass killing in which a state or other authority intends to destroy a group, as that group and membership in it are defined by the perpetrator" (Chalk and Jonassohn 1990, 23). In both North Korea and Zimbabwe, the state defined its victim groups.

In North Korea, certain groups that fit the UNGC categories of race, religion, ethnicity, or nationality were targeted for extermination, many starving to death in prison camps. Korean Christians were one such group, as adherence to Christianity was viewed as treason. Other religious believers besides Christians also appear to have been targeted. A second group was Japanese-Koreans. A third group was Korean-Chinese infants (Goedde 2010, 554), who were considered to "pollute" the pure Korean race. The forcible aborting of pregnant refugees who were returned to North Korea, and the murder of their infants, can be considered "ethnic infanticide," which constitutes killing of members of a distinct ethnic group (Park 2011, 11).

However, while these particular groups may fit the UNGC definition of victims, the majority of those subjected to state-induced famine in North Korea did not. Rather, the regime committed politicide. The famine of the 1990s and the continuing risk of starvation in the twenty-first century affected all North Koreans except the core inner elite; even members of the military and the Korean Workers' Party were at risk. Moreover, disproportionate incarceration of members of the so-called hostile class might be considered a form of politicide; certain categories of people deemed to be politically unreliable were at substantially increased risk of penal starvation. Yet politicide is not legally an aspect of genocide, despite arguments by some scholars that the law should be changed (Jacobs 2010, February 17, 4).

Some scholars believe that Zimbabwe was a perpetrator of genocide. In 2008 Gregory Stanton, then President of the International Association of Genocide Scholars, and Helen Fein, then Executive Director of the Institute for the Study of Genocide, sent a letter to *The New York Times* (which was not published), arguing that Robert Mugabe was committing genocide by attrition (Stanton and Fein 2008). The term "genocide by attrition," they argued, fell under Article 2, (c) of the UNGC. Genocide by attrition "decimates group members by several methods, including creating conditions undermining physical and mental health that regularly result in death of part of the group and demoralization and atomization of the remainder." Methods of genocide by attrition include "starvation, denial of heating fuel and clean water, overcrowding, overwork and exhaustion, and the consequent epidemics and diseases" (Fein 1993, 30–31).

In making their case for genocide by attrition in Zimbabwe, Stanton and Fein cited two major events. The first was the cholera epidemic of 2008–09. This epidemic was caused in large part by the breakdown of Zimbabwe's infrastructure, itself caused by severe neglect, corruption, and lack of funds. Moreover, most Zimbabwean medical professionals had fled the country by 2008. Between August 2008 and mid-July 2009, 98,592 cholera cases were reported in Zimbabwe, resulting in

4,288 deaths (Office for the Coordination of Humanitarian Affairs 2009, July 15, 1).

One might argue that while these deaths were undoubtedly an avoidable tragedy, their relatively low numbers did not suggest genocide. However, international case law has determined that deaths in the hundreds of thousands or millions are not necessary to a finding of genocide. The International Criminal Tribunal for the Former Yugoslavia ruled in 2001 that the massacre of almost 8,000 Muslim men and boys in Srebrenica, Bosnia in 1995 was an act of genocide, as they constituted a significant part of the Muslim population of that region of Bosnia (Southwick 2005, 189; Wilson 2005, 934–39). In 2013, a court in Argentina accepted the argument that the deaths and disappearances of almost 30,000 people during the junta rule of 1976–83 constituted a genocidal attack on the Argentinian people as a whole (Riveiro et al. 2013; for background see Feierstein 2006).

The second event that Stanton and Fein cited as genocide in Zimbabwe was Operation Drive Out Trash, the 2005 expulsion of urban residents. In her definition of genocide by attrition, Fein included denial of shelter "with intent to discriminate against the victim group" (Fein 1993, 12). It does seem that Mugabe's intent in instituting Operation Drive Out Trash was to discriminate against the group he defined as opponents of his regime. However, many of the expelled residents returned to the cities and rebuilt their homes; some moved to other parts of Zimbabwe; and some were presumably refugees in South Africa, Botswana, and elsewhere. While they undoubtedly experienced severe hardship, including lack of access to food, it is difficult to argue that the expellees were victims of genocide. A better term to describe their suffering is mass atrocity, a term used frequently in the academic literature to describe situations that resemble genocide or genocidal episodes but do not fit the legal definition of genocide (Zimmerer 2009).

The UNGC, Article 1, obliges states to prevent and punish the crime of genocide, but even if it could be shown that Zimbabweans were enduring famine in the early 2000s, the famine was not legally genocide. Those who died from hunger or related causes such as cholera were persecuted on the basis of their real or perceived opposition to the Mugabe regime, not their membership in any of the four groups protected by the UNGC. Mugabe's opponents were, rather, victims of politicide. Evidence for politicide includes not only the disease, expulsions, farm invasions, and politically biased distribution of food discussed in Chapter 5 but also systematic murders, torture, and rapes of Mugabe's opponents. A term used within Zimbabwe itself was "smart genocide," in which "There's no need to directly kill hundreds of thousands, if you can select and kill the right few thousand" (Godwin 2010, 109).

Schabas notes that "the concept of genocide has been extended to acts that compromise the survival of a group" (Schabas 2006, 102), but to claim genocide in Zimbabwe one would have to consider what "survival" of a group meant in the Zimbabwean context. White Zimbabwean farmers no longer constituted a group, "white citizens of Zimbabwe," many having emigrated, but others moved to urban areas of Zimbabwe. Shona and Ndebele people still constituted ethnic groups within Zimbabwe, despite massive refugee movements. Their survival as such was not threatened, though it might well have been had not the world community distributed food in Zimbabwe. The group, "opponents of Mugabe's rule," also still existed, despite massive persecution.

Some scholars and activists accused Israel of near genocide during the early twenty-first century. A group of scholars of genocide issued a statement in February 2009 declaring that both Israel's attack on Gaza in December 2008 and "its wider policies" had been "too alarmingly close [to genocide] to ignore" (Genocide Scholars and Professionals 2009, February 24). The respected Israeli human rights organization, B'Tselem calculated that from September 29, 2000 to May 31, 2013 6,829 Palestinians and 1,104 Israelis had been killed in the conflict (B'Tselem 2013, May 31): this is a ratio of about six to one and indicates the conflict's uneven nature. However, the Palestinian deaths were not results of genocide or of a single genocidal massacre: rather, they were the results of intermittent attacks on Palestinian targets. As discussed below, it is possible that Israel was guilty of crimes against humanity in its attacks on Gaza, but the accusation of genocide is far-fetched.

On the other hand, Israel's policies regarding food contributed to high rates of malnutrition in both the West Bank and Gaza (WBG). Thus, those who charged Israel with genocide might argue that it was "Causing serious bodily . . . harm to members of the group" and "Deliberately inflicting on the group conditions of life calculated to bring about its physical destruction in whole or in part," conforming to Article 2, b and c of the Genocide Convention. However, reports of malnutrition among the Palestinian population did not refer to deaths from starvation. Moreover, official Israeli policy appeared to be to ensure that Gazans consumed the minimum number of calories they needed to stay healthy, even though in practice this minimum was often not attained. A policy based on adherence to international health standards is a far cry from policies that deliberately provide a group of people with less than the necessary amount of food.

A more sensible way to address faminogenesis and state food crimes is via the category of crimes against humanity.

Crimes against Humanity

Marcus argued in 2003 (Marcus 2003, 279–80) that although aspects of intentional and reckless faminogenesis were already crimes under various international laws, faminogenesis should nevertheless be formally codified. A treaty prohibiting faminogenesis would not have to prove that such crimes were directed against a "national, ethnical, racial or religious group as such," as under the UNGC. It could simply refer to state-induced famine of part of the population under the state's authority.

Until such time as state-induced famine is recognized as a specific crime in international law, however, it falls under crimes against humanity as defined in the Rome Statute of the International Criminal Court (ICC). Since July 1, 2002, individuals can be charged before the ICC with genocide, crimes against humanity, or war crimes, but only for crimes committed since that date. Crimes against humanity are defined as certain acts "committed as part of a widespread or systematic attack directed against any civilian population, with knowledge of the attack" (International Criminal Court 1998, Article 7, 1). One of these acts is extermination, defined among other aspects as "intentional infliction of conditions of life, inter alia the *deprivation of access to food* and medicine, calculated to bring about the destruction of part of a population" (International Criminal Court 1998, Article 7, 2, b, emphasis mine).

As in the UNGC, intent is an important aspect of this crime. Thus, had the ICC been in existence in the 1990s and had Kim Jong Il of North Korea been indicted for the crime of extermination, the ICC would have had to determine whether he intended to kill 3 to 5 percent of North Korea's citizens or whether he was merely reckless in continuing his economic policies even when it was obvious that they caused starvation. Kim apparently said in 1996 that North Korea only needed 30 percent of its people to survive in order to construct a "victorious" North Korean society, suggesting a very high tolerance for mass death among those for whom he was responsible (Terry 2001). Indeed, it might seem that the combination of resistance to economic reform; complete denial of civil and political rights; diversion of food aid to support the Korean Workers' Party, the military, and the elite; and discrimination against some provinces in provision of food constituted evidence of intent. Nevertheless, none of these elements provides the smoking gun suggesting that Kim wanted to kill his own population, and his frequent appeals for international food aid suggested the contrary.

Grace Kang argued that food deprivation in North Korean prison camps could be considered an act of murder or extermination, reinforcing the argument that Kim Jong Il should have been referred to the ICC (Kang 2006, 79–80). Similarly, Debra Liang-Fenton argued that "The North Korean government is actively involved in committing crimes against humanity with respect to both its food policy leading to famine and its treatment of political prisoners"; these were crimes against humanity because the government knowingly engaged in policies that caused hunger and starvation (Liang-Fenton 2007, 69). However, as of the time of writing North Korea was not party to the ICC; thus, had he still been alive, Kim Jong Il would have had to be referred to the court by the United Nations Security Council (UNSC), as would his successor Kim Jong Un. Furthermore, any such indictments could refer only to crimes committed since July 1, 2002.

In 2013, the United Nations Human Rights Council established a Commission of Inquiry (COI) into North Korea, and on February 7, 2014 the United Nations General Assembly released the COI's report (COI: United Nations General Assembly 2014, February 7). The COI listed numerous ways that North Korea committed crimes against humanity, including, but not limited to, extermination, murder, enslavement, torture, imprisonment, rape, forced abortions, enforced disappearances, and knowingly causing starvation. It specifically referred to the use of food as a political weapon, and noted that North Koreans were still suffering from severe malnutrition. It also referred to the "re-emergence in testimonies of cannibalism" in 2006 (COI: United Nations General Assembly 2014, February 7, p. 157, par. 528). The COI called on the UNSC to refer the responsible North Korean officials – government, military, and security officials, including Kim Jong Un – to the ICC for trial. Thus, while a charge of genocide in North Korea would be hard to prove, there was overwhelming evidence that North Korea committed crimes against humanity.

Similarly, there was overwhelming evidence that Robert Mugabe and his coterie had committed massive crimes against humanity in Zimbabwe. Widespread hunger deliberately or recklessly caused by government actions qualifies as an act of extermination under the Rome Statute. "Deportation or forcible transfer of population" is also a crime against humanity (International Criminal Court 1998, Article 7, 1, d). The 2005 evictions could be considered such a crime, although Zimbabwe might argue that the people expelled had not been lawfully present in the areas from which they were evicted, as required by the ICC definition of unlawful deportation (International Criminal Court 1998, Article 7, 2, d). The threat of prosecution before the ICC might have been an inducement for senior Zimbabwean leaders to give up power and facilitate a democratic transition: alternatively, such a threat might have encouraged them to plan a military coup and directly take over the government once Mugabe died, so that their own government could not refer them to the ICC. Mugabe himself was reported in late 2011 to be afraid that he might be hanged should he give up power (WikiLeaks Press 2011, December 1, 2).

In 2005 Australia and New Zealand called for Mugabe to be referred to the ICC (NZHerald 2005, July 2), and in 2006 Zimbabwean non-governmental organizations and charities also called for his indictment (Zhakata 2006, January 27). Zimbabwe, though, was not a party to the ICC: it signed the Rome Statute in 1998 but as of 2015 had not ratified it. Thus, as in the case of North Korea, the UNSC would have had to refer Mugabe to the ICC, an unlikely event especially as China, with substantial interests in Zimbabwe, would probably have vetoed any such referral.

The threat of indictment before the ICC might have helped persuade Mugabe to share power. His allies in the Southern African Development Community (SADC) and the African Union (AU) could have promised him a comfortable retirement and no referral for trial at the ICC, or protection from actual transport to the Court, in return for his immediate resignation. Mugabe was already laboring under a travel ban to the EU and the US (discussed in Chapter 9), and was threatened by the principle of universal jurisdiction, which asserts that states can try individuals for crimes against humanity even if the crimes were not committed on the state's territory or against or by that state's citizens (International Justice Resource Center accessed December 19, 2014).

For example, a South African court ruled in 2012 that the South African Police Service was obliged to investigate Zimbabwean officials who had travelled to South Africa for crimes against humanity committed within Zimbabwe against Zimbabwean nationals (Supreme Court of Appeal of South Africa 2012). In so doing, the Court relied on the principle of universal jurisdiction. However, had the South African government followed through on this ruling, it might have undermined diplomatic efforts to persuade Mugabe and other senior government members to modify their actions within Zimbabwe, especially in the run-up to the 2013 election. Here, the "peace versus justice" dilemma appears. To obtain internal peace and move to a democracy, international authorities might have had to negotiate immunity from prosecution for the most powerful Zimbabweans, rather than risk a military coup or a civil war among various factions of the military and/or ZANU-PF after Mugabe died (Tendi 2010, September 1).

In any event, there was considerable resentment in the AU as a whole against the ICC, which by 2015 had still not indicted anyone from outside Africa. The AU was particularly angry because in 2009 the ICC had indicted a sitting head of state, President Omar Al-Bashir of Sudan (Magliveras and Naldi 2013, 423; International Criminal Court 2009). However, in December 2014 the ICC suspended its investigation of Al-Bashir, its prosecutor citing lack of co-operation from the UNSC as the reason for so doing. Al-Bashir was quoted as saying "The Sudanese people have defeated the ICC and have refused to hand over any Sudanese to the colonialist courts" (Abdelaziz 2014, December 14). The ICC also dropped its case against President Uhuru Kenyatta of Kenya for inciting ethnic violence in the run-up to the 2008 Kenyan elections: In this case the prosecutor cited lack of co-operation by the Kenyan government, as well as harassment and intimidation of witnesses (Bowcott 2014, December 5). Given this African climate of hostility to the ICC, Mugabe and other senior Zimbabweans could easily exploit accusations that the Court was racist.

Some Israeli leaders might also have been referred to the ICC. The Goldstone Report concluded that Israel might be found in a competent court to have committed crimes against humanity during the 2008–09 Gaza war (Goldstone 2009, 284, par. 1335). Since Israel was not party to the ICC, however, such a referral would have had to be by the UNSC (Barnette 2010, 20). The Permanent Five members of the UNSC (the United States, Britain, France, Russia, and China) all opposed considering the Goldstone Report (Morgan 2010, 162), Russia and China probably because of their general aversion to international interference in states' internal affairs, and the US because of its strong alliance with Israel. Another legal problem would have been whether the Palestinians, or any entity representing or purporting to represent them, had the status of a state and could therefore take their case against Israel to the ICC; while legal arguments in favor of viewing Palestine as a state existed, in 2010 they were still quite weak (Worster 2011).

In 2001, twenty-eight survivors of a massacre at the Sabra and Shatila refugee camps in Lebanon had attempted to indict Ariel Sharon, Prime Minister of Israel from 2001 to 2006, for genocide and crimes against humanity, via the mechanism of universal jurisdiction. The massacre occurred in 1982 during a civil war in which Israel was allied with Christian Phalange groups. Although the Phalange militia was the direct perpetrator of the massacre of approximately 1,000 people, Israeli troops under Sharon's command were accused of having assisted it by surrounding the camps and blocking all exits for three days (Tafadar 2003). Thus, plaintiffs against Sharon argued that he had had command responsibility (King-Irani 2003, 21). The case was filed in 2001 in Belgium, which at the time had recognized universal jurisdiction for war crimes, crimes against humanity and genocide, but it was withdrawn in 2003 under

US and Israeli pressure on Belgium (Byers 2005, 142). In any event the case against Sharon was based on violations of civil/political rights, massacres, and targeted killings, not the right to food.

Refugee Law

Under international law, an individual fearing torture or extra-judicial execution is considered a refugee, but a person fearing starvation is not. The 1951 Convention Relating to the Status of Refugees defines a refugee as a person who "owing to well-founded fear of being persecuted for reasons of race, religion, nationality, membership of a particular social group or political opinion, is outside the country of his nationality and is unable or, owing to such fear, is unwilling to avail himself of the protection of that country" (United Nations 1951, Article 1, A, 2). This definition excludes those who might be considered "economic" refugees, fleeing a country because of malnutrition or starvation caused by intentional or reckless economic policies imposed by governments with no regard for citizens' welfare.

"As classically understood, the 1951 Convention refugee definition would likely not be terribly sympathetic to the claims of persons in flight from famine or food deprivation" (Hathaway 2014, 329). However, recent jurisprudence in some Western countries including Canada, the United States, Australia, and the United Kingdom has widened the definition of a refugee to include individuals fleeing severe violations of their human rights such as violation of their right to food. In one British case involving a Zimbabwean refugee claimant, the court ruled that "discriminatory exclusion from access to food" constituted persecution (Hathaway 2014, 333).

Until such time as these judicial decisions become the basis of an international reinterpretation of the law, however, the classic definition of a refugee guides many policy decisions. Furthermore, refugee law at present applies only to members of the particular groups enumerated in its definition, that is, people seeking refugee status for reasons of race, religion, nationality, membership of a particular social group or political opinion (Hathaway 2014, 330). Many of the people fleeing North Korea and Zimbabwe were not members of any of these groups but were fleeing starvation and/or malnutrition. Yet unless refugee law is changed to consider state-induced famine a political condition, refugees from faminogenesis will not enjoy the right to asylum.

North Korean refugees in China exemplify this problem. By 2009 between 100,000 and 300,000 North Koreans were living illegally in China, having fled North Korea (Park 2010, 261). China became party to the UN Convention on Refugees in 1982; thus, it was obliged to protect refugees fleeing North Korea because of political or religious persecution. This should have entailed setting up a refugee adjudication process and allowing the UN High Commission for Refugees access to North Koreans in China (Cohen 2010, September 14). China should also have protected refugees who had had contact with South Koreans, Christian missionaries, or aid workers while in China, as they were likely to be punished more harshly than other returnees should they be sent back to North Korea (Human Rights Watch 2007, March, 4). China was also obliged to protect those many North Korean refugee women and girls who were coerced into becoming sex workers or were sold as "brides" to Chinese men, to make sure that they were not persecuted if they were returned to North Korea (Muico 2005).

Despite these obligations, China signed an agreement with North Korea in 1986 to return "illegal entrants" (Goedde 2010, 557), sending back about 10 percent of those in China every year (Park 2010, 260). It permitted North Korean agents to operate in North-East China to intimidate, abduct, and murder refugees (Becker 2005, 27). It imposed arrest quotas on Chinese border police, fined anyone helping refugees a substantial sum (Becker 2005, 38, 23), and offered a reward of $500 to any Chinese citizen who turned in a North Korean refugee (Park 2010, 273). China justified these actions by claiming that North Koreans entering China were not political refugees but economic migrants (Chan and Schloenhardt 2007, 224).

Yet most of these refugees were fleeing state policies that deprived them of food and imprisoned them if they were caught trading in, cultivating, or foraging for food. Moreover, the government's discriminatory distribution of food, for example by denying it to members of the hostile class, constituted political persecution (Chan and Schloenhardt 2007, 230–31). Since starvation was a result of political decisions made by their government, North Korean "economic migrants" were in fact political refugees (Kim 2008, 213). Yet refugee activists were limited to the argument that even if North Koreans had not originally been political refugees, they became political refugees *sur place* (in place) once they entered China, when threatened with the torture, imprisonment, executions, and starvation that would follow their return to North Korea (Cohen 2010, September 14).

Refugees from Zimbabwe to South Africa had an easier time than those from North Korea to China. Slightly over one million Zimbabweans were thought to be in South Africa in 2007 (Crush and Tevera 2010, 5); most were not refugees in the legal sense and many were not refugees even informally. The pattern of movement to South Africa was one of "mixed migration" (Polzer 2008, 1), in which some people moved there (semi)-permanently to escape political persecution and/or economic difficulties, while others, especially from border regions, frequently returned home. These return trips by individuals bringing cash, goods, and food were – along with remittances in cash or kind, especially food – the mainstay of their malnourished families. Families that received remittances were generally better fed than those who did not (Tevera et al. 2010; Maphosa 2007, 128).

Like all sovereign states, however, South Africa, along with its neighbor, Botswana, balked at accepting every potential refugee who approached or crossed its borders. Botswana built electric fences to keep out Zimbabwean refugees, while South Africa placed military guards along the Zimbabwean border (Central Intelligence Agency 2008). Refugees put an enormous strain on neighboring countries' resources and competed with citizens for jobs, causing brief flare-ups of ethnic violence against Zimbabwean migrants in South Africa in 2008 and 2015 (Hammer 2009a, February 12, 28; Economist 2015, April 25). South Africa deported about 200,000 Zimbabweans per year (Polzer 2008, 8), and the vast majority of those seeking official asylum were rejected (Polzer 2010, 382). In any event, most Zimbabweans did not avail themselves of the opportunity to seek formal refugee status, for lack of information and/or resources (Bloch 2010, 236).

South Africa's general approach to undocumented migrants from Zimbabwe was fragmented, in part because it had to consider how its policies regarding Zimbabwean migrants/refugees might affect its role as a mediator between Mugabe and his opponents (Polzer 2008, 2, 16). South Africa could have availed itself of a clause in the 1969 Organization of Africa Unity Convention on Refugees, which applied the term refugee to a person fleeing "events seriously disturbing public order in either part or the whole of his country of origin or nationality" (Organization of African Unity 1969, Article 1, 2). Using this clause it could have conferred a group status of refugee on Zimbabwean migrants but as of 2008 had not done so (Polzer 2008, 19–20). Moreover, once the Unity government was established in Zimbabwe in 2009, it became easier for other countries to deport refugees on the grounds that the conflict within Zimbabwe had ended, especially as Zimbabwe did not appear to systematically imprison, torture, and execute returned refugees, as did North Korea.

Aside from refugees and migrants, there were upwards of a million internally displaced Zimbabweans in 2008. These included workers from expropriated farms; people who could not find new homes after they were expelled from cities by Operation Drive Out Trash (Potts 2010); and several tens of thousands of people fleeing state-sponsored violence after the March 2008 elections (Internal Displacement Monitoring Centre 2008, August, 4). The government's motive for these last displacements appeared to have been to remove possible opposition voters from their voting districts; indeed, the expulsions were referred to as "Operation Mayhoterapapi (Where Did you Put Your [Voter] Cross?") (Internal Displacement Monitoring Centre 2008, August, 14). These internally displaced people were not protected by international refugee law, even though many were fleeing overt political persecution. Ironically, in October 2009 Zimbabwe signed the newly minted African Union Convention for the Protection and Assistance of Internally Displaced Persons in Africa (African Union 2009).

The status of Palestinian refugees in the West Bank and Gaza (WBG) differed from what is normally thought to be the refugee situation. While one might think of refugees solely as people fleeing immediate persecution or threat thereof, the population of those officially considered to be Palestinian refugees – in WBG and elsewhere – included the descendants of those who fled or were expelled from Israel in 1947–48 or later. Thus, the official Palestinian refugee population, reaching about five million by 2012, was much larger than the numbers of people who had left Israel in earlier decades (Baer 2015, 49). This definition included Palestinian refugees and their descendants who held citizenship in other countries such as Jordan. Under the 1951 Refugee Convention, individuals who attain citizenship in a country other than the one they fled are not considered to be refugees, nor are descendants who hold citizenship (Lindsay 2012 Fall, 88). The broad definition of what constitutes a Palestinian refugee was a tool in the creation of a Palestinian identity, and contributed to the sense of crisis surrounding Palestinian/Israeli relations, especially as the United Nations Relief and Works Agency for Palestinians gradually evolved to become an advocacy rather than strictly a refugee relief organization (Al Husseini 2010).

Many Palestinian refugees hoped that they would eventually be able to return to their – or their ancestors' – former homes in Israel. Yet even in the event of a peace treaty, Israel was unlikely to accede to this demand as to do so would upset an already uneasy demographic balance in Israel in which Jews were numerically predominant but would not be so if too many (in Israel's eyes) Palestinians returned (Lustick and Lesch 2005). Some Israeli politicians believed that Israel should be proclaimed a Jewish state, in which this ethno-religious group should always be numerically predominant.

For those without citizenship anywhere, including both refugees and indigenous residents in the WBG, the Palestinian refugee problem was essentially one of statelessness. Palestinians in the WBG did not have a state to call their own, to represent them internationally, although by 2015 many countries had recognized Palestine as a state. The solution to this problem lies in the diplomacy which may eventually result either in the creation of one bi-national Jewish/Palestinian state or, more likely, in a separate independent Palestinian state. International refugee law does not provide guidance for this protracted problem, yet Palestinians might well continue to endure malnutrition until they have their own state, which can restore their land and water to them.

Venezuela until 2015 was not a major source of refugees and those who did flee fell under the legal definition of refugees fleeing persecution because of their political opinion, as opponents of Chávez or Maduro. These refugees tended to be professionals and wealthier individuals who had been threatened or persecuted because of their opposition to the two leaders. Between 2004 and 2010, for example, about 4,500 requests by Venezuelans for political asylum were granted in the US (Fox News Latino 2011, June 24), whereas from 1996 to 1999, before Chávez became President, only about 70 Venezuelans became refugees in the US (Refugee and Immigration Ministries n.d.). Within Latin America, the United Nations High Commission for Refugees identified 9,548 refugees from Venezuela in early 2014 (UNHCR 2014). There was no mass movement of Venezuelans fleeing food shortages; thus, current refugee law was sufficient to cover the Venezuelan case. However, just as violation of civil and political rights is often a harbinger of violation of economic human rights, so also increases in numbers of political refugees are often harbingers of increases in numbers of "economic" refugees.

Israel: The International Law of Occupation and the Apartheid Debate

As an occupying power, Israel was ruled by international humanitarian law rather than by international human rights law. The international law of occupation is regulated by the 1949 Fourth Geneva Convention (FGC). However, Israel denied that it was an occupying power (Williams 2006, 201) and that its control of WBG violated international humanitarian law. Rather, it claimed that the FGC did not apply to these two areas as they had not been the territory of any legal sovereign before they were conquered in 1967 (Khen 2011, 77, note 62). Thus, according to Israel, Palestinians in these two areas were not entitled to the protections normally afforded to citizens of conquered sovereign entities (Benvenisti 2004, 109). Israel claimed that, nevertheless, its "administrative practices [were] consistent with [the FGC's] relevant humanitarian provisions" (Farer 1991, 40).

Over-riding this argument, the United Nations Security Council in Resolution 471 (1980) defined Israel as an occupying power (United Nations Security Council 1980, June 5, article 2). The international consensus was that Israel's control of the West Bank was a form of "belligerent occupation" (Kretzmer 2009, 311; Khen 2011, 57–58, 65). This consensus existed even though belligerent occupation formally consisted of "control of the territory of one state by the forces of another state" (Gasser 2009, 468), and the West Bank was not technically the territory of any state, as Israel had argued. As the occupying power, Israel was obliged to make sure that Palestinians were not deprived of their basic needs (Ziegler et al. 2011, 181).

Article 49 of the FGC prohibits forcible transfers and deportations of populations from occupied territories. It also prohibits transfers of part of the occupier's own civilian population into the territory it occupies (Geneva Convention 1949). Supplementing the Geneva Conventions, the ICC also lists "the transfer, directly or indirectly, by the Occupying Power of parts of its own civilian population into the territory it occupies" as a crime (International Criminal Court 1998, article 8,2,b, viii). Thus, movements of Jewish settlers to WBG, taking over land and water which Palestinians had used to feed themselves, were illegal. Israel claimed that Jewish settlement in the West Bank was the result of individual choice, but the government actively encouraged settlements (Roberts 1990, 83, 85). In any case, any purchase of land by settlers, even if purchased from an individual who was ostensibly willing to sell, was also illegal (Loucaides 2004, 679). Thus, the 69 percent of settlements built on private Palestinian land as of 2008 had no legal standing (Gordon 2008, 272, n. 37).

Except for military needs, expropriation of private property by an occupying power is also illegal under international humanitarian law. The 1907 Hague Convention, Article 46, states that "Private property... cannot be confiscated" (Loucaides 2004, 678). The FGC further outlaws destruction of property in occupied areas (Geneva Convention 1949, Article 53; Loucaides 2004, 679). The ICC also outlaws as a war crime "extensive destruction and appropriation of property, not justified by military necessity and carried out unlawfully and wantonly" (International Criminal Court 1998, Article 8, 2, a, iv). Thus, destruction and appropriation of Palestinian property to make way for settlements and nature reserves was illegal. The Israeli Supreme Court ruled in at least one case that requisition of private property for settlements was illegal, but as of 2009 had refused to rule on the question of whether the settlements as a whole violated Article 49 of the FGC (Kretzmer 2009, 321). Israel maintained that settlements improved its security and were therefore legal under international law (Loucaides 2004, 679, fn. 14).

Other aspects of international humanitarian law also apply to Israel. Article 59 of the FGC mandates that an occupying power must ensure that the occupied population has sufficient water and food (Geneva Convention 1949). Occupiers are, moreover, obliged to ensure equitable distribution of groundwater between themselves and the inhabitants of the area they occupy (Benvenisti 2004, 129).

Israel also refused to accept a 2004 advisory opinion regarding its construction of the Separation Wall. Responding to a request for an opinion from the United Nations General Assembly (UNGA), the International Court of Justice had advised that it was illegal for Israel to build any part of the Wall within occupied Palestinian territory, and that Israel should therefore remove all parts not built on its own territory (International Court of Justice 2004, July 9; Williams 2006, 198; Falk 2005, 47). Israel did not comply with that advice and continued to build the Wall on occupied territory.

A debate exists about whether, and how, international law applied to the Israeli blockade of Gaza from 2007 to 2010. On May 31, 2010 Israel attacked a Turkish ship, the *MV Mavi Marmara*, which was carrying activists trying to take humanitarian aid to Gaza: in the ensuing fight eight Turkish citizens and one Turkish-American were killed (Migdalovitz 2010, June 23, 2–3). The authors of a UN-commissioned report on the incident argued that at least the naval aspect of the blockade was a legitimate security measure, whose implementation "complied with the requirements of international law" (Palmer Report 2011, September, ii, p. 4). However, a comment on this report by five independent UN Human Rights Rapporteurs claimed that the blockade was illegal as it constituted collective punishment against Palestinian civilians for the actions of some of their political leaders, depriving them of their human rights (United Nations High Commissioner for Human Rights 2011, September 13). These Rapporteurs did not, however, claim that Israel imposed the blockade in order to starve the residents of the Gaza Strip, which would be illegal under the international law of blockades (Buchan 2012, 270). The Geneva Conventions state that blockades "cannot be so restrictive as to block foodstuffs necessary to support the civilian population" (DeFalco 2009, 21). In any event the international reaction against Israel's attack on the *MV Marmara* was so severe that it eased – but did not end – the blockade (Gisha 2012, October 17).

A separate avenue by which some activists and scholars attempted to address Israeli actions in WBG was by reference to the crime of apartheid. Apartheid is outlawed by Article 7, 1, j of the Rome Statute of the ICC, and is defined in Article 7, 2, h as "inhumane acts . . . committed in the context of an institutionalized regime of systematic oppression and domination by one racial group over any other racial group or groups and committed with the intent of maintaining that regime." Some critical scholars maintain that this is a correct description of Israel's policies in so far as it maintained a racially determined regime of systematic oppression and domination by Jewish Israelis over Arabs both within Israel itself and within WBG (Bakan and Abu-Laban 2010; Yiftachel 2009; Gordon and Cohen 2012, 8). Israel's reply to this charge, however, was that it did not oppress or dominate Palestinians in WBG because they were members of a different racial group, but because they were a danger to its security (Shulman 2014, May 22, 30; Sabel 2011, 26). In any event, the 1973 International Convention on the Suppression and Punishment of the Crime of Apartheid refers to measures taken to "prevent a racial group . . . from participating in the political, social, economic and political life *of the country*" (United Nations General Assembly 1973, Article II, c, italics mine). Thus, the Convention does not refer to practices that characterize occupation of one geographical entity by another.

It is unnecessary to engage in a debate over whether Israel's policies in the WBG constituted apartheid when from the legal point of view its actions are covered by war crimes and crimes against humanity, as well as violation of the international law of occupation. These are the crimes for which some Israeli leaders might in principle have been indictable. In the meantime, Palestine was acknowledged by the UNGA on December 4, 2012 as a non-member observer State in the UN (United Nations General Assembly 2012, December 4, Article 2), and on December 31, 2014 it joined the ICC (Beaumont 2014, December 31). In January 2015 the then Prosecutor of the Court, Fatou Bensouda, acting on a referral by Palestinian representatives, announced that she would begin an examination of whether there had been potential war crimes committed in Gaza; this preliminary examination, however, would investigate potential crimes by both Israelis and Palestinians (Beaumont 2015, January 16). It was not known whether the Prosecutor would focus specifically on the right to food.

Penal Starvation

There appears to be no international law specifically prohibiting what I labeled in Chapter 4 as penal starvation. A positive obligation exists on the state to make sure that all its citizens enjoy the right to food. The United Nations Committee on Economic, Social and Cultural Rights has ruled that whenever individuals or groups are unable to enjoy the right to adequate food via their own means, the state is obliged to directly fulfill that right (Human Rights Watch 2007, March, 10). With regard to imprisoned citizens, The United Nations' Standard Minimum Rules for the Treatment of Prisoners specify that "Every prisoner shall be provided . . . with food of nutritional value adequate for health and strength" (United Nations 1977, Article 20).

These rules can be read to protect not only "normal" individual prisoners, but also large groups of incarcerated people deliberately subjected to rations below subsistence level. This positive obligation to provide food, however, fails to penalize states or their leaders that deliberately starve large numbers of prisoners as a matter of policy or of common – and encouraged – practice. Nor is penal starvation specified as an act of cruel, inhuman, or degrading punishment in the Convention against Torture (United Nations General Assembly 1984), although it is extremely cruel and degrading to force individuals to beg, scrounge, smuggle, steal, kill, and even become cannibals in the search for food. One might argue that deprivation of food, as an act of extermination as described in the Rome Statute, is sufficient to cover the particular case of prisoners who are deliberately starved, but this practice is so horrendous that it deserves its own law prohibiting the practice and specifying punishments for those who engage in it. These punishments should apply to anyone who starves prisoners of whom they are in charge, not only to those who give orders.

The totalitarian states discussed in Chapter 2 practiced penal starvation. Dikötter estimates that during China's Great Leap Forward there were eight to nine million prisoners every year in prison camps, where they were sometimes fed sawdust and wood pulp (Dikötter 2010, 291, 282). Cannibalism was common: starving prisoners dug up the bodies of the newly dead and ate their flesh or sold it to others in return for clothing or tobacco, both seller and buyer pretending not to know the meat was actually human (Pu Ning 2007, 380–81). With 1–2 percent of the population incarcerated at any time during the entire Maoist era and a mortality rate of about 5 percent, Margolin estimated that twenty million Chinese died during imprisonment (Margolin 1999b, 498). Prisoners were systematically underfed in part to make them more easily vulnerable to brain-washing "re-education" sessions. As was to be the case later in North Korea, the amount of food one was given depended on one's ability to work; the Chinese practice of "reform through labor" meant twelve-hour working days on one or two sparse meals (Margolin 1999b, 510). Such prisons still existed at the time of writing, although reports in 2013 suggested the Chinese government had decided to abolish them (Amnesty International 2013).

Compared to China, there were few official prisoners in Cambodia under the Khmer Rouge (KR) as the entire country was, in effect, one gigantic prison using slave labor to produce rice. Moreover, perceived enemies of the KR were usually killed immediately rather than being imprisoned. As in China and North Korea, however, those who were formally imprisoned received even lower rations than the rest of the population, and prisoners' average life expectancy was three months (Margolin 1999a, 612). Rations consisted of watery rice, hardly enough to sustain prisoners engaged in agricultural labor (Ngor 1987, excerpted in Hollander, 447).

Among the contemporary cases described in this book, North Korea stands out for its systematic starvation of prisoners. Zimbabwean prisoners also starved, although not, it appears, as a matter of actual policy as in North Korea. Yet there is still no international law identifying and outlawing systematic penal starvation. One might argue that such a law is not necessary, as the Rome Statute identifies deprivation of food as an aspect of persecution. Kim Jong Il could have been charged before the ICC for starvation of prisoners as he was personally responsible for prisons, which were run by the National Security Service, which reported directly to him (Hawk 2003, 26). But given the limited capacity of the ICC to try any but the most serious cases of genocide, war crimes, and crimes against humanity, a document outlining the penalties for penal starvation should supplement the Standard Minimum Rules for Treatment of Prisoners.

The Standard Minimum Rules do not address large-scale deliberate incarceration of perceived enemies of the state or deliberate or reckless disregard of prisoners' nutritional needs. At minimum, the Rules require a supplement explaining the punishments that international law would impose on prison officials and the government agents that oversee them who neglect prisoners' rights. Such punishments, moreover, would have to include more than the threat of trial before the ICC. They could, for example, include censure by international organizations of prison officials or denial of the right of such officials to attend international conferences. Shaming might ameliorate inadvertent or incompetent starvation of prisoners, but more severe punishments would have to be specified for intentional starvation.

Emerging "Soft Law": The Kimberley Process

There is no agreed definition of soft law, but in general it is thought to stretch from new norms and regulations not yet entrenched into formal law to international covenants and treaties which, while technically binding upon the countries that sign them, are not enforceable (Fajardo accessed December 3, 2014).

One aspect of soft law applies to the deprivation of livelihoods in Zimbabwe that prevented many people from earning a living to feed themselves and their families. Established in 2003, the Kimberley Process could be used to regulate small-scale diamond miners' loss of livelihood as a result of takeovers of diamond mines by the state and military. This Process was devised at an international conference of governments, non-governmental organizations, and diamond industry representatives in the diamond center of Kimberley, South Africa, to ensure that diamonds produced in situations of conflict and exploited by conflict leaders could not be sold on the international market (Nichols 2012). Originally, it was aimed at diamonds from Sierra Leone, then in the throes of a civil war.

Zimbabwe was a relatively late producer of diamonds, which were discovered at Marange in 2006. The government and military almost immediately took over the diamond fields, displacing small diamond diggers. The government and military were also alleged to employ miners in slave-like conditions and to employ child labor (Human Rights Watch 2009c, 39), as well as using torture and rape to displace the small-scale miners and villagers who lived on the diamond fields (Nichols 2012, 650). As a result of these conditions, activists turned to the Kimberley Process to ensure that diamonds from the Marange fields did not reach the international market. This attempt failed, however, when Zimbabwe diamonds were certified in 2010 as conflict-free (Nichols 2012, 651). Many diamonds were sold to India and to China, the latter country one of Mugabe's allies, even though both countries were participants in the Kimberley Process (Nichols 2012, 678).

There was considerable debate among the Kimberley participants as to whether the Process had jurisdiction over the Marange diamonds, with some participants proposing a new definition of "conflict" diamonds to refer to diamonds from "areas where mining is based on the systematic violation of human rights," which would have covered Zimbabwe's diamonds (Nichols 2012, 681). Mugabe argued to the contrary that "blood diamonds" were diamonds that emerged from civil wars and there was no such war in Zimbabwe. This was indeed the case: the Kimberley Process did not refer to diamonds whose production entailed violations of human rights outside conflict situations. Rather, conflict diamonds were defined as "rough diamonds used by rebel movements or their allies to finance conflict aimed at undermining legitimate governments" (Human Rights Watch 2009c, 53). Moreover, the fact that an allied government, the Democratic Republic of the Congo, chaired the Kimberley Process in 2011 (Mail and Guardian Online 2011, June 21) made it easier for

Zimbabwe to escape the Process' censure. Internally, the government skillfully utilized human rights rhetoric to claim that a ban on sale of Marange diamonds deprived Zimbabweans of necessary income and therefore of the capacity to enjoy their economic human rights (Nyamu-rundira 2011, December 22). In so doing it ignored its own violations of the rights of small diamond diggers, including their capacities to provide for their own economic rights and the economic rights of their families.

Conclusion

Very little in this chapter pertains to Venezuela. Whatever the policy errors that Chávez and Maduro made, shortages of food in that country had not resulted by 2015 in famine, although it appeared that malnutrition was becoming a problem, as noted in Chapter 6. Even if malnutrition were widespread, the worst famine crime with which they could have been charged was incompetence, not an indictable offense no matter how one argues that faminogenesis should be considered a crime under international law. Certainly, Chávez and Maduro were not indifferent to Venezuelans' food needs, trying to rectify shortages through distribution of subsidized food and regulation of producers and distributors whom they considered to be depriving Venezuelans of affordable food. States possess the sovereign right to be incompetent; it is not a crime to institute policies that undermine market efficiency. While redistribution of property without adequate compensation may violate the international human right to own property, the most that could be done by any United Nations human rights committee would be to "name and shame" the Venezuelan government, along with attempts at shaming by human rights bodies of the Organization of American States.

There remains the problem of intentional and reckless faminogene-sis, as in North Korea and Zimbabwe. Even if it had been possible to indict the Kims and Mugabe under international law, such indictment of individual leaders would not address the real problem, the existence of entire regimes that deprive significant sections of their own popula-tions of food. Chapter 9 addresses the "sticks and carrots" problem of how both international and internal politics complicate efforts either to impose sanctions on food-depriving regimes or to assist the starving and malnourished via food aid.

9   Sticks and Carrots
Sanctions and Food Aid

States frequently try to persuade or coerce each other to change their behavior toward their citizens or accept outside intervention for humanitarian reasons. States' actions can include positive measures such as diplomatic engagement and foreign aid, or negative measures such as moral condemnation, sanctions, and – in the last instance – military force. Since 2000 an international consensus has been evolving that states are obliged to protect citizens of other states when they suffer extreme violations of their human rights.

In 2001 the Canadian government sponsored the International Commission on Intervention and State Sovereignty. This Commission concluded that there were sometimes just causes for military intervention against a sovereign state, and advocated a responsibility to protect, colloquially known as R2P. The threshold for such intervention was "serious and irreparable harm," defined as large-scale loss of life or large-scale ethnic cleansing, whether or not with genocidal intent, as the product of deliberate state action, state neglect, or state failure. Like the Rome Statute of the International Criminal Court, however, the Commission's report did not identify state-induced famine as a specific crime (International Commission on Intervention and State Sovereignty 2001, xii).

In 2005 a report by Kofi Annan, then Secretary-General of the United Nations, discussed whether states had the right, or even the obligation, to use force "to rescue the citizens of other States from genocide or comparable crimes" (Annan 2005, par. 122, p. 33). In 2006 the United Nations Security Council (UNSC) adopted a resolution on R2P, but most of its clauses referred to the responsibility of a state to protect its own people. Only clause 26 referred to the UN's own responsibility, noting that "the deliberate targeting of civilians and other protected persons, and the commission of systematic, flagrant and widespread violations of international humanitarian and human rights law in situations of armed conflict, may constitute a threat to international peace and security," and reaffirming the readiness of the UNSC "to consider such situations and, where necessary, to adopt appropriate steps" (United Nations Security Council 2006, April 28). Actual armed intervention was still, however, a last step, not to be taken lightly. Moreover, the UNSC Resolution referred only to situations of armed conflict, not to criminal behavior by states. Both in its objectives and its mechanisms, humanitarian intervention had not yet reached the point at which it could protect citizens against state-induced famine and other food crimes.

It is easier to say that something should be done to stop mass atrocities than to actually take action: most options are fraught with ambiguities about actors, procedures, and outcomes. In the case of state food crimes, there are two major possibilities. The first is to take punitive measures such as sanctions, and the second is to offer food aid. In this chapter I focus on sanctions and food aid: In none of the four cases described in Part II was military intervention to protect the rights of citizens deprived of food seriously considered. I first consider the political difficulties that hamper international attempts to protect the right to food in North Korea, Zimbabwe, Venezuela, and the West Bank and Gaza (WBG). I then discuss the general problem of food aid as it is found in North Korea, Zimbabwe, and WBG, and as it might be found in Venezuela in the future. I begin with the political difficulties of imposing sanctions, because those difficulties also affect the likelihood of food aid's being effective.

Failure to Protect: Humanitarianism vs. Strategic Considerations in North Korea

Overwhelming considerations regarding East Asian and world-wide nuclear security took precedence over North Koreans' food security throughout the early 2000s. North Korea tested nuclear bombs in 2006, 2009, and 2013. Five countries – the United States, South Korea, China, Japan, and Russia – had been trying to negotiate with North Korea since the 1990s to contain the nuclear threat (Bajoria 2012, February 29), at the same time as they tried to encourage economic change that would increase the supply of food. These actors adopted alternating policies of containment and engagement, but North Koreans' human right to food was always secondary to concern about the nuclear threat.

The ins and outs of these negotiations are too complicated to explain here (for detailed histories, see Bluth 2008; Kim 2011): Suffice it to say that North Korea sometimes agreed to negotiate with some or all of these five interested parties, but other times it refused. It made commitments, for example to de-commission nuclear facilities, then reneged or claimed to have taken the promised action when it had not done so. It joined the

Treaty on the Non-Proliferation of Nuclear Weapons in 1985, then left it informally in 1993 (French 2007, 197) and formally in 2003 (Bluth 2008, 118). It allowed inspectors from the International Atomic Energy Association into the country, then thwarted their activities or expelled them. It appeared oblivious to sanctions imposed by the UNSC.

Thus, North Korea conducted a policy of brinkmanship, threatening escalation of its nuclear program to obtain concessions or aid but withdrawing from the brink whenever it thought that the US might get fed up and attack it, as it had attacked Iraq in 2003. Moreover, North Korea was aware that after Libya gave up its nuclear weapons in 2003, the US and NATO assisted the opposition to institute regime change in 2011. To prevent the US or other countries from promoting regime change in North Korea the government threatened nuclear or conventional attacks on South Korea (Kim 2011, 120). Yet it appeared willing to trade its nuclear capacity for a formal peace treaty with, and formal recognition by, the US.

North Korea also engaged in other activities that took precedence over its citizens' food rights in the eyes of the international community. It committed terrorist actions such as assassinating South Korean cabinet ministers in 1983 (Bluth 2008, xiii). In March 2010 it sank the South Korean ship, the *Cheonan*, killing forty-six people, and also attacked a South Korean military base on Yeonpyeong Island. As a result, South Korea referred North Korea to the International Criminal Court (ICC) for investigation of possible war crimes. In June 2014 the Office of the ICC Prosecutor concluded that it did not have jurisdiction over the two incidents, owing to complicated legal reasoning emerging from the fact that North and South Korea were still technically at war, having signed an armistice in 1953 but never having signed an actual peace treaty (International Criminal Court 2014, June).

North Korea possessed illegal chemical and biological weapons (Bluth 2008, 156–59), and as of 2012 was thought to be the world's third-largest possessor of chemical weapons after the US and Russia (Nuclear Threat Institute 2012, August). Moreover, it appeared that by 2005 it was developing missiles that might hit Hawaii or even the mainland US West Coast (Becker 2005, 161; Bluth 2008, 87). It also exported arms, particularly to enemies of the US such as Iran, and possibly Syria (Becker 2005, 159–60; Bluth 2008, 160). It threatened to export nuclear technology or might already have done so, not only to other states but also to non-state entities (Kim 2011, 130; Moore 2014). North Korea also trafficked in illegal drugs to earn foreign currency (Bernstein 2007, March 1, 39): "Office 39," a branch of the ruling Korean Workers' Party, was dedicated to importing luxury goods for the elite, for which it paid with profits from drugs and counterfeit American currency (Landler 2010, August 30).

The US veered between hardline policies and softer measures to contain the North Korean strategic threat. President G.W. Bush declared North Korea a terrorist state in 2002 (Bush 2002, January 29, 3) but pledged to remove this designation in 2008, when it appeared that North Korea was co-operating in talks to reduce its nuclear program (Moon 2008, 263). Removal from the list of terrorist states meant that North Korea could join international institutions such as the World Bank (Economist 2008, September 27, 17). In 2004 the US Congress passed the North Korean Human Rights Act (Goedde 2010, 560), authorizing the government to give $20 million to individuals and organizations helping North Korean refugees, to help finance broadcasts to North Korea, and to give immigrant visas to North Korean defectors (Kim 2011, 127). One purpose of US sanctions was to block the flow of luxury goods to the North Korean elite; however, the North Koreans forged trade documents and changed the names of the trading firms under sanctions.

In early 2011 North Korea made overtures to the US, proposing to resume searches for the remains of 8,000 American prisoners of the Korean war: One reason for this proposal may have been that the US paid the full cost of such searches in American dollars (Starr 2011, January 18). Yet in February 2013 North Korea further provoked the US as well as the broader international community by conducting a failed nuclear test (United Nations Security Council 2013, January 22). Thus, all these interests prevented the US from adopting a straightforward policy to promote the right to food in North Korea.

South Korea might be assumed to have been wholeheartedly in favor of supporting North Koreans' right to food, but there too, security considerations took precedence. North Korea possessed conventional weapons that could severely damage South Korea's capital, Seoul, even if it did not use nuclear weapons (Bluth 2008, 139). South Korea's security concerns were, however, counterbalanced by its desire for reunification. According to South Korean law, all North Koreans were citizens of South Korea, but in fact, South Korea feared a refugee overflow (Bernstein 2007, March 1, 37). South Korea also feared the high costs of reunification: one estimate was $US 900 billion over four decades (Economist 2010, May 29, 25). South Korea also wanted to re-unite families that were split after the Korean War and rescue some elderly South Korean prisoners of war still held in North Korea, as well as an estimated 500 of its citizens whom North Korea had abducted (Human Rights Watch 2010b, 329).

South Koreans actively debated whether humanitarian or strategic interests should take priority in their North Korea policy. Some believed the best strategy was to continue humanitarian aid and family reunions: These advocates of engagement believed that contact with and knowledge of South Korea could strengthen North Koreans' opposition to the Kim regime. Others advocated economic engagement in the hope that it would result in political change. There was some opportunity to invest in North Korea – thus providing North Koreans with jobs and income, which would improve access to food – however, both South Korean corruption and North Korean policies such as denying visas to South Korean investors made such investment difficult. Yet other South Koreans believed a hard line, including cutting off food aid, was the best reaction to the North Korean threat.

Presidents Kim Dae Jung and Roh Moo Hyun, who respectively ruled South Korea from 1998 to 2003 and 2003 to 2008, encouraged a policy of engagement, including investment in the North and limited reunification of families. But President Lee Myung-bak, elected in 2008, ended all economic aid (Laurence and Kim 2012, January 16) and family reunifications, and was generally very critical of North Korean human rights violations. The president as of February 2013, Park Geun-hye, offered a policy of "trustpolitik" by which South Korea would offer concessions in return for real reform by North Korea (Economist 2013, May 11), but was stymied in that aim when North Korea conducted its third nuclear test less than two weeks before she took power.

China's policy was similarly inconsistent. On the one hand, China protected North Korea, viewing it as a buffer state between itself and South Korea, Japan, and Taiwan (Bluth 2008, 120). China also invested in North Korea and established joint economic zones with it. In general, China wished to counterbalance US influence on the Korean Peninsula and ensure North Korean stability to undermine any risk of massive refugee outflows to its own northern region (Kim 2011, 135–57).

On the other hand, China appeared impatient with North Korea's violations of international rules; for example, North Korea counterfeited Chinese as well as US currency (Moore 2008, 10). North Korea also conducted nuclear tests close to China's border in 2006 and 2009, causing environmental damage (Lim 2012, May 17). Along with Russia and the US, China consistently discouraged North Korea's nuclear program, arguing that small states did not need nuclear weapons. It did not veto UNSC sanctions on North Korea after the 2006 and 2009 nuclear tests (United Nations Security Council 2006, October 14, 2009, June 12), and in 2013 it supported UNSC sanctions (United Nations Security Council 2013, March 7). Chinese residents close to the test locations apparently worried about nuclear fallout in 2013 (Epstein 2013, February 21), a concern China might not be able to ignore as its citizens gained a greater political voice. China feared a general war and possible nuclear arms race in Northeast Asia, which would involve not only itself, the Koreas, and Japan, but also the US (Moore 2008, 13).

Japanese-North Korean relations were also fraught. In 1998, North Korea shot a test missile over Japan (Kim 2011, 140); it also kidnapped Japanese citizens to work as translators or language instructors (Bluth 2008, 125). North Korea claimed $12 billion in compensation for the Japanese occupation of Korea from 1905 to 1945, but Japan would not consider paying unless North Korea ceased its threatening activities (Kim 2011, 166). Many ethnic Koreans living in Japan sent remittances to their kin in North Korea, a valuable source of hard currency for the regime which Japan periodically threatened to ban (Bluth 2008, 74). For its part, North Korea feared the US military presence in Japan (Kim 2011, 166).

Finally, after an initial lack of interest in North Korea after the end of the Soviet era, Russia under Putin reasserted its friendship with the Kim regime. Russia was interested in becoming an influential actor in the northeast Asian region and hoped to build a railway line from its Far East through both North and South Korea. Above all, it wanted to counter both American and, to a lesser extent, Chinese interest in the region (Kim 2011, 159–64).

All these national interests affected, and sometimes superseded, any concern these five countries might have had for North Koreans' food security. The overwhelming fear of North Korea's nuclear program, combined with the disparate foreign policy interests discussed above, made it difficult to decide on strategies to promote North Koreans' human right to food. The UNSC sanctions on North Korea after its 2006, 2009, and 2013 nuclear tests pertained principally to weapons, weapons-related materiel, and luxury goods without which the elite might be less likely to support the Kim regime. The UNSC was careful to note that the sanctions were not meant to harm the civilian population of North Korea (United Nations Security Council 2006, October 14, Article 9a; United Nations Security Council 2009, June 12, Article 19; United Nations Security Council 2013, March 7, Article 18); thus, it imposed no restrictions on food exports or food aid to that country.

As debates about various forms of involvement with North Korea took place, one option was simply to wait for domestic change to produce an active demand for human rights, including the right to food. News of the prosperity of China and South Korea filtered into North Korea via returned refugees and traders who travelled illegally to China and returned with smuggled videos and DVDs; indeed, it was believed that perhaps 500,000 North Koreans had spent some time in China by 2009 (Lankov 2009, 99). It also seemed that North Korea was becoming more willing to engage with the international community (Bellamy 2015, 229–30); in particular, it was somewhat more co-operative with World Food Programme (WFP) and FAO food missions in the twenty-first century and was also willing to discuss its obligations under the Convention on the Rights of the Child to prevent child malnutrition (Moon 2008, 268).

In the meantime, however, in North Korea "loose nukes" trumped human rights. One might think that its famine crimes constituted a clear case for invocation of R2P, but no state had invoked this principle regarding North Korea. As long as it possessed or threatened to possess nuclear weapons, the risks of invasion were too high. The right to life of everyone within range of North Korean weapons was a constant source of tension that conflicted with humanitarian efforts to fulfill North Koreans' right to food.

Failure to Protect: Sanctions vs. Rhetoric in Zimbabwe

During the first decade of the twenty-first century various sanctions were imposed on Zimbabwe. Sanctions were imposed because of its violations of human rights and the democratic process, not specifically because of its violations of the right to food; however, restoration of human rights and preservation of democracy would have assisted Zimbabweans to obtain food. The sanctions not only failed but also provided the regime with a rhetorical tool to divert blame for its mismanaged economic policy.

A standard assumption is that when humanitarian pressure is deemed necessary, those political entities closest to the offending state should take responsibility first, as they are least likely to be seen as outsiders trying to violate sovereignty. The closest country to Zimbabwe, politically as well as geographically, was South Africa. The closest regional political entities were the Southern African Development Community (SADC) and the continental African Union (AU). Neither criticized Mugabe's leadership in Zimbabwe.

Thabo Mbeki, President of South Africa from 1999 to 2008, protected Mugabe from sanctions by the AU (Phimister and Raftopoulos 2004), claiming before the 2005 elections that "Nobody in Zimbabwe is likely to act in a way that will prevent free and fair elections being held" (O'Malley 2005, March 30). This reflected a general unwillingness by many presidents of African countries to acknowledge violence in Zimbabwe. In 2005, the AU resisted calls from the US and Britain to criticize Operation Drive Out Trash (BBC News 2005, June 24). In 2006, it refused to make public a report critical of Zimbabwe's human rights record, which had been prepared two years earlier by the AU Commission on

Human and Peoples' Rights (IRIN Humanitarian News and Analysis 2006, July 8). In May 2007, the African bloc at the UN successfully nominated Zimbabwe's Environment Minister, Francis Nhema, to chair the UN Commission on Sustainable Development, despite allegations that he had ruined a previously successful white-owned farm that he had received during land redistribution (Deutsche Presse-Agentur 2007, September 4).

Attitudes among some African leaders began to change in 2007. The AU's then President, John Kufuor of Ghana, called the situation in Zimbabwe "very embarrassing" (Associated Press 2007, March 14); Botswana, Kenya, Zambia, and Tanzania also criticized Mugabe (Hammer 2008b, August 14, 4; Africa Research Bulletin 2008, July 1–31, 17600). Nevertheless, the AU welcomed Mugabe to its summit in June 2008, issuing a weak statement that it hoped he and opposition leader Morgan Tsvangirai would successfully come to an agreement on a unity government. At that meeting the AU also appealed to all "states and all parties concerned to refrain from any action that may negatively impact on the climate of dialogue" (African Union 2008, July 1). Confirming the almost universal African disapproval of any punitive actions by non-African states, SADC at its 2009 meeting demanded that the West lift its targeted sanctions (discussed below) against Mugabe and his inner circle (Elliott 2009, September 29).

In 2009, Jacob Zuma was elected President of South Africa. Before his election Zuma had been quite critical of Zimbabwe. His supporters in the South African dockworkers' union had refused to allow a Chinese ship carrying arms for Zimbabwe's security forces to land at Durban in April 2008 (Evans 2008, 104), and once he was elected President he stressed the importance of respect for human rights and good governance in a visit to Zimbabwe in August 2009 (Economist 2009, September 19, 52). His criticism, however, was muted: at the 2009 SADC summit, he referred to the power-sharing agreement between Mugabe and Tsvangirai as a "positive development," without criticizing the murders, tortures, and rapes after the 2008 election or Mugabe's many attempts to keep Tsvangirai from wielding real power (Zuma 2009). By 2011, however, Zuma had become more cognizant of the need for change in Zimbabwe, reporting to SADC that Mugabe and his political party, the Zimbawe African National Union-Patriotic Front (ZANU-PF) should honor the 2009 Global Political Agreement (Economist 2011, June 25).

The uncritical attitudes of SADC and the AU to Mugabe reflected other African leaders' respect for his role in the anti-colonial struggle against the former British colonizer, along with his support for the anti-apartheid struggle in South Africa: He was considered one of the "grand old men" of the African liberation movement. In 2002, Mbeki claimed that attempts in the British Commonwealth (see below) to ostracize Mugabe were "inspired by notions of white supremacy" (Taylor and Williams 2002, 558). Mbeki may have had other reasons to oppose outside interference, such as fear that civil war might break out if Mugabe were pushed too far, resulting in an even larger influx of refugees into South Africa than had already occurred (Soko and Balchin 2009, 40).

Many SADC members felt that the West had unfairly demonized Zimbabwe because of the land seizures from white owners (International Crisis Group 2005, 19). In 2005, South African Foreign Minister Nkosazana Dlamini-Zulu argued that there was an "element of racism" in the Zimbabwe debate, saying that "the hullaballoo is about black people taking land from white people" (International Crisis Group 2005, 17). South Africa's ruling political party, the African National Congress, defended Mugabe's decision in 2000 to reject Britain's offer of an extra £36 million to facilitate land reform, agreeing that Britain's conditions that prices had to be fair and the rule of law had to be respected were unreasonable (Taylor and Williams 2002, 554, 559).

Mugabe himself regularly attributed attempts to force him to change his policies to "white," "Western," or "imperialist" interference. At the UN World Food Summit in Rome in November 2009, he accused "certain countries whose interests stand opposed to our quest for the equity and justice of our land reforms," claiming that these countries were neo-colonial powers who had imposed unilateral sanctions in order to undermine Zimbabwe's land reforms and make it dependent on food imports (Mugabe 2009, November 17, 3). In 2011 Zimbabwe assumed its turn as chair of the AU's Peace and Security Council (Bell 2011, May 30), further buttressing Mugabe's reputation, demonstrating resentment against Western sanctions, and undermining the Council's credibility (SADOCC 2011, May 27). In 2014, Mugabe was elected Chair of SADC, and in early 2015 he was appointed Chair of the AU (Al-Jazeera 2015, January 30).

The fear of being charged with neo-colonialism may be one reason why Western and UN actions against Mugabe were relatively ineffective. The Commonwealth Organization is a group of countries formerly under British rule. It suspended Zimbabwe from membership in 2002 (Nading 2002, 763); in return, Mugabe withdrew Zimbabwe from the organization, charging that his expulsion was caused by white racism (Calderisi 2006, 93). By 2015, Zimbabwe had not returned to the Commonwealth.

Britain imposed sanctions on Zimbabwe as early as 2000, cutting certain types of aid while retaining others, such as funds for HIV/AIDS treatment; it also imposed an arms embargo on Zimbabwe (Taylor and Williams 2002, 555). In 2002, the European Union (EU) began a series of targeted sanctions, including bans on arms and any equipment that could be used for internal repression, as well as financial sanctions and travel bans on individual Zimbabweans (Pillitu 2003, 454–55). In 2004 the EU imposed a travel ban and asset freeze on ninety-five Zimbabweans, including Mugabe (United Kingdom Parliament 2004, March 2), extending its sanctions in 2008, the election year (Africa Research Bulletin 2008, July 1–31, 17602). Despite these sanctions, however, Mugabe was invited to and attended the EU-Africa Summit in 2007 (Evans 2008, 185).

In 2008 the Group of 8, a gathering of leading industrial powers, expressed its "grave concern" about the violence surrounding Zimbabwe's election, as well as about the general humanitarian situation and the refusal by Zimbabwean authorities to allow non-discriminatory access to all humanitarian agencies (G8 Leaders 2008, July 8). Also in 2008, the US tightened a travel ban on 250 Zimbabwean individuals and corporations and forbade Americans to do business with them: These sanctions remained in force as of December 2013 (Office of Foreign Assets Control 2013, December 18). EU and US policies also included restrictions on loans, credit and development assistance, including from international financial organizations (International Crisis Group 2012, February 6).

In 2008 the US and UK introduced a resolution in the UNSC to freeze the assets of Mugabe and thirteen senior Zimbabwean government and security officials, ban them from travel outside Zimbabwe, and impose an arms embargo on Zimbabwe. Russia and China vetoed the resolution on the grounds that under Chapter VII of the United Nations Charter, the UNSC is supposed to take action against states only when there is a threat to international peace and security (United Nations Security Council 2008, July 11), which they argued did not exist in this instance. In vetoing the UNSC Resolution, China and Russia were defending their own interests. China was investing in Zimbabwe (Taylor 2008, 74–77) and had supported Mugabe by building him a $9 million palace (York 2006, March 4): Its general approach to human rights in Africa was to support national sovereignty and oppose interference in states' internal affairs (Taylor 2008). Moreover, China opposed sanctions on sovereign states because any precedent could affect its own authority in Tibet. Russia had similar concerns.

South Africa, one of the UNSC non-permanent members in 2008, also voted against the US and UK resolution, arguing that problems in Zimbabwe were best left in the hands of regional organizations and that the AU summit in 2007 had asked for all sanctions against Zimbabwe to be lifted (United Nations Security Council 2008, July 11, 5). Zimbabwe's information minister claimed that the UNSC resolution was a form of "international racism disguised as multilateral action" (BBC News 2008, July 7). Thus, as of mid-2008, a weak statement deploring violence and denial of civil liberties and expressing concern about the grave humanitarian situation in Zimbabwe remained the only official UNSC response (United Nations Security Council 2008, June 23). No subsequent resolutions on Zimbabwe were introduced in the UNSC.

In any event, sanctions might have backfired. Mugabe and his colleagues very skillfully used sanctions as a propaganda tool, arguing that they were the cause of Zimbabweans' economic problems, depriving Zimbabweans of their "socio-economic rights" as well as their right to property (in formerly white-owned land) (Nyamurundira 2011, December 22; Nkomo 2011, September 15). For example, the then governor of the Zimbabwe Reserve Bank, Dr. G. Gono, issued a document (probably in 2008 or 2009) blaming sanctions for all of Zimbabwe's economic woes, including steep declines in foreign investment and the unwillingness of the International Monetary Fund to grant it loans (Zimbabwe Reserve Bank accessed January 26, 2015). Mugabe frequently claimed that the sanctions were illegal and the reasons for them false; "we . . . are subjected to unparalleled vilification and pernicious economic sanctions, the false reasons alleged being violations of the rule of law, human rights, and democracy" (Mugabe 2011, September 22). Zimbabweans were not informed that most sanctions were imposed only against certain individuals and economic entities, not against the Zimbabwean people or economy as a whole. Thus, it was easy for them to be persuaded by the rhetoric that sanctions were part of a "neo-colonial and imperialist regime-change agenda" (Tungwarara undated, 111).

Perhaps realizing that they were not efficacious, in 2010 Botswana, Zambia, and South Africa advocated ending the sanctions, on grounds of the formation of the unity government after the 2008 elections (Bell 2010, December 2; Agence France-Presse 2010b October 5). SADC also lobbied for removal of sanctions, ostensibly because they were hurting the entire Southern African economy. Despite these arguments, the EU renewed its sanctions in 2010. But in 2012 the British Foreign Minister announced that Britain wanted to lift many of the sanctions, to bring Zimbabwe back into the community of nations (Oborne 2012, July 18). The EU then suspended sanctions, despite pleas from white farmers not to do so until they were compensated for their expropriated land (Sengupta 2012, October 8). At this point the then United Nations

High Commissioner for Human Rights, Navi Pillay, had visited Zimbabwe and called for removal of sanctions on the grounds that they had unintended side effects that were hurting the poor, such as discouragement of foreign investments (BBC News 2012, May 25). In response, in 2014 the EU lifted most of its sanctions against individuals, although sanctions against Mugabe and his wife remained (HM Treasury 2014, February 25).

Aside from their opposition to sanctions, African regional organizations also eschewed other measures available to them to ameliorate human rights abuses in Zimbabwe. The Constitutive Act of the AU, Article 4, refers to the "right of the Union to intervene in a Member State pursuant to a decision of the Assembly in respect of grave circumstances, namely: war crimes, genocide, and crimes against humanity" (African Union 2000, Article 4, (h)). Thus even armed intervention was not an unthinkable option, as crimes against humanity were common in Zimbabwe, especially murders and tortures of opposition members. In 2008, Morgan Tsvangirai, the opposition leader, asked for an African police force to be sent to Zimbabwe (Verma 2008, July 1), and some Zimbabwean civil society groups also called for armed intervention by the AU to control Zimbabwean private militias and security forces (Ecumenical Zimbabwe Network 2008, June 25). But even if the AU had wished to actively intervene, it was already over-stretched with troops in Burundi and Sudan (Williams 2007, 270).

Had armed intervention from outside Africa been considered, the AU would probably have defended Zimbabwe, asserting the principles of state sovereignty and African solutions for African problems. The UN was in any case overstretched in Africa, with troops in Congo, Darfur, and Somalia in 2008, the peak year of crimes against humanity in Zimbabwe (International Crisis Group 2008, December 16, 10). In any event, without actual civil war and the threat not only of regional spillovers but also spillovers to the Western world, such as piracy, terrorism, or uncontrollable refugee flows, it was highly unlikely that any non-African military force would intervene to protect Zimbabweans from their oppressive government.

Zimbabwe certainly fit the criteria of R2P; the harm to its population was serious and irreparable, and was the product of state action. Yet despite the rhetoric about the responsibility to protect people from their own abusive governments, there seemed to be no responsibility to protect the people of Zimbabwe. Commentators who discussed R2P in Africa during the height of the Zimbabwean crisis consistently mentioned Burundi, Congo, Somalia, and Darfur but ignored Zimbabwe (Powell and Baranyi 2005; Kuwali 2009, March). Speakers at a seminar in January 2009 organized by the Global Centre for the Responsibility to Protect concluded that military intervention was not an effective means to protect Zimbabweans, although they did urge other measures such as referring some members of the regime to the ICC (Global Centre for the Responsibility to Protect 2009, January 30). The reluctance to invoke R2P was in part a result of the fact that the principle was meant – in so far as it was taken seriously at all – to apply only to conflict zones, as clause 26 of the 2006 UNSC Resolution noted, not to countries where people quietly starved without any open warfare.

Venezuela: When Non-Interference Is a Better Option

Whereas North Korea and Zimbabwe implemented deliberate policies that undermined their citizens' right to food, and Israel's security and settlement policies resulted in malnutrition among Palestinians, Venezuela under Chávez exhibited, at worst, incompetent management of the food supply buttressed by denial of civil and political rights. As I argued in Chapter 8, states possess the sovereign right to be incompetent, and it is quite common for elected left populist regimes such as Venezuela's to exhibit incompetence by interfering with markets to protect the interests of the poor. In practice if not in law, states also possess the sovereign right to undermine civil and political rights. The only check on such practices is soft and unenforceable international law – and then only when states have signed and ratified the relevant instruments. By 2015, however, Nicolás Maduro was engaging in policies that constituted reckless indifference to Venezuelans' food needs.

In Venezuela under Chávez, positive measures such as diplomatic engagement and offers of assistance would have been appropriate to promote the right to food, but negative measures such as sanctions (leaving aside armed humanitarian intervention) would have been unwise. In particular, it was not appropriate for the US to try to undermine the Venezuelan government, especially given its twentieth-century interventions in Central and South America to subvert left-wing governments and prop up right-wing military dictatorships, including those guilty of genocide, mass torture, incarcerations, and disappearances. Yet the US regarded Chávez as an enemy from the beginning of his tenure in office and endorsed the 2002 illegal attempted coup (Shifter 2006, 56). US hostility to Chávez was all the more unreasonable given that some of Venezuela's predecessor regimes during the period of the Punto Fijo pact had also mismanaged the economy, relying too heavily on oil revenues, overvaluing the currency, tolerating high inflation, and imposing price controls. The difference, however, was that predecessor governments had not attacked private property, as Chávez did. Not without reason, then, Chávez feared a US invasion (Marcano and Barrera Tyszka 2006, 291).

US moves to punish or overthrow Chávez merely reinforced many Latin Americans' mistrust of the "imperialist" US. This mistrust stemmed not only from memories of US interventions in the twentieth century but also from fear of US-led globalization in the twenty-first century (Hellinger 2011, 48). Many influential politicians believed that Latin America's relative backwardness was caused by its economic dependence on the US (Lapper 2006, 16): Many pro-Chávez Venezuelans also assumed that the US's chief interest in their country was access to their oil (Hellinger 2011, 55). They were particularly angry at US support for the 2002 attempted coup (Lapper 2006, 8).

Rather than try to overthrow left populist, anti-capitalist regimes such as Chávez's and Maduro's, a better strategy for the international community was to encourage and reward good governance in Latin America, in states such as Chile and Brazil that promoted social welfare and equality while respecting democracy and the rule of law and operating within the boundaries of market economies (Castaneda 2006, 42). In post-Chávez Venezuela, this might have meant encouraging Maduro to rescind those arbitrary measures that undermined democracy, the rule of law, and civil and political rights. It would also have meant encouraging a gradual return of property to those from whom it had arbitrarily been taken, or at least fairly compensating the owners; any further redistribution of property would have had to be conducted according to the rule of law. It would have been important to retain the real improvements that had occurred in nutrition, education, and health care while dismantling arbitrary measures.

However, the US did not take this path. In early 2015 it imposed sanctions on unnamed Venezuelans accused of perpetrating human rights abuses during 2014's civil unrest; the sanctions banned them from obtaining US visas and froze their assets, thus resembling sanctions against North Korean and Zimbabwean officials (Obama 2015, March 9). The ostensible reason for the sanctions was that the situation in Venezuela constituted a threat to US national security, but the sanctions may actually have been a quid pro quo measure to satisfy Republicans who opposed President Obama's decision to establish normal diplomatic relations with Cuba (Economist 2014, December 6). The sanctions also represented a significant change from Obama's own early policy to stress dialogue and multilateral diplomacy when dealing with leftist Latin American states, including Venezuela (Hellinger 2011, 46). For many Venezuelans, the sanctions were evidence of the US's continuing imperialist influence, and Maduro skillfully played on anti-US feelings to improve his popularity, as Mugabe had done in Zimbabwe. In April 2015 Maduro threatened to present a petition against the sanctions with ten million signatures to President Obama at a Summit of the Americas in Panama, although it appeared that many Venezuelans had been coerced into signing the petition (Vyas 2015, April 8). In the event, he did not present it, leading to doubts as to its existence (Martel 2015, April 13).

Diplomatic means, naming and shaming, and various other "soft" measures seemed more appropriate to dissuade Maduro from continuing to undermine Venezuelans' rights than US sanctions. Such measures might have sent a signal that peaceful opposition to Maduro must be allowed. Moreover, had democracy been restored, the opposition might have had leeway to demand economic reforms that would alleviate food shortages. Such "soft" diplomatic measures might also have taken into account the inequality and social exclusion (Lapper 2006, 38) which many Venezuelans had suffered before Chávez took power, and his early success in improving access to food before his economic mismanagement and political authoritarianism undermined it.

The Organization of American States (OAS) adopted this milder approach throughout Chávez's and Maduro's presidencies, insisting on preservation of human rights in Venezuela and on Venezuelans' right to elect their own leaders. Thus, the OAS condemned the 2002 attempted coup against Chávez as an assault on democracy (Organization of American States 2002, April 13), but in 2009 the Inter-American Commission on Human Rights issued a highly critical report on human rights abuses in Venezuela (Inter-American Commission on Human Rights 2009, December 30). The Inter-American Court on Human Rights also defended the rights of individual Venezuelans, including the opposition leader Leopoldo López, jailed in 2014 despite the Court's having ruled in 2011 against a government decision barring him from holding office for six years (Economist 2014, February 22, 31). None of these actions, however, appeared to have any effect on the policies of either Chávez or Maduro. Instead, in 2012 Venezuela withdrew from the Inter-American Commission on Human Rights (Kornblith 2013, 52).

The OAS took a principled stance on human rights in Venezuela, upholding universal and regional standards without falling prey to the anti-leftist rhetoric that characterized the American attitude. Its position also contrasted with the AU's uncritical rhetorical support for Robert Mugabe. On the other hand, the OAS did not threaten to expel Venezuela, preferring to keep it within the regional fold. Unfortunately, its even-handed approach did not appear as of 2015 to have modified the

Venezuelan government's increasingly repressive approach to its political opposition.

Israel: Legitimate Security Concerns vs. Palestinians' Right to Food

Any possible call for coercive humanitarian intervention to protect the right to food of Palestinians in WBG, be it via sanctions against Israel or via actual armed force, would have been complicated by two factors.

First, however tragic the malnutrition of large percentages of the Palestinian population was, it did not reach the threshold needed for humanitarian intervention of the kind envisaged by R2P; namely, large-scale loss of life or large-scale ethnic cleansing. Second, Israel had legitimate security interests that applied to its relations with the WBG. Hamas, the ruling political party in Gaza as of 2007, was reluctant to recognize Israel's right to exist as a state and persisted in attacking it with rockets. That proportionately far more Palestinians than Israelis died in this conflict did not obviate Israel's right to defend itself against these attacks. While some might argue (as I do) that in the long run Israel's national security depended on making peace with the Palestinians and co-operating to create an independent Palestinian state, others viewed the Palestinians as a constant short-term threat. In the twenty-first century, this latter group dominated Israeli government and policy circles.

Moreover, despite the fact that Israel did not meet its legal obligations as an occupying power under international humanitarian law, as discussed in Chapter 8, it enjoyed strong support from the Western world. The US viewed Israel as an outpost of democracy in the Middle East and a bulwark against past, present, or future US enemies such as Iraq and Iran. Israel received a very high proportion of US military aid, $3.1 billion in 2012, second only to Afghanistan (USAID 2012): There was also a very strong pro-Israel lobby within the American Jewish community (Ron 2003, 141; Mearsheimer and Walt 2007). Many Christians also supported Israel either for eschatological reasons (the Second Coming of Christ would not occur until the Jews had resettled the Holy Land) or out of guilt at the Christian world's unwillingness to assist Jews during the Holocaust.

Despite this support, in 2005 some Western civil society organizations began a campaign for boycott of Israel, divestment from Israeli firms, and sanctions against Israel (the BDS movement), to pressure it to reform its policies in the WBG. By 2009 this international movement had found traction among many Western university students, some universities, some churches, some trade unions, and a variety of influential public figures, including some Jews (Bakan and Abu-Laban 2009, 43–46). By 2011 it had many more adherents, including, for example, a Norwegian pension fund that sold its share in Israeli firms and several Belgian municipalities that boycotted a bank that had business dealings in Israel. There were also civil society campaigns for arms embargoes against Israel, and for imposing aid conditionality on Israel or cutting off its military aid (Steinberg 2011, 31, 37, 42).

By 2015 the BDS campaign had not received official support from any Western governments, in part because of anti-boycott laws passed in the 1970s, for example in the US, although some municipalities in some Western countries supported divestment. The Organization of Islamic States had organized its own boycott of Israel immediately after the 1948 Arab-Israeli war, and some radical non-Western countries – including Venezuela under Chávez – took symbolic steps such as expelling Israeli diplomats (Bakan and Abu-Laban 2009, 33–37, 45). In reply, in 2011 the Israeli government passed a law outlawing advocacy of a boycott of either Israel or the West Bank settlements: Penalties included, *inter alia*, denial of tax exemptions, and exclusion from the right to bid for government contracts (Greenberg 2011, July 22). Israel's Supreme Court upheld this law in April 2015 (Economist 2015, May 2, 39).

While it is tempting to compare the BDS campaign to the international social movement from the 1960s to the 1990s to end apartheid in South Africa, international interests differed in the two cases. By the 1960s South Africa's overt legal regime of racial discrimination was offensive to all countries, including its erstwhile Western allies. Moreover, there was a strong social movement within South Africa for sanctions against the apartheid regime. By contrast, the US was a strong strategic ally of Israel, and memories of the Holocaust undermined concerns about Israeli settlements in the WBG. American support for Israel continued to be strong despite the 2008–09 and 2014 attacks on Gaza. In any event, it is not clear that the international sanctions movement did have the positive effect in ending apartheid that some advocates of the anti-Israel BDS movement appeared to believe it had had (Alsheh 2016).

Even if civil society boycotts and divestments became much more widespread than they were by 2015, Israel would probably be able to find its way around them, just as South Africa found its way around boycotts and divestments in the 1970s and 80s. For example, Israeli companies exporting products from the West Bank settlements apparently re-labeled them to suggest they were made in Israel proper, after some supermarkets and other organizations in Europe announced that they would boycott settlement products (Agricultural Guiding and Awareness Society et al. 2013, 19, 22). Moreover, as the BDS movement became more widespread, Israel's resolve to defend itself against a movement that many Israeli Jewish leaders considered anti-Semitic would probably strengthen.

The Politics of Food Aid

Article 28 of the Universal Declaration of Human Rights (UDHR) states that "Everyone is entitled to a social and international order in which the rights and freedoms set forth in this Declaration can be fully realized," implying that such an order must be created by states. States have obligations to each other and to the citizens of other states to ensure the right to food; according to Article 11, 2, b of the International Covenant on Economic, Social and Cultural Rights (ICESCR) they are obliged to "ensure an equitable distribution of world food supplies in relation to need." This Article suggests that states must take affirmative steps to secure the human right to food of people living outside their own borders (Gibney 2008, 95).

The 1986 United Nations Declaration on the Right to Development mandates all states to assist underdeveloped countries (United Nations General Assembly 1986, Articles 3 and 4). Moreover, General Comment 12 (1999) of the UN Committee on Economic Social and Cultural Rights maintains that "States parties should take steps to respect the enjoyment of the right to food in other countries, to protect that right, to facilitate access to food and to provide the necessary aid when required" (Committee on Economic Social and Cultural Rights 1999, Article 36). The Food and Agriculture Organization's (FAO) 2004 Voluntary Guidelines on the right to food suggest international responsibility to protect the right to food, grounding this in the principle that "developed countries should assist developing countries in attaining development goals" (Food and Agriculture Organization 2005, Chapter III, par. 4, 33). There is no specific obligation, however, to prevent faminogenesis, nor is there any obligation to donate food aid, which is still a voluntary matter. The general assumption is that food aid should be temporary, dealing with crisis situations (Moreu 2011, 245, 247), not a prop for governments that intentionally or recklessly impose domestic policies that deprive their own citizens of food.

In its 2004 Guidelines the FAO advised food recipient states, in their turn, to ensure that humanitarian agencies had "safe and unimpeded access to the[ir] populations" (Food and Agriculture Organization 2005, Chapter II, Guideline 15.3, 27). General Comment 12 also includes the obligation not to prevent access to humanitarian food aid (Committee on Economic Social and Cultural Rights 1999, Article 19). States that cannot protect their citizens' right to food are expected to permit entry of food from abroad and to ensure that it is distributed in a non-discriminatory fashion. Yet there are concerns about the effects of giving food aid to countries that are gross violators of human rights, as North Korea and Zimbabwe illustrate.

Food aid to North Korea was not distributed in a non-discriminatory fashion: Rather, it was used to feed party members and the urban elite, while non-party members and rural or remote North Koreans, especially in the northeast, continued to be malnourished (COI: United Nations General Assembly 2014, February 7, p. 189, par. 626). The state also discriminated in distribution of food aid to the "wavering" and "hostile" classes discussed in Chapter 4 (Cohen 2013, 4). Food aid was also diverted to the military; some refugees said they had witnessed military trucks carrying away food aid, while in other cases food aid was ostensibly distributed among the population at large, but recipients were forced to return the food to the state as soon as international monitors had left the country (COI: United Nations General Assembly 2014, February 7, pp. 183–84, par. 609). Several reputable NGOs discontinued operations in North Korea because of the conditions the government imposed (COI: United Nations General Assembly 2014, February 7, p. 190, par. 628).

Food aid also had political implications. Even if the aid did reach ordinary North Koreans, it released funds that the regime could instead spend on arms (COI: United Nations General Assembly 2014, February 7, pp. 196–97, par. 646): South Korean conservatives feared that food aid merely strengthened the North Korean military (Kim 2011, 174). At the height of the 1990s famine, North Korea was spending 26 percent of its GNP on the military; thus, international food aid permitted the regime to develop its missile and nuclear programs (Leitenberg 2012, 2). Food aid could also be used for general balance of payments support (COI: United Nations General Assembly 2014, February 7, p. 198, par. 652). Finally, food aid might delay those necessary reforms without which North Korea would always rely on other countries and outside agencies for food (Noland 2007, 216). The aid might also have helped to keep the regime in power by feeding people who might otherwise have rebelled.

Along with other countries, especially South Korea and China, the US periodically supplied food to North Korea, hoping that it would feed the most vulnerable but aware that it might instead feed the elite, members of the Korean Workers' Party, and the military. The US and its allies were interested in North Koreans' food security but had no mechanisms to provide it that could escape the regime's cynical manipulation of its starving population. Indeed, the regime might not have been able to survive at all without the aid concessions that its nuclear brinkmanship extracted from the US, South Korea, China, and Japan. Thus, these countries allowed themselves to be manipulated into providing food aid, although they frequently demanded hard security concessions in return.

In early 2012, the US concluded a deal with North Korea under which the latter country would renounce its nuclear ambitions and stop testing missiles in return for 240,000 metric tons of food (Ide 2012, February 29), which would have covered almost 60 percent of the 2011–12 shortfall (FAO/WFP 2011, November 25, 4). Barely two weeks after the deal was concluded on February 29, North Korea announced plans to test a missile: The US responded by withdrawing its offer of food aid (Ide 2012, March 28).

After the February 2012 deal collapsed, the question arose whether the US was justified in withholding food aid. One argument was that food aid was strictly humanitarian and should not be subject to negotiations over arms or nuclear technology: The people of North Korea should be fed regardless of other interests, as long as monitors were admitted to ensure the food reached those for whom it was intended. An additional justification of this approach was that monitors would be able to "engage" with the North Korean people (Editors 2012, March 22). In reality, however, monitors were rarely admitted, so that this condition effectively prevented much food aid. North Korea might have feared a hidden agenda of regime change in the Americans' attempts to monitor food aid.

Just as aid agencies in North Korea were afraid to speak out about human rights violations in case they were denied access to the starving, so aid agencies in Zimbabwe faced a similar dilemma. The Mugabe regime manipulated access to Zimbabwe and restricted recipients of food aid, favoring its own supporters over supporters of the opposition. For example, in the immediate aftermath of the 2005 urban expulsions, police were reported to be seizing food provided by international agencies (Romero 2007, 279); the government refused to co-operate with the United Nations in an emergency appeal for aid for victims of the expulsions (Human Rights Watch 2006b, 156). In early 2011 the agriculture minister barred UN agencies and NGOs who had hoped to participate in food and crop assessment surveys, objecting to the "negative information" they had disseminated in the past (IRIN: Humanitarian News and Analysis 2011, March 16). Again in 2012, UN agencies that could assess the need for food were denied access to Zimbabwe on grounds of national security (IRIN Humanitarian News and Analysis 2012, May 21). When food was imported by international organizations, for example the World Food Programme (WFP), ZANU-PF-affiliated officials such as district councilors and traditional leaders manipulated lists of the most needy families to exclude those thought to be supporters of the opposition Movement for Democratic Change (MDC) (Physicians for Human Rights Denmark 2002, November 20, 26).

The Zimbabwean government also blocked non-governmental organizations from distributing food (Radio VoP 2012, February 16; IRIN: Humanitarian News and Analysis 2012, February 17). For example, the Catholic Church of Zimbabwe was blocked from importing food for the Bulawayo district in 2002 (Physicians for Human Rights Denmark 2002, November 20, 20). Some CARE (a humanitarian NGO) officials were "terrified to talk:" "We don't want to say anything to jeopardize the feeding... The government can suspend our operations at any time. And then these people will starve" (Godwin 2010, 284).

The situation in WBG presented different problems than those in North Korea and Zimbabwe. Food aid policies to WBG were too complex to review in detail in this section, especially as they varied as the political situation changed. Diplomatic openings between Israel and Palestinian leaders resulted in opening to humanitarian aid, while conflicts and their aftermath resulted in tightened controls on food aid and passage of the aid from Israel to WBG.

To take one example, after Hamas took power in Gaza in 2007, not only did Israel impose a blockade, as discussed in Chapter 7, but the United States and other Western countries also cut off direct aid to Gaza via its government, preferring to channel it through international and non-governmental organizations. The purpose of this new policy was to pressure Hamas to recognize Israel, renounce violence, and honor previous agreements with Israel (Goldstone 2009, par. 188). This boycott of Hamas was endorsed by the members of the Quartet (the US, Russia, the EU, and the United Nations) who had joined together in 2002 to try to facilitate an agreement between Israel and the Palestinians (Qarmout and Beland 2012, 33). Nevertheless, food aid continued to flow into WBG; by 2010 about 80 percent of Gazan families relied on foreign aid, while 79 percent of families in those parts of the West Bank under Israel's formal control lacked enough food (Roy 2012, 82).

The siege policy that Israel imposed after Hamas was elected may not have completely prohibited imports of food to Gaza, but it did restrict imports of fuel and cooking gas, as result of which, for example, most Gazan bakeries closed in December 2008 because they lacked both cooking gas and flour (Myers 2009, 118). The United Nations Relief and Works Agency (UNWRA), responsible for distributing food rations to refugees in Gaza, found its supplies limited whenever Israel closed the borders or restricted the numbers of trucks permitted to enter (Myers 2009, 118; Ma'an News Agency 2011, February 19). Attempts by Hamas to expropriate aid shipments further undermined the international policy of sending aid to non-governmental organizations in Gaza (DeFalco 2009, 12, note 14).

Another problem was the constant need for the international community to rebuild infrastructure it had already financed, for example after Israel's attacks on Gaza in 2008–09 and 2014. NGOs had to consider whether it was worthwhile to rebuild physical infrastructure which might simply then be demolished again (Ma'an News Agency 2011, February 19), nor was there any financial penalty on Israel for frequently destroying roads, infrastructure, homes, and other buildings (Feldman 2009, 33). This put the donor community in a dilemma: how often should it rebuild, essentially permitting Israel free reign to destroy infrastructure? In 2010, for example, the US pledged to donate $5 million to wastewater collection systems and water distribution infrastructure in Gaza (Migdalovitz 2010, June 23, 10), in part to repair the damage incurred in the 2008–09 war.

Thus, the international community faced the question of whether it was actually subsidizing the occupation, when it was Israel's responsibility to ensure that Palestinians' nutritional needs were fulfilled (Qarmout and Beland 2012, 35). By constantly pouring in aid, donors to WBG were averting what might otherwise have been a much more severe catastrophe that might either have resulted in more international pressure on Israel to change its rights-abusive policies (Mountain 2011, September 22), or more internal unrest and rebellion against Israel. International donors' subsidies to the occupation lessened the urgency of a settlement between Israel and the Palestinians (Taghdisi-Rad 2011, 199), transforming what was actually a political problem into a supposedly non-political humanitarian one (Feldman 2009, 24).

The US and other donors cut off direct aid to Hamas because it was designated a terrorist organization that did not respect the principles of democracy, human rights, and good governance on which aid was conditioned, and because, as the Goldstone report quoted above argued, it did not renounce violence, it did not recognize Israel's right to exist, and it refused to adhere to interim peace agreements with Israel. While in the long run such aid conditionality might make it easier for Gazans to assert their civil and political rights – and their need for economic human rights – against Hamas' notoriously undemocratic governance, immediate restrictions on general aid exacerbated Palestinians' need for food. The US, for example, withheld aid as a punishment for Palestinians' seeking membership in the UN in 2011 (Roy 2012, 84), although President Obama lifted these restrictions in 2012 (Fox News 2013, March 25). Even if the withheld aid did not include food aid, it undermined Palestinians' capacity to make a living; for example, when aid which was meant to help pay Palestinian civil servants' salaries was withheld (Kestler-D'Amours 2013, February 28).

As in the cases of North Korea and Zimbabwe, moreover, corruption in WBG might have reduced residents' access to food aid. Rigorous research on corruption in WBG is difficult, owing to its sensitive nature, but polls in the 1990s showed widespread belief among Palestinians that their leaders were corrupt (Turner 2006, 745–46). After 2006 there were many reports in the Arabic press of corruption among Hamas leaders, running into billions of dollars (Jerusalem Post 2014, July 20). However, some of these reports might have emanated from the Palestinian Authority's rivalry with Hamas, and therefore have been fabricated or exaggerated (Sayigh 2010, 6). Nevertheless, one cannot rule out the possibility of corruption in the distribution of food aid. Corruption in other kinds of aid – such as selling cement meant to be used to rebuild homes after Israel's 2014 incursion into Gaza – also affected access to food, as without kitchens it was difficult for people to prepare proper meals for their families (Beaumont 2014, December 25). Controls imposed by Hamas on NGOs in Gaza (Sayigh 2010, 3–4) – like controls imposed on NGOs in North Korea and Zimbabwe – may have detrimentally affected their ability to distribute food.

By early 2015, food shortages in Venezuela were becoming extremely severe. From the beginning of his tenure in office in 2013, Nicolás Maduro had been preoccupied with the shortages and was increasingly relying on allied countries to supply food (Hummel 2013, June 17). Yet despite these shortages and civil unrest, in an act of populist bravuro Venezuela sent food aid to Gaza in mid-2014 (Middle East Monitor 2014, September 15). Given Maduro's reluctance to change policies that were causing the shortages, malnutrition among Venezuelans might well increase in the near future, resulting in calls for assistance from international organizations such as the WFP. But if the WFP were invited to assist Venezuelans, it would have to consider whether the food it contributed was being equitably distributed, or whether discriminatory allocation of food on political grounds was continuing or intensifying. And if NGOs volunteered to provide food, the same concern might be magnified, especially if the NGOs were viewed as American stooges.

Conclusion

The complexities of both sanctions policies and food aid show how difficult it is for outsiders to resolve or ameliorate state food crimes, despite international laws concerning the universal responsibility of states to protect the right to food. As the discussions above regarding North Korea and Zimbabwe show, sanctions are often symbolic, with little or no real effect (Evans 2008, 114). Food aid in general is not merely a "neutral" act of benevolence but is influenced by wider political exigencies and can have unexpected side effects.

Political exigencies such as the conflicting interests of Israel and Palestine, and the left populist defense of Venezuela's policies, also undermined the ability of the international community to pressure states whose policies violated the right to food. All food aid was subject to the criticism that it might help keep the rights-abusing regime in power, delaying possible reforms or rebellion by the affected population. Like most other human rights, the right to food is principally an internal matter, requiring efficient market economies and good governance. Above all, as Chapter 10 will show, protection of the "economic" human right to food requires internal protection of civil and political rights.

10   Interdependent Human Rights

In Chapter 3, I discussed Sen's argument that there are no famines in functioning multiparty democracies. Sen argues for the importance of civil and political rights to prevent famine but focuses his argument on freedom of the press, freedom for opposition political parties to function, and the ability of citizens to vote their governments out of power (Sen 1999, 178–82). While I agree with Sen's stress on these important rights, the cases I selected for this volume show the equal importance of other civil and political rights, including the rule of law, the right to citizenship, and mobility rights. Both property rights and the right to work, which might be viewed more as economic than civil and political rights, are also key to protection of the right to food. Thus, Sen's initial thesis must be expanded to take a careful look at the entire gamut of human rights and their effect on individuals' right to food. Human rights are interdependent.

Civil and Political Rights

The victims of state-induced famines in Ukraine, China, and Cambodia were ruled by totalitarian governments that denied them all civil and political rights. Neither in those countries was there any semblance of the rule of law. Nineteenth-century Irish peasants were colonial subjects of Britain, without the rights that Sen finds so crucial. While they may have had some right to criticize Britain and to protest the government's actions through a (quasi) free press, they could not vote their government out of power: In Ireland only landlords and the middle classes were represented in the British Parliament. Aboriginals starving in the Canadian West in the 1870s did not possess even these minimal rights to criticize their rulers, nor did they have access to the courts to protect them against deprivation of their land, property, and food. Indeed, well into the twentieth century Aboriginals living on reserves were prohibited from voting and from organizing in defense of their own interests. And Germans after the November 1918 Armistice were officially enemies of the government that starved them, without any capacity to influence its policies except through their diplomats.

The case studies in Part II also demonstrate the necessity of civil and political rights for protection of the right to food. North Koreans enjoyed no civil and political rights; Zimbabweans' civil and political rights had been systematically undermined as of 2000, if not before; and Venezuelans' civil and political rights had been progressively undermined since Hugo Chávez took power. Palestinians did not enjoy civil and political rights within Israel itself or within the West Bank and Gaza (WBG). Nor did their ostensible representatives, Fatah and Hamas, grant them fair trials, freedom from torture, freedom from arbitrary execution, or the political right to criticize their own governments.

North Korea became party to the International Covenant on Civil and Political Rights (ICCPR) in 1981; however, it withdrew from it in 1997. Despite its withdrawal from the ICCPR, however, in a façade of legality the regime several times introduced constitutional changes that were supposed to – but did not – protect human rights. In 1998, a constitutional revision introduced *habeas corpus*. Revisions in 2004 prohibited arrests and detention not in accordance with the law; required warrants for arrest; and introduced other such procedural guarantees (Haggard and Noland 2009, 17). In 2009, the Constitution was revised ostensibly to protect human rights (Song 2010, 113). For example, Articles 65 to 68 of the revised Constitution ostensibly protected equal rights, including the right to vote; freedom of speech, press, assembly, demonstration and association; and freedom of religion (Democratic People's Republic of Korea 2009, trans. Steve S. Sin). At the same time, however, the principle of "military first" allocated resources to the military before any other sector of society (Song 2010, 93).

Yet denial of citizens' civil and political rights was a key cause of starvation in North Korea. If North Koreans had actually enjoyed freedom of speech, press, association and assembly, they would have been able to tell their rulers what was happening and perhaps persuade them to introduce new policies. Instead, citizens were tortured, imprisoned or executed for pointing out that government decisions caused them to starve. There was no indication that North Korea respected the rights written into the 2009 Constitution. Elections were unheard of, so that North Koreans were under the totalitarian control of the Kim dynasty. Nor did North Koreans have recourse to independent courts, which had never existed in their country.

Zimbabwe also illustrates the proposition that realization of the right to food relies on protection of civil and political rights. Despite its ratification of the ICCPR in 1991, all of Zimbabweans' human rights were under attack during the human rights freefall of the early twenty-first century. In order to expropriate the property of large-scale farmers, the government undermined the rule of law; used racist rhetoric; and turned a blind eye to – if not actually encouraging – assaults on, torture, and murder of the farmers themselves. Zimbabweans had been progressively deprived of their civil and political rights since independence in 1980. All "free" elections since 1980 were marred by intimidation and violence (Kriger 2005). The independent judiciary was undermined despite its valiant attempts to protect citizens' human rights (Gubbay 1997). Mugabe also undermined the free press and used murder, torture, and rape to intimidate and punish his opponents. This deprivation of civil and political rights was a central cause of the barely averted famine in Zimbabwe: Neither wealthy white farmers, nor farm workers, miners, or urbanites expelled from their dwellings had any legal recourse within Zimbabwe, nor could they protest government actions or vote their government out of office, as the intimidation that prevented the opposition leader, Morgan Tsvangirai, from entering the run-off elections in 2008 showed.

Given the absence of rule of law within Zimbabwe, pan-African courts might have helped to mitigate human rights violations. However, a case brought before the Southern African Development Community (SADC) Tribunal in 2008 by white Zimbabwean farmers demanding compensation for the land they had lost illustrates the fragility of rule of law in Africa. The Tribunal found in favor of the farmers, ruling that the Zimbabwean government had violated the SADC treaty by denying them access to Zimbabwean courts and by engaging in racial discrimination (Southern African Development Community Tribunal 2008, November 28; Nathan 2013, 871). In response, the SADC heads of state suspended the Tribunal first for six months in 2010, then for another year, on the grounds that it had been improperly constituted in the first place, rather than force Zimbabwe to uphold the ruling in favor of white farmers (Mugabe 2012, November 2; Bell 2011, June 3). In 2012, SADC decided to reconstitute the Tribunal but permit complaints only by states, disallowing individual complaints (Nathan 2013, 886).

The Zimbabwean High Court ruled in 2010 that the SADC Tribunal's decision in favor of the white plaintiffs was not enforceable in Zimbabwe (Bell 2010, September 1). Violence against white farmers continued in 2010 and 2011 (Newsday 2011, November 10), as did expropriations of their land. Despite the pro-Mugabe policies of Thabo Mbeki and Jacob Zuma's ambivalent attitude to Mugabe, however, the South African judiciary decided to enforce the Tribunal decision even though SADC had suspended it. Several white Zimbabwean farmers sued in South Africa for Zimbabwean government property to be expropriated and sold to compensate them for the legal costs that the SADC Tribunal had said should be awarded to them. The Pretoria High Court accepted this argument, ruling that Zimbabwe had signed the SADC Treaty and could not renege on its obligations (Nathan 2013, 879). Two of the dispossessed farmers tried to take their case to the African Court of Human and Peoples' Rights, naming all SADC heads of state as respondents (Bell 2012, February 16), even though Zimbabwe had not ratified the protocol establishing the Court. However, the African Court ruled in 2014 that it had no jurisdiction over the SADC Court (Bell 2014, March 5).

Venezuela ratified the ICCPR in 1978, but both Chávez and Maduro progressively undermined civil and political rights. Originally elected democratically, Chávez manipulated the electoral process, intimidated his opponents, and imposed restrictions on the media so that all later elections were suspect. He progressively undermined the rule of law, freedom of the press, and independent trade unions. Thus, Chávez continued those policies that undermined production of and access to food without facing criticism or opposition from his people. He won the 2012 election partly by mobilizing the resources of the state, such as finances and television time, in his favor and partly by threatening civil war if he did not win. By 2015 Maduro was resorting to outright political violence in order to quell opposition, in the face of increasing food shortages.

Israel was obliged to respect the human rights of Palestinians in WBG: it signed the ICCPR in 1966 and ratified it in 1991. Article 2, 1 of the ICCPR mandates that a state respect human rights "within its territory and subject to its jurisdiction;" therefore, Israel was obliged to protect the civil and political rights of the population of WBG (Goldstone 2009, p. 78, par. 297). But Palestinians did not enjoy civil and political rights in those parts of the West Bank directly ruled by Israel: They were subject to Israeli military rule and courts and had very limited opportunity to put their cases before Israel's civilian courts. At various times in various ways their own elected Palestinian rulers also undermined those rights. This made it very difficult for them to fight against the illegal expropriation of their land by settlers.

The Right to Citizenship

Citizenship is formally a legal status that individuals can use to access rights and goods in the states of which they are nationals: Citizens also have obligations to the state such as to pay taxes; obey the law; and in some states to perform military or national service. In democratic states, citizenship also has a political or sociological sense as "that set of practices (juridical, political, economic, and cultural) which define a person as a competent member of society, and which as a consequence shape the flow of resources to persons and social groups" (Turner 1993, 2). Legal citizenship in and of itself does not always imply the right and capacity to be an efficacious member of the polity; this depends on the set of civil and political rights that the formal, legal citizen enjoys – or does not enjoy. The individual may be formally under the protection of the state to which she belongs, but that has no meaning in totalitarian states like North Korea and little meaning in dictatorships such as Zimbabwe or quasi-dictatorships such as Venezuela.

Citizenship is a relatively modern invention, stemming from states' desires in the late nineteenth and early twentieth centuries to control who entered their territory (Torpey 2000). Before the formalization of citizenship, only certain categories of residents were considered to be part of the body politic, even in embryonic democracies such as nineteenth century United Kingdom. Thus, when Irish peasants and Canadian Aboriginals starved, they could not call upon British or Canadian authorities to regard them as fellow citizens worthy of their concern. Nor were foreigners accorded any status whatsoever: Starving Germans could not call upon Allied citizens to treat them as equals after WWI. The colonized and the enemy could draw only on goodwill and charity, not the equal respect or sense of collective obligation expected among fellow-citizens. Well into the twentieth century, most people who resided in colonies were subjects, not citizens. Several colonial powers, including Britain, tried unsuccessfully to argue that the Universal Declaration of Human Rights (UDHR), which in its Article 15 protected the right to a nationality, should not apply to residents of colonies (Burke 2010, 40).

Nor in the great totalitarian famines did citizenship have any meaning. Citizenship in Ukraine, China, and Cambodia meant that the state legally controlled its subjects, not that it had any obligations to them. People like Denise Affonço, who claimed French citizenship, could sometimes call on the protection of foreign governments (Affonço 2007), but those without such legal protection were completely without human rights. Citizenship in totalitarian states is a negative attribute; it means that the individual is utterly rightless.

It might seem farcical to speak of citizenship rights in North Korea where, in effect, no one was a citizen in the sense of an active citizenry capable of influencing the policies of the government. In so far as it existed at all, citizenship seemed in North Korea to be a perquisite of racially "pure," able-bodied members of the "loyal" class. North Korea killed racially "impure" half-Chinese babies; discriminated against and imprisoned Japanese-Koreans; and also imprisoned disabled people. The state also classified the population on the basis of perceived loyalty, or lack thereof, to the regime. Thus, even formal legal citizenship rights were allocated according to discriminatory criteria while active, participatory citizenship rights were unknown, as all civil and political rights were violated in practice if not in theory.

Ironically, however, North Koreans did enjoy formal citizenship rights in South Korea, where legally all Koreans, from South or North, were citizens. The very few North Koreans who escaped to South Korea were able to assert their citizenship rights. Should reunification ever seriously be a possibility, however, and a large inflow of North Koreans result, South Korea might change its policy. North Koreans' citizenship rights in South Korea could be at risk if the North Korean regime falls.

Both Zimbabwean whites and some people of African, but not strictly Rhodesian/Zimbabwean, descent lost their citizenship rights after 2000. A 2001 amendment to the Citizenship of Zimbabwe Act stripped nearly three million people of citizenship on the grounds that they had a legal possibility of dual nationality. The amendment pertained to almost all white Zimbabweans as well as to migrants and their descendants from other African countries, who, Mugabe thought, were likely to support the opposition (Mashingaidze 2011, 272). In 2013, Zimbabwe's registrar-general announced that only those who could prove that both they and both their parents had been born in Zimbabwe would be allowed to vote (Fields 2013, April 18). This excluded many white Zimbabweans; indeed, Mugabe, using increasingly racist rhetoric, described whites as "just visitors" (Chadenga 2013, July 26). Under indigenization laws, moreover, whites were barred entirely from some businesses, such as bakeries and beauty parlors (Economist 2010, April 24). Thus Zimbabwe joined several other African countries that had laws restricting citizenship to members of certain ethnic groups (Open Society Institute 2009, October 21). It is significant in this regard that the 1981 African Charter of Human and Peoples' Rights does not contain a right to a nationality.

Nor is this surprising: it is common in formerly colonized countries to find discrimination against "racially" or ethnically differentiated populations whose origins are in the former colonial power. Indeed, even ethnic outsiders who are not from the former colonial power may see their rights eroded. In some early post-independence African countries, racially based citizenship laws were used to expel ethnic Asians, as from Uganda, and Lebanese, as from several West African countries, as well as to expel persons of African descent whose ancestors were from other countries (Howard 1986, 99–107). If members of such ethnically differentiated populations choose to stay in a newly independent country and become citizens under the new regime, they ought to be treated as equals to the formerly colonized populations. Yet Mugabe insisted that white Zimbabweans did not deserve citizenship, saying in 2002, "The white man is not indigenous to Africa. Africa is for Africans, Zimbabwe is for Zimbabweans" (quoted in Meredith 2007, 203).

Dietrich's description of Nazi Germany's treatment of Jews as "the legal conversion of citizens into aliens" (Dietrich 1981, 453) applies clearly to the Zimbabwean case. Deprivation of citizenship is often a first step to much worse treatment. Many white farmers were subjected to extra-judicial torture and murder both by the state and by individuals acting with impunity. Many emigrated, realizing that their status in Zimbabwe was extremely precarious. While the farmers themselves were not victims of malnutrition or starvation, their emigration decreased the supply of food, contributing to the malnutrition and starvation of their black fellow-citizens. Economic decline is a typical result when entrepreneurial minorities are expelled from a country. And many black residents of Zimbabwe who might have previously considered themselves citizens, and who found themselves without employment after the land seizures, discovered that they were not eligible for redistributed land.

Finally, Palestinians in WBG did not enjoy citizenship in those territories, though some may have held citizenship elsewhere, such as in Jordan; as of the time of writing this chapter Gaza and the West Bank did not comprise an independent state, and their governments could not confer citizenship on their residents. Palestinians lived in a legal citizenship limbo, able to acquire so-called passports that were little more than travel documents (Baer 2015, 60). Nor, as residents of occupied territories, were they entitled to citizenship rights within Israel. Meantime, Israel's Law of Return permitted "persons of Jewish origin all over the world, even if they have never set foot on Israeli soil," to "return" there and take up citizenship, but "It denie[d] such entry to its former Arab residents and their descendants, the Palestinians" (Baehr 1990, 105). Many settlers in the West Bank were Jewish immigrants to Israel who had availed themselves of the Law of Return, only to then participate in the theft of Palestinians' land.

As discussed in Chapter 8, on November 29, 2012 the United Nations General Assembly voted to grant Palestine non-member state status, with 138 of 193 member states in favor, but significantly excluding Canada, the US, Australia, New Zealand, and most of Europe (Charbonneau 2012, November 29). Citizenship in a legally recognized state might give Palestinians some protection against Israeli thefts of their property and other human rights abuses. Meantime, they were effectively stateless.

A stateless person is one "who is not recognized as a citizen of any state" (United Nations 1960; Belton 2015, 31).

By contrast to North Korea, Zimbabwe, and WBG, citizenship rights did not seem to become a problem in Venezuela under Chávez and Maduro. The criteria of discrimination in Venezuela were wealth and poverty – as defined by Chávez – rather than ethnicity. Landowners and others deprived of their property were not labeled outsiders, although in typical populist fashion Chávez did rail against foreign corporate owners. Rhetoric by his successor, Maduro, did border on exclusionist, but since there was no easy way to identify potentially excludable classes by ethnicity or religion, it seemed doubtful that the property-owning classes would be deprived of citizenship.

Mobility Rights

The UDHR protects mobility rights in Article 13: "1. Everyone has the right to freedom of movement and residence within the borders of each State. 2. Everyone has the right to leave any country, including his own, and to return to his country." This right is repeated in the ICCPR, Article 12, 1, 2, and 4: "Everyone lawfully within the territory of a State shall, within that territory, have the right to liberty of movement, and freedom to choose his residence." Moreover, "Everyone shall be free to leave any country, including his own," and "No one shall be arbitrarily deprived of the right to enter his own country." These laws, however, leave potential emigrants and refugees in a dilemma; while they have the right to leave their own country they do not have the right to enter any other, as North Koreans fleeing to China learned.

States jealously guard their sovereign right to determine under what conditions non-citizens may enter their territory. Moreover, most totalitarian and dictatorial states restrict freedom of movement within their own borders through the use of internal passports and travel documents. In Ukraine in the 1930s, starving peasants were not permitted to move to cities in search of food; in China in the 1950s and Cambodia in the 1970s, citizens were obliged to live where they were assigned by the state. North Koreans enjoyed no mobility rights; during the famine of the 1990s starving people were imprisoned for moving around the country to find food, and city dwellers were punished for going to the countryside where their rural relatives might have had a little more food than they did.

Conversely, mobility rights also include the right to stay where one lives rather than being expelled. Rather than take care of the starving Irish, Britain encouraged their emigration during the nineteenth century.

White Zimbabwean farmers were expelled from their farms while urban Zimbabweans were expelled *en masse* from their neighborhoods in 2005, and rural gold and diamond diggers were expelled from their work locations. Some Venezuelan ranchers and farmers were also expelled from their properties.

In the West Bank, Jewish settlers, with government connivance, expelled many Palestinians from their homes, farms, and vineyards. At the same time, Israel rendered mobility much harder by building restricted highways, thus restricting contact among Palestinians as well as frequently cutting them off from their own farms. Israel may have deliberately made life difficult for Palestinians in WBG in order to encourage as many of them as possible to migrate to other countries, as many middle-class and professional Palestinians had already done (Baer 2015, 52). This, then, would constitute a voluntary form of ethnic cleansing, allowing Jewish settlers to retain control of their stolen land. Extremely limited mobility both within WBG and between it and the outside world encouraged international migration of Palestinians.

Property Rights

The right to own property is neglected in much of the human rights literature, yet it assists individuals to enjoy their subsistence rights, either directly by cultivating food on their own land or indirectly by providing income from property that they can use to purchase food. In this sense, the right to own property is one of Sen's entitlements; property helps people grow food or produce other products that they can sell to buy food (Sen 1981). The right to own property can, therefore, also be considered an aspect of the right to development, in so far as possession of land is necessary for the physical survival that eludes so many people in less developed countries (Nading 2002, 786). Yet the three communist countries discussed in Chapter 2 in which famine occurred had already deprived their citizens of their property, especially but not only property in land, or were in the process of so depriving them. In colonial Ireland, peasants did not own the property they needed to feed themselves and often had to pay very high rents to their landlords; in Western Canada, Aboriginals had no protection against settler or state theft of their land.

In Zimbabwe white farm owners and urban residents were denied property rights; in North Korea no one was allowed to own private property; in Venezuela Chávez introduced arbitrary attacks on private property; and in the West Bank the Israeli government, military, and settlers stole Palestinian land. In each of these cases property rights emerged as key to protection of individuals against starvation and real or potential malnutrition.

Article 17 of the UDHR states: "1. Everyone has the right to own property alone as well as in association with others. 2. No one shall be arbitrarily deprived of his property." There was, however, much discussion among the drafters of the UDHR about this right. They disagreed over whether it should refer only to personal property and if so, what personal property meant, as opposed to a more expansive meaning of property including shares in corporations. The section "alone or in association with others" was a compromise to permit both capitalist forms of joint ownership and Soviet forms of collective ownership (Morsink 1999, 139–52).

The right to own property was not included in the two subsequent international human rights Covenants, the ICCPR, and the International Covenant on Economic, Social and Cultural Rights (ICESCR), so it is not clear in which category it ought to fit. It might best be considered an economic human right in so far as it is about the ownership of material assets, even though it is rarely, if at all, mentioned in the literature on economic human rights. Both Covenants prohibit discrimination on the basis, *inter alia*, of property (ICCPR, Article 2, 1; ICESCR, Article 2, 2), but they do not include the actual right to own it. The omission of a right to own property from these Covenants was not a result of opposition from the communist bloc but rather of disagreement between those who proposed a right to own any form of property and those who proposed a right only to own personal property, similar to the discussion that preceded the formulation of the UDHR. There was also much discussion when the two Covenants were being drafted about what would constitute fair compensation in the event a state were to deprive a citizen of property in a non-arbitrary manner, as permitted by the UDHR in Article 17, 2 (Schabas 1991).

The question of fair compensation pertains to both Zimbabwe and Venezuela, where the state deprived particular categories of people of property. It might also apply to North Korea if the regime were to change to a democracy and former property-owners or their descendants to claim compensation, as happened in eastern Europe after the end of communism. Under the international law of occupation, Israel is not supposed to have deprived West Bank Palestinians of property under any circumstances – even supposedly willing sale – except military necessity. Any peaceful settlement of the Israeli-Palestinian conflict would have to include compensation for Palestinian property lost in the WBG since 1967, if not for property lost in Israel itself during the 1947–49 Nakba.

Among regional documents, the 1948 American Declaration of the Rights and Duties of Man, Article 23, guarantees "[the] right to own such private property as meets the essential needs of decent living and helps to maintain the dignity of the individual and of the home." Venezuela deprived some people of this right by confiscating farms and ranches, but it would be difficult to argue that these confiscations meant an attack on decent living and human dignity, as other livelihood options were available to those who lost this property. In any case, as noted in Chapter 6, Venezuela withdrew from the human rights treaties of the Organization of American States. The African Charter on Human and Peoples' Rights, Article 14, states that "The right to property shall be guaranteed. It may only be encroached upon in the interest of public need or in the general interest of the community and in accordance with the provisions of appropriate laws," but as seen above, this did not prevent SADC from suspending the tribunal that ruled in favor of the property rights of white Zimbabwean farmers. As of the time of writing, there was no regional Asian human rights document that might protect North Koreans' right to property.

In 1990 the UN General Assembly passed a Resolution defending the right to own property, which it acknowledged "contributes to the development of individual liberty and initiative." This Resolution called for further measures to protect: "a) Personal property, including the residence of one's self and family; b) Economically productive property, including property associated with agriculture, commerce and industry" (United Nations General Assembly 1990, Articles 5, 3 a and b). The Resolution passed without a vote but did not generate much further interest, leaving the right to own property in abeyance. Had it been seen as a definitive statement of the right to property, the Resolution might have helped to protect Palestinians' rights against settlers in the West Bank, who would not have been permitted to take over their land and farms. It might also have provided some protection for white farmers in Zimbabwe and Venezuelan farmers and ranchers from arbitrary expropriations of their land and homes. However, in all three cases such protection would have been normative at best, unlikely to affect actual practice.

Those 700,000 Zimbabweans who were displaced in 2005 by Operation Murambatsvina also lost their property. The authorities argued that these urban dwellers had no rights to property as they were squatters living illegally on land they did not own; however, some international legal cases suggest that proof of formal ownership is not necessary to protect property, especially when people are arbitrarily deprived of it without notice (Romero 2007, 282–83). Although the African Charter on Human and Peoples Rights guaranteed the right to property, we cannot assume that judges of the African Court of Human Rights would rule in favor of squatters were such a case presented to them.

The right to own property is included in the emerging movement for an international declaration of peasants' rights (Edelman and James 2011, 86). If a peasant's land is securely his own, he can feed himself and his family in normal times, only relying on the state or other agencies in emergencies. In the event that North Korea in the future permits small-scale farming as well as, or to replace, collective farms, its peasant farmers will need entrenched property rights so that they can invest in their land without fear of arbitrary expropriation by the state.

In earlier work, I suggested that it is time for a separate international Convention on the Right to Own Property. I proposed that such a convention should include a clause stating that "Everyone has the human right to own property:" this right is completely lacking in North Korea. I also proposed that "Everyone has the right to seek and acquire property without discrimination;" this applies particularly to white farmers in Zimbabwe. Another proposed clause was "No collectivity may be deprived of property because of its collective ethnic, national, or racial identity;" this applies to Palestinians whose collective rights to own land in the West Bank were under attack. The clause "No one (either individual or collectivity) may be deprived of property without due process of law and without adequate compensation as determined by law," applies to Zimbabwe, Venezuela, and WBG. Finally, my proposed clause, "No one (individual or collectivity) may be deprived of property on discriminatory grounds" also applies particularly to Zimbabwe (Howard-Hassmann 2013, 193).

A draft convention on the right to own property should include punishments for violation of that right. Massive, discriminatory, and arbitrary violation of the right to own property in Zimbabwe since 2000 resulted in severe deterioration of the food supply, causing widespread malnutrition and disease, if not actual famine. It also resulted in individuals' losing their houses and businesses, thus becoming unable to support themselves and their dependents in the cities. Similarly, arbitrary deprivation of property in Venezuela resulted in deterioration of the food supply. As Schaber suggests, "Massive violations of people's property rights, particularly when they affect their fundamental rights, should be prosecuted": The International Criminal Court (ICC) is the appropriate venue for such prosecution (Schaber 2011, 194). Israel's massive expropriation of Palestinians' property in the West Bank may be one reason why Israel objected when the Palestinian Authority referred Israel to the ICC in late 2014.

Laws against massive violations of property would also apply when expropriation is limited in a discriminatory manner to particular categories of owners, as in the case of white farmers in Zimbabwe. Thus, I proposed two additional clauses to a convention on the right to own property: "Massive, arbitrary expropriation of property that causes famine or mass malnutrition is a crime against humanity," and "Massive, arbitrary expropriation of property on grounds of race, religion, ethnicity or nationality that causes famine is a crime of genocide" (Howard-Hassmann 2013, 194). These clauses in a new convention would strengthen the normative international regime on the right to own property, prohibiting large-scale state or settler appropriations of land from productive owners, whether large-scale landowners, as in Venezuela and Zimbabwe, or smaller agriculturalists and peasants, as in the West Bank.

The Right to Work

For many if not most people, the right to own property is irrelevant. They have none; rather, their immediate concern is to work for pay in order to acquire the goods, including food, that they need. Article 23, 1 of the UDHR states that "everyone has the right to work, to free choice of employment, to just and favourable conditions of work and to protection against unemployment." A negative interpretation of this right – implying obligations on the state to respect it and to protect individuals from interference with it – would mean that it is a right to work without discrimination as the result of an individual's racial, ethnic, or gender identity; his political beliefs; or his class position. A positive interpretation of the right to work – implying that the state must fulfill it – might mean that the state must provide a job to everyone who wants one. In the four cases investigated in this book, only the negative aspect of the right to work is in question. The four governments of Zimbabwe, Israel, North Korea, and Venezuela either deprived people directly of their work or deprived them of the conditions necessary to find it.

Assaults on livelihoods characterized Zimbabwe from 2000 onwards. White landowners found themselves dispossessed of their property, so that they could no longer run their farms. More importantly from the perspective of the right to work, an estimated 150,000 to 200,000 black farm workers lost their jobs. Those who were migrant workers from other African countries, or had been deprived of their Zimbabwean citizenship, were not eligible for redistributed land on which they could work either as subsistence or cash crop farmers. The 700,000 urban victims of Operation Murambatsvina lost their livelihoods, as also did small diamond diggers and gold panners. In all these cases, the government deprived people either of the conditions necessary for work or of the work itself. Only in the case of land redistribution were some Zimbabweans provided with new conditions that would facilitate their working.

Israel indirectly deprived residents of WBG of their right to work by depriving them of their conditions of work. One such condition was the right to own property; without property in their land, Palestinians in the West Bank could not support themselves by farming. Nor could they easily – if at all – work land from which they were cut off by the seam zone, or which it was difficult to access because of segregated highways on which they were not permitted to travel. Palestinians also lost livelihoods when migration to Israel in search of work was cut off by strictly enforced border controls (Farsakh 2000). In legal terms, however, individuals do not enjoy the right to work in any state but their own, as they do not have the right to enter and reside in any country except their own (Weissbrodt 2015, 27). To argue that Palestinians should have the human right to work in Israel might imply acceptance of Israeli sovereignty over WBG, implying that Palestinians are or ought to be Israeli citizens. It is also worth noting that the boycott movement discussed in Chapter 9 might have the effect of depriving Palestinians who work for Israeli firms in the West Bank of employment, thus furthering their impoverishment.

The government of Venezuela did not directly attack the right to work. Some individuals, however, found it difficult to retain their livelihoods because of government actions. Land invasions of farms and ranches deprived owners and their employees of work. Price controls drove some small entrepreneurs out of business, while others found their businesses closed because of alleged price speculation.

North Korea ostensibly provided work for all its citizens, indeed compelling them to work in mass campaigns to cultivate crops or build monuments honoring the Kim dynasty. Even starving prisoners were compelled to work. Here, work was provided but without any choice of work and often without pay. Private enterprise was forbidden and petty market activities strictly controlled. North Korea therefore violated the UDHR's stipulations that the right to work included free choice of employment and just and favorable conditions of work. It further violated laws against forced labor and slavery (Howard-Hassmann 2016 in press). Forced labor and slavery contributed directly to violations of the right to food, as prison camps were designed intentionally to starve enslaved inmates. Nor were forced laborers fed enough to ensure freedom from hunger and adequate nutrition.

North Korea's resort to forced labor and slavery resembled its pre-decessor totalitarian states' violations of the right to work. While the Soviet Union, China, and Cambodia all expected their citizens to work and claimed to provide them with jobs, work was often performed under conditions that violated free choice of work and just and favorable conditions of work. All three countries subjected even "free" citizens (those not in prison camps) to long hours and atrocious working conditions. The absence of free (not state-controlled) trade unions in the Soviet Union, along with the absence of all other civil and political rights, meant workers could not protest poor working conditions, a situation that also existed in China, where in the early post-revolutionary period individuals were assigned jobs by the state, often in regions far from their families. Cambodia was a giant slave-labor camp.

As for the situation of Irish subjects of Britain in the nineteenth century, property laws favoring landlords, along with high rents, prevented peasants from working on the land. During the famine the British forced adult male recipients of "relief" to perform degrading, often useless tasks, often miles from home. Canadian authorities forced similar "work" onto starving Aboriginal men. In both cases, the purpose of such policies was ostensibly to prevent the victims of starvation from becoming overly dependent on charity. While Ukrainians, Chinese, and Cambodians were victims of communist ideology, Irish and Aboriginals were victims of a free-market ideology that assumed that merely leaving the market to itself would eventually result in enough work to support those famine victims who still survived.

The right to work is usually considered an economic rather than a civil/political human right. It is intimately connected with the right to own property, which might also be considered an economic rather than a civil or political human right. But elements of the right to work clearly have civil/political implications, especially the stress on non-discrimination as a basis for civil and political rights. The UDHR in Article 2 forbids discrimination *inter alia* on the basis of race, color, political opinion, or property (presumably meaning property ownership). White landowners in Zimbabwe were deprived of their right to work because of their race, color, and political opinion, since most supported the opposition to Mugabe; victims of Operation Murambatsvina were also deprived of work because of their real or presumed support of the opposition. Venezuelan trade unionists and civil servants lost their jobs because of their opposition to Chávez, especially after the attempted coup of 2002 and after signing the 2004 recall referendum. The UDHR in Article 4 also explicitly forbids slavery, which was practiced in North Korea; indeed, in such a controlled economy one could argue that the entire population was, in effect, enslaved. As discussed in Chapter 8, deprivation of work and property in the WBG falls under the international law of occupation rather than international human rights law.

Thus, separation into neat categories of civil/political, or economic human rights is not possible; both in their definitions and in their actual protection and practice, they are intertwined. For this reason it is difficult to assign categories of "indifference" or "incompetence" as sufficient to explain deprivation of food in cases like Venezuela or Israel/WBG, where there were no policies designed explicitly to actively deprive citizens or subjects of food, as there were in North Korea and Zimbabwe. In all four cases citizens and subjects were deprived of all or some civil and political rights. State food crimes causing famine or high rates of malnutrition cannot be considered unforeseen consequences of food, property, or work policies when the elites that rule those states consciously deprive those under their control of civil and political rights.

Denial of Civil and Political Rights and the Question of Intent

Marcus argues that both intentional and reckless faminogenesis should be deemed crimes under international law. In Chapter 8, I detailed the weaknesses of international laws on genocide and refugees as they pertained to faminogenesis. I also noted the absence of any international law forbidding penal starvation. Only the law on crimes against humanity refers to deprivation of food as an aspect of extermination.

One difficulty in including faminogenesis in international law is the question of intent. Convictions for genocide require some evidence of intent to commit it, although judgments on cases at the International Criminal Tribunals for Yugoslavia and Rwanda now permit inference of intent from actions (Schabas 2006, 98, 101). Denial of civil and political rights, however, is not viewed in and of itself as evidence of faminogenic intent. Yet faminogenic regimes such as North Korea and Zimbabwe deny all civil and political rights in order to protect themselves against criticism and against possible rebellion or other types of political protest. Systematic denial of civil and political rights is often a first step to famine and is often the precipitating factor for refugees from famine. Refugees differ in their ability to see the handwriting on the wall, but some will take the early prohibition on civil and political rights as enough evidence to induce them to flee.

Unfortunately, there is not yet any international legal regime that can call political leaders to account for violations of civil and political rights. Until and unless those violations reach the level of genocide, war crimes, or crimes against humanity, states still possess sovereign immunity. They may no longer possess what Leo Kuper referred to as the sovereign right to commit genocide (Kuper 1981, 161), but they do possess the sovereign right to prohibit those human rights that might protect their citizens from state-induced starvation or massive malnutrition. There is no pro-active law that can punish leaders for actions that they take quite deliberately to repress civil and political rights, knowing that their actions assist them to intentionally impose famine or recklessly continue policies that create famine. It is time to assume that all political decisions to prohibit or limit civil and political rights are intentional, and to find new ways to call states or their leaders to account at the early stage of faminogenesis, rather than wait until a sufficient number of people has been murdered or starved before turning to punitive institutions such as the ICC.

The four cases discussed in Part II differ radically from advanced liberal democracies that routinely protect civil and political rights and in which, as Sen suggests, there are no famines. Nevertheless, there can be malnutrition even in advanced liberal democracies where most citizens, most of the time, enjoy most of their civil and political rights. I term this type of malnutrition a state food crime by the process of neglect, and discuss it in Chapter 11.

11 Liberal Democracies and the Right to Food

The Right to Adequate Food in Liberal Democracies

This book deals specifically with prevention and punishment of state-induced famine, or faminogenesis, especially in North Korea and Zimbabwe. It also discusses severe state-induced malnutrition in the West Bank and Gaza (WBG), and state-induced food shortages in Venezuela. However, it does not discuss policies affecting access to food defined more broadly, especially in democratic market economies.

Yet many individuals are malnourished even in rich, democratic states. Indeed, one might add to Marcus' four categories of food deprivation presented in Chapter 1 another category, that of neglect. This neglect can be seen, for example, in the extent of food insecurity in Canada and the United States. In Canada in 2011–12, 5.8 percent of households were judged to be moderately food insecure, in the sense that the quality and quantity of their food was compromised, while another 2.5 percent of households were judged to be severely insecure, in the sense that their food intake was reduced (Statistics Canada 2013). In the US in 2013, 13.6 percent of households were judged to have low food security, in the sense that they could "get by" with coping strategies, while 5.9 percent of households were judged to have very low food security, in the sense that their food intake was reduced (Coleman-Jensen et al. 2014). It should surely be of concern that approximately one in twelve Canadian households and one in five American should have suffered from such serious food insecurity.

While I do not adhere to a relativist stance that finds false rights-violating equivalencies between developed democracies and underdeveloped non-democratic states, I do maintain that developed democracies could do a better job of protecting their citizens' rights to adequate nutrition. One respect in which they fail is by not providing enough welfare – indeed, by more accurately providing "illfare" (Sen 1981, 30) – to those who cannot fend for themselves. Policies and income supports ostensibly to protect the poor often leave them so poverty-stricken that they cannot purchase the food they need after paying their rent and other necessary expenses. Other ways democratic states fail their poorer citizens are through low minimum wages that prevent some citizens from earning enough money to purchase the food they need, and by not protecting the trade union rights of workers who need to be able to bargain collectively in order to earn enough to buy their food.

These are problems that undermine the right to food in my own country, Canada. That food insecurity exists in Canada does not undermine Sen's claim that there are no famines in functioning multiparty democracies (Sen 1999, 178), but it does draw our attention to malnutrition. As Sen states regarding rich countries in periods of high unemployment, "but for the social security arrangements there would be widespread starvation and possibly a famine" (Sen 1981, 7). This suggests that liberal democracy, human rights, and indeed market economies may all be necessary to promote and fulfill citizens' right to adequate nutrition, but they are not sufficient.

Peter Baehr, to whom this book is dedicated, pointed out the inconsistency of supporting civil and political rights – as liberal democracies do – while not paying attention to economic human rights. When criticizing the US for not accepting the principle of economic human rights, he wrote, "How can one reject such notions as the rights to food, shelter, clothing, and health, yet continue to accept the right to life as a human right?" (Baehr 2001, ix). Economic human rights are integral aspects of the human right to life. "There can be little doubt that hunger, lack of adequate housing and the lack of sufficient health care are serious infringements of human dignity. In many cases, they coincide with a violation of the fundamental right to life" (Baehr 2001, 40).

The role of the international community in furthering the right to food in developed, rights-respecting democracies is limited. Malnutrition in countries such as Canada is not severe enough to warrant resort to international food aid or international criminal law. And national law is frequently out of the question, as even countries that have ratified the International Covenant on Economic, Social and Cultural Rights (ICESCR) often do not consider economic human rights to be justiciable, nullifying the option of legal action in defense of the right to adequate nutrition. For example, economic human rights are not included in Canada's 1982 Charter of Rights and Freedoms (Government of Canada 1982). Indeed, when the Charter was being drafted the then Liberal Minister of Justice (later Prime Minister) Jean Chrétien explicitly rejected a motion by the opposition New Democratic Party (a left-leaning social democratic party) to include the rights in ICESCR in the Charter. Chrétien declared "I am waiting soon for an amendment to inscribe in the Constitution the apple pie and the recipe of ma tante Berthe [my aunt Bertha], and I do not think we can put everything there" (Robertson 1990, 196).

Canada regularly submits reports to UN agencies such as the Human Rights Council, including on poverty and the right to food (e.g., United Nations General Assembly 2013, February 8, 13–15). Comments on these reports (e.g., United Nations General Assembly 2013, February 7, p. 11, pars. 54, 56, 57) can shame Canada, but shaming does not necessarily result in policy changes. These minimal international monitoring and reporting mechanisms cannot promote adequate nutrition without political action from below within the countries concerned. Remedy of state neglect of citizens' rights to adequate nutrition in advanced industrial democracies rests in citizens' effective use of their human rights. In developed capitalist democracies citizens can use their rights to freedom of speech, association, and press to organize against governments that do not do enough to protect the right to adequate nutrition, and they can vote their governments out of office. Citizens can also use their mobility rights within their own country to move to areas where they are more likely to obtain work at good wages rather than relying on welfare cheques. They can use their property to cultivate food or use it in other ways to earn income with which to buy food. And they can create civil society organizations and social movements in which they use their civil and political rights to try to enforce changes in law and public policy.

Yet there are still barriers that render it difficult for the poor to assert their rights. That Canadians do not starve to death is a consequence of their long history of living in a democratic, relatively rights-protective country. That, nevertheless, some of Canada's poor are food insecure is in large part a consequence of their being unable effectively to assert their rights. The poor lack the resources of wealthier Canadians; they lack the social capital, education, time, and funds necessary to assert their legal rights and use the political rights to which they are formally entitled (Howard-Hassmann 2003, 178–99). This is particularly so regarding Canada's indigenous population.

Aboriginals' Right to Food in Canada

In Chapter 3 I discussed famine among Aboriginal peoples in Canada's West during the 1870s. The consequences of their conquest by a supposedly democratic settler state last to the present.

Even in the twenty-first century malnourishment was significantly higher among Aboriginal Canadians than among the general Canadian population. In 2012, 28.2 percent of Canada's Aboriginal households were food insecure, as opposed to 12.6 percent of all households, for a ratio of 2.2:1. Of the 28.2 percent, 5.1 percent were marginally insecure, 14.8 percent were moderately insecure, and 8.3 percent were severely insecure, as opposed to comparable figures of 4.1, 6.0, and 2.6 percent for all Canadian households (Tarasuk et al. 2014, 24–25).

A nutrition survey conducted in 2004 found that 33 percent of off-reserve Aboriginal households were food insecure, compared to 9 percent of other Canadians. In part, this insecurity was attributable to the higher prevalence of risk factors among Aboriginals than among non-Aboriginals, including higher rates of reliance on social assistance and higher rates of lone parenthood. Yet even controlling for these risk factors, Aboriginal households' rates of food insecurity were 2.6 times higher than non-Aboriginal households' rates (Willows et al. 2008, 1152). In 2001, the human development index score for non-Aboriginal Canadians was 0.880, while for Aboriginals it was only 0.765 (Indian and Northern Affairs Canada 2008, slide 9). In 2009 Canada's indigenous population ranked at about the same level on the Human Development Index as Belarus, Malaysia, and Panama (Daschuk 2013, ix).

Some of this malnourishment might be a consequence of the high cost of transporting nourishing food to remote Aboriginal communities in the far north; for example, in 2012 residents of the northern territory of Nunavut (including non-Aboriginals) spent $14,815 per person per year on food, or 25 percent of their total expenditures, as compared to the average of $7,262 in Canada overall, or about 11 percent of total expenditures (Food Banks Canada 2012, section 1). A 2007–08 study of preschoolers aged three to five in Nunavut found that 56.1 percent were food insecure, among whom 31 percent were moderately insecure and 25.1 percent severely insecure (Egeland et al. 2010, 243).

Another major cause of Aboriginals' continued food insecurity was the residual effects of the residential school system imposed on Canadian Aboriginal peoples. Residential schools were boarding schools run by the government or by various Christian missions under government authority, where during most of the twentieth century many Aboriginal children were confined, often against their parents' wishes. A scandal that broke in 2013 illustrates this neglect; the Canadian media was awash with stories about malnourishment of Aboriginal children in nutrition experiments. The source of the media's information was an article by historian Ian Mosby, who described experiments in Indian residential schools from 1948 to 1952. In an ostensible attempt to improve Indian children's nutritional status, researchers gave nutritional supplements to some children in some schools but left other students and schools without such supplements as control groups. They also denied some children dental care in order to observe the effects of malnourishment on the children's teeth and gums (Mosby 2013, 158–64). Yet the children who were the subjects of these controlled nutritional experiments were already malnourished. As one former school resident put it, "I was always hungry. And we stole food. I remember stealing bread." Another recounted, "[W]e cried to have something good to eat before we sleep. A lot of the times the food we had was rancid, full of maggots, stink" (Truth and Reconciliation Commission of Canada 2015, 71–72). Hunger combined with rampant tuberculosis and other illnesses in residential schools caused many child deaths (Milloy 1999, xv), similar to the child deaths in North Korea in the 1990s and 2000s.

The researchers who left the "control" children malnourished while feeding others experimental nutritional supplements were trying to find ways to improve Aboriginal peoples' diets without addressing long-term structural problems. These structural problems included erosion of Aboriginal people's traditional diets and inadequate funding both of schools and Aboriginal reserves by the relevant government departments. Indeed, even though food was hardly adequate in the residential schools, some Aboriginal parents voluntarily sent their children to them because there was even less food at home, especially in winter (Haig-Brown 1988, 86). Meantime, at least until WWI, the government denied rations to Aboriginal parents who refused to send their children to these appalling schools-cum-prisons.

Yet parents had no say over how the children were treated in these schools, whose notorious purpose was to "take the Indian out of the child." Moreover, the schools did not permit preparation for higher education; boys were generally trained only for manual and girls for domestic labor, most children being obliged to leave at sixteen, or before they would have graduated from high school (York 1989, 23–24). Thus, Aboriginals were deprived of the educational tools necessary to make a living to feed themselves and their families. The long-term effects of the residential schools, the last of which was not closed until 1996, also undermined Aboriginals' capacities to function in the wider society. Having been removed from their families as children, forbidden to speak their native tongue, and subjected to long-term physical and sexual abuse, many Aboriginal adults found it difficult to obtain and hold down a job.

Another reason for food insecurity and malnutrition among Aboriginal Canadians was reduced access to traditional or "country" foods – especially meat. Nutritionists have determined that country food is much healthier than the processed foods that Aboriginal people are likely to eat, especially in remote northern areas where it is difficult to import or cultivate fresh foods such as dairy products, fruits, and vegetables. Loss of land and historic limitations of rights even to use the land supposedly reserved for Aboriginal people is one major cause of lack of access to traditional foods. Another is loss of culture, especially loss of transmission of hunting skills over the generations; the kidnapping of children and their confinement in residential schools meant that they could not learn from their elders how to fish and hunt. Other factors include lack of funds to finance the expenses connected with hunting and fishing (Power 2008, 96). Thus, poverty and the "transition away from local nutrient-rich traditional food resources" combined to impose a "dual nutritional burden" on Aboriginal Canadians (Egeland et al. 2011, 1746).

Exacerbating these difficulties was an on-reserve school system that received less than 70 percent of the funds provided for students attending provincial schools (Chiefs' Assembly on Education 2012, October 1–3, 2). Indeed, the then United Nations Special Rapporteur on the rights of indigenous peoples, James Anaya, urged in 2013 the necessity "to ensure that funding delivered to aboriginal authorities for education per student [be] at least equivalent to that available in the provincial educational systems" (Anaya 2013, October 15, 2). Without good education and with much higher rates of unemployment than the general Canadian population, many Aboriginal individuals became homeless or were incarcerated. Indeed, in 2010–11 Aboriginals constituted about 27 percent of the adults in provincial and territorial custody, and 20 percent of those in federal custody, yet they were only about 3 percent of the total Canadian population (Dauvergne 2012, 11). Thus, unable to fully enjoy the right to work or the right to education, and often incarcerated, Aboriginal adults found it difficult to acquire the wherewithal to provide a healthy diet to their children.

In 2012 the then United Nations Special Rapporteur on the right to food, Olivier De Schutter, visited Canada. He included a section on Aboriginal peoples' right to food in his report, noting in particular the difficulties of using traditional means such as hunting and gathering to obtain food. Problems included "limited availability of food flora and fauna; environmental contamination of species; flooding and development of traditional hunting and trapping territories; lack of equipment and resources to purchase equipment necessary for hunting/fishing/ harvesting; and lack of requisite skills and time" (De Schutter 2012, 8). Sadly, instead of formally replying to his comments, the federal government dismissed De Schutter's report, calling him an "ill-informed academic" (Galloway 2013, October 4). Then Health Minister, Leona Aglukkaq, herself an Aboriginal Canadian, said that De Schutter's report had "no credibility" (Lofaro 2013, March 4).

This is a shameful record for a wealthy democratic country with a functioning multiparty democracy and one in which all human rights are supposedly guaranteed to all citizens In the next section, I discuss the liberal democratic prerequisites to ensure the right to food, above and beyond those that Sen stressed, but these prerequisites are never sufficient when some categories of individuals are marginalized in the very liberal democracies of which they are citizens.

Prerequisites for the Right to Food

Citizens of developed democracies possess a "modern equivalent of feudal privilege – an inherited [or naturalized] status that greatly enhances one's life chances" (Carens 1995, 230). They are winners of the birthright lottery (Shachar 2009) not only in the sense that they have the good fortune to be citizens of rich countries but also in the sense that, enjoying full civil and political rights, the rule of law, mobility rights, property rights, and the right to work, they can act upon their citizenship to demand protections of their economic human rights by the state. Nevertheless, the poor, citizens who live on welfare or who earn only the minimum legal wage, are often those least able to pressure governments. The two prerequisites to the right to food that I discuss below – democracy and market economies – are not sufficient to protect it.

In general, there is no rights-protective country that is not also a democracy. Democratic political systems, in which political parties compete for office, free and fair elections are held, and parties relinquish the reins of government if they are defeated, help to protect, promote, and fulfill the right to food. The three cases of Ukraine, China, and Cambodia discussed in Chapter 2 illustrate how easy it is for totalitarian governments to induce starvation, but the cases discussed in Chapter 3 show how even democratic states can cause malnutrition or starvation through colonialism or war.

Of the four contemporary cases discussed in Part II, North Korea never had a democratic political system. Zimbabwe was ostensibly democratic after independence, but elections were rigged, sometimes violently, even before Mugabe started to centralize power and undermine all opposition. Under Chávez's rule, Venezuela remained a formal, elections-only democracy, but Chávez rigged funding, restricted his opponents' media access, intimidated voters, and even threatened civil war if he did not win elections. Restrictions on democratic rights intensified under Maduro. Palestinians had no say in who was elected to govern Israel and hence themselves, as they were not Israeli citizens. They did have a say in choosing the governments of Gaza and the West Bank, but these governments were characterized by corruption, mismanagement, and severe violations of civil and political rights.

In any case, formal electoral politics are only a small part of what is required to create a rights-protective society. Secure rule of law must underpin the democratic system. In a country under the rule of law, the government is subject to the judiciary, which is independent and free of government control. Under totalitarian rule in the Soviet Union, China, and Cambodia there was no rule of law. In early democratic Britain and its colonies, rule of law protected landlords and settlers against peasants and indigenous peoples, while no law of war protected German victims of Britain's food blockade. Rule of law was also missing in all four of the contemporary cases discussed in Part II. Rule of law never existed in North Korea. Mugabe progressively undermined the rule of law in Zimbabwe, as did Chávez and Maduro in Venezuela. And Palestinians in the West Bank lived under precarious Israeli military rule, with very little recourse to Israeli civilian courts.

Aside from democracy and the rule of law, there are several other social institutions that any society that protects human rights must have. There is no human right, as such, to these institutions; nevertheless, without them, it is difficult to protect human rights. Foremost among them is simply a functioning government. A functioning government requires a military that is subject to civilian control and a police force upon which it can rely to enforce its laws but which is restrained by human rights principles and practices. Personnel in these social institutions must be trained not to starve their prisoners and not to destroy citizens' access to food. In North Korea, by contrast, the military and police were trained to use food as a weapon against their own citizens, and to starve political prisoners. Israel, internally a liberal democracy, permitted – indeed perhaps encouraged – its soldiers to destroy Palestinians' water supplies, vital to the right to food, and permitted the military to destroy houses and farms without reference even to the minimal rule of military law. Meantime Mugabe in Zimbabwe and Chávez and Maduro in Venezuela used their militaries for their own personal purposes and also established private militias to enforce their wishes.

Rights-protective governments also need bureaucracies that honestly and efficiently administer their territory. In North Korea, bureaucrats were actually party functionaries whose actions were determined entirely by the need to demonstrate loyalty to the Kim dynasty. The bureaucracy in Zimbabwe was perverted into personal servants of Mugabe and his clique. Instead of fairly distributing food to all who needed it, it favored supporters of Mugabe's political party and denied food to those seen as his enemies. In Venezuela, Chávez usurped bureaucratic authority by taking complete control of the national development fund and by ordering the national oil company and central bank to divert funds to the social-welfare missions that he had instituted. Residents of WBG were subject not only to Israeli military control but also to corrupt and often abusive bureaucratic control by Hamas and the Palestinian Authority.

Rights-protective governments must also pay attention to economic human rights, even when they do not acknowledge those rights in law. Most Western democratic governments have incorporated principles of economic justice, emerging from both liberal and social-democratic conceptions of what citizens need and what the duties of states are. Even the United States, among Western democracies one of those least likely to provide welfare, health, and other benefits (Wilkinson and Pickett 2009), acknowledges responsibility for its citizens' welfare (Donnelly 2007). Much of what functioning governments do in democracies promotes economic human rights. For example, governments maintain the sanitation systems and clean running water that underpin their citizens' health and long life expectancy. Most democratic Western governments consider provision of social benefits to be fundamental obligations. But as Chapters 3 and 7 on Britain/Canada and Israel/Palestine show, democratic governments do not necessarily extend these obligations to those whom they have colonized.

People living in developed democracies also enjoy the benefits of market economies, while most of the worst cases of state-induced famine have occurred in non-market states. The Soviet Union, China, and Cambodia completely abolished market relations. In Ukraine in the early 1930s, the Soviet authorities destroyed a self-supporting peasant economy, as did the Chinese after the Communist takeover in 1949 and the Khmer Rouge in Cambodia from 1975 to 1979. In all three countries, authorities also instituted other anti-market policies, including the complete abolition of private property. These policies effectively caused the de-development of their economies. North Korea abolished market relations as soon as it became independent in 1948. All agriculture was collectivized, peasant farmers losing their property rights in land, livestock, and tools. North Korea also abolished private industry and private trade, turning over both to state regulation. The modified reforms instituted in the late 1990s and early 2000s were unsuccessful, as they were erratic, incomplete, and did not provide any legal or regulatory security to those who might have wanted to engage in private production and trade. In any case, after 2005 many reforms were revoked.

Zimbabwe did not abolish its market economy; however, the dispossession of white farmers constituted a de facto attack on normal market relations in the country. The production of food staples deteriorated drastically, while those who took over confiscated farms often either did not know how to turn them into productive entities, or chose not to. Some small peasant farmers were able to produce for subsistence on redistributed land, but others lacked access to the seed, credit, and expertise that would enable them to produce food. While after 2009 market relations were somewhat stabilized with the introduction of the dollar as a national currency, threats to indigenize the economy by requiring minimum percentages of ownership by black Zimbabweans discouraged foreign investment. Foreign direct investment can have significantly positive effects on national economic development and can encourage human rights through complicated spin-off effects (Howard-Hassmann 2010, 49–65).

In Venezuela, Chávez and Maduro undermined market transactions. They arbitrarily and inconsistently confiscated productive land, even though the original intent was that the state would confiscate only idle land. Price controls effectively instituted a dual market system for food, rendering some items very cheap while others became more expensive: controls also created food shortages. The government's decision to institute differential foreign exchange rates for essential and non-essential goods resulted in illegal manipulatory behavior by importers, who would import food at low exchange prices and sell it at higher prices.

Israel is the outlier in this discussion, as it had a well-functioning capitalist market economy. However, Israel was engaged in a colonial takeover of the West Bank. As part of that takeover, it put severe constraints on Palestinians' capacities to engage in market transactions, confiscating their land and undermining their mobility. Israel also blockaded Gaza, which could not control its own imports of food. In the face of Israeli restrictions on food crossing into their territory, Gazans resorted to smuggling food through tunnels from Egypt, risking their periodic closure by Egyptian authorities. Even when they could establish farms and businesses within Gaza, businessmen suffered from severe constraints and faced considerable financial and material losses whenever there was an Israeli military incursion.

It seems, then, that a free market economy is necessary to prevent starvation. Citizens must enjoy their property rights; they must be permitted to choose their work and establish businesses if they wish; they must be allowed to buy and sell in the market; a tradable currency must exist. They must also be free to exercise their mobility rights in search of jobs and to have access to jobs without discrimination. If they enjoy these rights, they are far less likely to be dependent on rations or coupons handed out by the state, as in North Korea, or on food provided only to those considered loyal to the regime, as in Zimbabwe. Citizens must not be subject to a command economy that tries and fails to plan every item that is produced or used. Command economies deny their citizens the entitlements they need to obtain food: these entitlements consist of the capacity to produce food for themselves and the capacity to earn money to buy food (Sen 1981). By contrast, market economies do provide these entitlements to most of their citizens.

Markets must not be idealized, however, and no government should leave entirely to the market the provision of its citizens' basic necessities. Ideological capitalism can cause severe malnutrition, even if it is less likely than ideological communism to cause outright famine. The willingness of market ideologues to leave individuals to strive or sink, to eat or starve, is an ideological stance as much as is communism: democratic, rights-protective governments must actively intervene to make sure that everyone eats enough and healthily. Market economies are never sufficient to ensure all citizens' right to food, and ideological attachment to free market relations can severely exacerbate famine. An ideology of the invisible hand of the market was one reason that the English government left the Irish to starve in the 1840s and the Canadian government left Aboriginal Canadians to starve in the 1870s.

Capitalism is not sufficient to guarantee protection of economic human rights such as the right to food. While market economies may produce the amount and range of goods and services necessary to fulfill human rights, they are often dominated by a capitalist class that acts in its own interest and has disproportionate influence over the state. Market economies require government regulation to ensure that the rich do not get richer while the poor are left behind. The neo-liberal late twentieth century model of a completely free market ignored the reality that all economies require government investment and regulation. Food riots erupted all over the world after the implementation of structural adjustment programs at the behest of the International Monetary Fund in the 1980s and 90s (Patel and McMichael 2009, 9–10). These programs encouraged governments to spend less on social welfare and on the civil service, open up their economies to foreign investment and competition, devalue their currencies, and institute better protection of private property. Some of these conditions would have helped to protect Venezuelans from the detrimental consequences of Chávez's and Maduro's economic policies, but without simultaneous concern for citizens' economic human rights, neo-liberal economic policies can undermine fundamental human security, including access to food.

The 2008–09 food crisis, when the prices of staple foods rose dramatically, also shows the dangers of unregulated capitalist markets. The causes of these price rises were complex, including temporary weather conditions, the increased use of food to produce biofuels, and increased consumption of meat. Other causes were market distortions in rich countries, including subsidies to farmers to produce food. Restrictions on food exports and speculation in food also drove up prices (Howard-Hassmann 2010, 76–78). Poor people living in developing countries spend as much as 50 to 80 percent of their income on food, so the crisis hit them particularly hard; indeed, the Food and Agriculture Organization estimated that in just one year, 2008–09, 150 million more people were going hungry. The crisis was caused in large part by world-wide deregulation of international financial transactions, including transactions related to the market in food. Food had been transformed into a purely commercial commodity, controlled in large part by transnational food corporations, with little or no regard for people's actual food needs (Clapp 2012, 4, 14–17).

Thus, people will not enjoy their right to food until non-state actors have human rights obligations, especially private international and nationally owned businesses. Indeed, international human rights emerged in Europe as a means to control not only the state but also the marketplace (Donnelly 2003, 57–70). Canada and the US show that a functioning and thriving market economy is no guarantor of economic human rights. State intervention is crucial to protect those who are not part of the market economy, such as the disabled or elderly, or who do not earn enough money in the marketplace to provide their own nutritional needs. Redistribution of wealth via taxation and various social welfare schemes is necessary to protect and fulfill economic human rights.

In the end, ideologies either of the market or of command economies will harm economic human rights. Even developed welfare states do not protect everyone's right to food, as the section above on malnutrition among Aboriginal Canadians shows. Much stronger international law, imposing obligations not only on governments but also on international organizations and private corporations, is necessary to ensure that everyone enjoys their right to food.

Extraterritorial Obligations Regarding the Right to Food

This volume is about how states cause famine and malnutrition within their own territories or territories under their control. It is not about how wealthy states might contribute to violations of the right to food outside their own territories, yet it is necessary to briefly acknowledge how this can occur. In particular, since most wealthy states (excluding some oil-rich countries) are also developed market economies, it is important to acknowledge how such states can contribute to food scarcity or to high costs of food through insufficient regulation of food corporations based in their territory, or by disregard of the human rights obligations of the international organizations to which they belong.

Obligations of one state to citizens of other states are usually referred to as extraterritorial obligations. International human rights law includes extraterritorial obligations: it applies not only to states' relations with their own citizens but also to their relations with citizens of other states. This aspect of international law has been relatively neglected until recently, yet it is entrenched in the earliest human rights documents (Gibney 2015). Article 28 of the UDHR states that "Everyone is entitled to a social and international order in which the rights and freedoms set forth in this Declaration can be fully realized," suggesting that one's rights are not restricted by one's membership in a particular state, but rather that all states are responsible for establishing and maintaining an international order in which all individuals' human rights are protected.

Article 2, 1 of the International Covenant on Economic, Social and Cultural Rights (ICESCR) specifies that "Each State Party to the present Covenant undertakes to take steps, individually and through international assistance and co-operation . . . to the maximum of its available resources, with a view to achieving progressively the full realization of the rights recognized in the present Covenant." This implies that assistance and co-operation is a positive obligation of states that sign the Covenant, and also that each state must use the maximum of its available resources to achieve progressively the full realization of human rights. States may not simply set aside a tiny proportion of their resources, as they see fit, to assist citizens of other states. Article 11, 1 of the ICESCR, the principal article on the right to food, also mentions extraterritorial obligations, stating that states party to the ICESCR recognize "the essential importance of international cooperation." Section 2, b of Article 11 notes that measures to ensure freedom from hunger must include steps "to ensure an equitable distribution of world food supplies in relation to need."

Moreover, according to Articles 3, 3 and 8, 1 of the 1986 United Nations' Declaration on the Right to Development, "states have the duty to co-operate with each other in ensuring development and eliminating obstacles to development." The right to development includes "equality of opportunity for all in their access to basic resources . . . [including] food" (United Nations General Assembly 1986). Thus, it can be inferred that states have a duty to protect the international food rights of everyone, not only of their own citizens: The obligation to respect the right to food has an extraterritorial dimension. States must, especially, "refrain from taking action that would compromise the right to food extraterritorially" (DeFalco 2009, 17). This particularly refers to international trade, and how states' actions restricting or regulating trade could affect the right to food of people outside their own borders. The Maastricht Principles on economic human rights, drafted by a group of international human rights lawyers in 2011, argued in Articles 4 and 24 that "All States . . . have extraterritorial obligations to respect, protect, and fulfill economic, social and cultural rights" and that such obligations extended to ensuring that non-state entities which they were "in a position to regulate" also respected human rights (Abraham et al. 2011). Such principles, drafted by groups of eminent international jurists, are sometimes the first step to evolving or specifying international human rights law.

The world is not composed only of states: the international food market is heavily influenced by international organizations (IOs) and transnational corporations (TNCs). The law regarding IOs is still evolving, but suggests that they do have some human rights obligations, although such obligations are much weaker than the obligations of states (Clapham 2006; Kinley 2009). A general principle is that if an action by a state is a human rights violation, then so is a similar action by an IO (Kent 2005b); as specialized agencies of the United Nations, the International Monetary Fund (IMF) and the World Bank are especially bound by the UN's commitment to human rights and international co-operation (Apodaca 2014, 355). Moreover, states are voting members of IOs and are responsible not to vote for policies that could undermine human rights, including the right to food (Niada 2006–07, 159–60).

This is not to suggest that there are any particular economic policies that international human rights law should endorse. For example, food sovereignty, discussed in Chapter 1, is not necessarily a better option for protection of the right to food than reliance on the international food market. Food sovereigntists rightly criticize the structural adjustment policies imposed by the IMF in the 1980s and 1990s on many less-developed countries in exchange for financial assistance. These policies had severe detrimental consequences for the right to food (Abouharb and Cingranelli 2007). Frequently the IMF obliged recipient states to turn to cash-crop export agriculture instead of subsistence agriculture or production for the internal market. This left peasant farmers extremely vulnerable to the fluctuating world market in food – and often to the TNCs that controlled it – resulting in malnutrition when cash crop prices fell and peasants did not earn enough money to buy food on the local market.

Yet people are not necessarily better off if they live in states that are self-sufficient in food rather than in states where farmers produce cash crops for export and buy imported food. Ravallion argues that "as a generalization, the view that export-crop production creates famines is questionable; if by producing a cash crop instead the rural poor can afford to buy more food, and the markets and infrastructure are adequate for getting the food to them from elsewhere, then that will reduce their vulnerability to famine" (Ravallion 1997, 1229). Much of the criticism of IOs for introducing and defending neo-liberal economic policies fails to take into account the actual economic justifications for their policies, and looks only at their failures, not their successes (Dicklitch and Howard-Hassmann 2007). This does not mean, however, that IOs should be exempt from human rights concerns, permitted to make economic policy decisions that disregard their effects on citizens, especially the poorest.

TNCs are the other significant set of actors in the world food market. States often insufficiently or incompetently regulate the national and international food markets, especially the TNCs that produce and market food. States are normally responsible for the domestic consequences of actions or inactions of TNCs, but this responsibility does not usually extend to the consequences of TNC actions or inactions in other states. Often these TNCs organize cartels that drive up the price of food while simultaneously lowering the prices they pay to food producers (Feunteun 2015).

TNCs are not yet under any legal obligation to protect human rights, yet they undermine the right to food by contributing to malnutrition and by indifference to the consequences of their policies. Attribution of culpability for malnutrition to TNCs is more difficult than attribution to states but is not impossible. In recent years there has been an emerging consensus that TNCs bear human rights responsibilities. In 2003 the UN Sub-Commission on the Promotion and Protection of Human Rights issued an extensive set of norms applying to transnational corporations (UN Sub-Commission on the Promotion and Protection of Human Rights 2003). More recently, the UN commissioned a report by Professor John Ruggie that more carefully elucidated the human rights responsibilities of these enterprises (Ruggie 2011; Aaronson and Higham 2013).

A move to hold officers of TNCs that undermine the right to food accountable under international law might render them more cognizant of the possible ways that monopolies and oligopolies, exorbitant prices of seeds or fertilizers, or other such policies contribute to nutritional insecurity. In the four contemporary cases I consider in Part II, however, TNCs were not culprits in faminogenesis or policies and practices that caused malnutrition. Indeed, had TNCs been allowed more latitude in Venezuela and Zimbabwe, citizens' rights to adequate nutrition might have been more successfully protected, as they might have been had TNCs had any right at all to operate in North Korea.

Just as TNCs were not implicated in the state food crimes I discuss in this volume, IOs were not implicated. No IO advised North Korea to institute its ruinous economic policies; indeed all would have advised against it, if given the chance. Nor did IOs advise Robert Mugabe to institute violent confiscation of white-owned farms, or Hugo Chávez to institute price controls on food. Neither were IOs implicated in the Israeli defense and settlement policies that had the effect of increasing malnutrition among Palestinians. IOs would have advised North Korea to adopt a market economy and Zimbabwe and Venezuela to restore those aspects of the market economy that their leaders had destroyed. IOs tried to assist Palestinians in WBG to maintain and strengthen their economies, despite the difficulties of living under effective Israeli rule (World Bank 2013, September 16; International Monetary Fund 2014, September 12).

Extraterritorial obligations also extend to the obligation to provide assistance in the realization of economic human rights. Developed Western countries have the resources to provide food aid to help the victims of their own states' policies, if they cause famine or malnutrition, but they often are unable to assist victims of other states' policies. As Chapter 9 shows, the politics of food aid render it difficult for states to protect the right to food of citizens of other countries. Food aid to North Korea may have been diverted to the military, to members of the elite, or to more loyal but less needy regions of the country. Provision of food aid may have released funds that the government then used to buy arms. Similarly, food aid to Zimbabwe alleviated some of the effects of the government's destructive policies but was subject to political manipulation as it was destined for Mugabe's supporters. And food aid to WBG may have relieved Israel of its responsibilities to those two territories. Meanwhile, any international attempt to protect the right to food of Venezuelans under Chávez or Maduro would have been considered a form of Western imperialism and unwarranted intervention.

Developed Western countries are frequently criticized for protecting their own citizens' right to food while neglecting their responsibility to ensure that citizens of other countries do not go hungry or suffer malnutrition. But not only developed countries are at fault in this regard. Some states neglect the right to food of citizens of other countries even when they could use international law to protect that right. The African Union's disregard of food crimes in Zimbabwe constituted a form of international indifference. When less-developed states could resort to international law to punish political leaders such as Mugabe, who undermine their citizens' right to food but do not do so, then they are neglecting the right to food as much as, if not more than, developed capitalist countries that fail to regulate IOs or TNCs. Moreover, under international law states also have a duty to accept food aid if circumstances so require. Thus, North Korea and Zimbabwe disobeyed international law by not accepting aid or by manipulating it. And by 2015, it could be argued, Venezuela had a duty to solicit food aid to rectify its severe food shortages.

The worst state food crimes – actual faminogenesis – are generated by internal state policies imposed by elites either as a means to their own material benefit, as in Zimbabwe; for ideological reasons as well as personal benefit, as in North Korea and Venezuela; or as a consequence of conquest and colonialism, as in WBG. As Chapter 12 discusses, a new international treaty controlling faminogenesis and deprivation of the right to food might help to alleviate these failures.

12   A New International Treaty on the Right to Food

For a New International Treaty on the Right to Food

I propose that there should be a new and distinct United Nations treaty to protect the right to food. Such a treaty would reiterate the relevant clauses in the UN Genocide Convention and the Rome Statute of the International Criminal Court (ICC). It would include new measures prohibiting penal starvation and prescribing punishments for those engaged in it. It would revise international refugee law to include as refugees those who flee state-induced famine. It would specify obligations of both donor and recipient states regarding food aid, specify when and how sanctions could be invoked against states committing food crimes, and specify new rules for the responsibility to protect victims of state-induced famine. Such a treaty on the right to food would both indicate the responsibilities of states – to their own and other states' citizens – and prescribe punishments of those who significantly violate these rights. Finally, it would reiterate the importance of civil and political rights to the "economic" human right to food.

In recommending a new treaty on the right to food I join David Marcus, who made such a recommendation in 2003. One of Marcus's aims was to specifically criminalize what he called famine crimes, defined as follows:

A person commits a first-degree famine crime when he or she knowingly creates, inflicts, or prolongs conditions that result in or contribute to the starvation of a significant number of persons.

A person commits a second-degree famine crime by recklessly ignoring evidence that his or her policies are creating, inflicting, or prolonging the starvation of a significant number of persons (Marcus 2003, 247).

Marcus argued that formal codification of famine crimes would debunk the myth that famines are the result of natural disasters and might force the international community to take action against them. He noted that under both the Geneva Conventions and international customary law, civilians were protected from famine in times of war but not peace

(Marcus 2003, 265–71). He agreed that the crime of extermination, defined in the Rome Statute of the ICC as "the intentional infliction of conditions of life, *inter alia* the deprivation of access to food and medicine, calculated to bring about the destruction of part of a population" (International Criminal Court 1998 Article 7, 2, b) did fit peacetime famine crimes well. However, he believed that the crime of extermination had "seen little jurisprudential development" (Marcus 2003, 273).

In general, Marcus argued, current international law and legal precedents, including adjudication of the questions of intent and knowledge, buttressed his argument for a new, comprehensive treaty prohibiting both intentionally and recklessly induced faminogenesis (Marcus 2003, 274–79). Although there are myriad obligations in international law to protect the right to food which apply not only to states but also to international organizations, transnational corporations, and indeed, private individuals (Niada 2006–07, 153–65), Marcus argued that precedents regarding famine crimes were "scattered throughout international criminal law," necessitating a more coherent approach. He maintained that "codification will convey expressive value that will force the international community to address outbreaks of famine appropriately." It would force the international community "to determine whether a famine had erupted as a result of criminal behavior," thus raising "the political stakes for ignoring famine." Marcus did not, however, suggest criminalizing failures to act by third parties, i.e., by outside states (Marcus 2003, 279–81).

One might argue that a separate treaty on the right to food is unnecessary, since the Rome Statute of the ICC already prohibits denial of food as an aspect of extermination. Indeed, on December 18, 2014 the United Nations General Assembly (UNGA) voted to submit the report of the Commission of Inquiry into North Korea discussed in Chapter 8, to the United Nations Security Council (UNSC), to "consider the relevant conclusions and . . . take appropriate action . . . including through consideration of referral of the situation in the Democratic People's Republic of Korea to the International Criminal Court and consideration of the scope for effective targeted sanctions against those who appear to be most responsible for acts that the commission has said may constitute crimes against humanity" (United Nations General Assembly 2014, December 18, Article 8).

This referral was unusual in that its rationale was not North Korea's program to develop nuclear weapons, but rather its possible crimes against humanity. Debating an earlier report by the UNGA Third Committee on North Korea, China and Russia had backed a defeated amendment proposed by Cuba to remove the suggestion that the UNGA accepted the Commission's view that crimes against humanity were being committed in North Korea, and also to remove the call to refer North Korea to the ICC. North Korea, in its turn, had angrily threatened to resume nuclear tests in response to the Third Committee resolution (Donath 2014, November 18). This case shows the difficulty of relying only on the ICC to enforce the right to food – or at least, the right not to be deliberately starved. It was unlikely that the UNSC would vote to refer North Korea to the ICC, as China and Russia would probably exercise their veto.

The international human rights regime does not make strong demands on the international system as a whole. Few mechanisms exist that can actually check human rights abuses. The UNSC can pass Resolutions regarding human rights abuses it deems to adversely affect international peace and security. It can also impose sanctions, although as Chapter 9 shows, as of 2015 it had not done so for deprivation of the right to food, even in the case of North Korea. The ICC can convict individuals of war crimes, crimes against humanity, or genocide, but only after they have already severely abused human rights. Regional human rights bodies are often stymied by member nations' political interests, as in the case of the failure of the Southern African Development Community to follow through on its own court's protection of the non-discrimination rights of white Zimbabweans. Thus, although individual states bear the responsibility to protect their citizens' human rights, the international system as a whole does not bear similar responsibilities.

This does not necessarily mean that a new treaty on the right to food might be useful. One might object to it on the grounds that it contributes to an ever-expanding panoply of human rights, which might eventually undermine the entire international human rights system. Posner argues that UN human rights treaties are overloaded, with the result that "In most countries people formally have as many as 400 international human rights" most of which are ignored or unenforceable (Posner 2014, December 4, 5). It might be the case that a shorter, more concrete set of rights would enable states to fulfill their obligations more efficiently. Nevertheless, many other rights have been expanded beyond their initial articulation in the basic human rights documents. For example, the 1979 Convention on the Elimination of All Forms of Discrimination against Women (United Nations General Assembly 1981) expands on the basic equality of the sexes found in the 1948 Universal Declaration of Human Rights. Nor does the expansion and specification of human rights pertain only to identification of particular groups of rights-holders, such as women. The 1984 Convention against Torture, for example, specifies in detail what torture is and who its agents are (United Nations General Assembly 1984).

A separate treaty on the right to food might result in identification of human rights violations undermining access to food before, not after, state-induced famine or malnutrition became widespread. As I have shown in this volume, violations of civil and political rights contribute to violation of the economic human right to food. Yet there is not yet any international legal regime that can call political leaders to account for violations of civil and political rights. The most that can be done is to name and shame states that violate these rights through the mechanisms of the Human Rights Committee and other treaty-monitoring bodies at the United Nations.

Until and unless violations reach the level of genocide and crimes against humanity, states still possess the sovereign right to violate those civil and political rights that might protect their citizens from state-induced starvation. There is no pro-active law that can punish leaders for actions that they take quite deliberately, knowing that their actions impose great harms such as famine or continue policies that inadvertently create it. There is no international human rights court that can deal with human rights violations before they reach extreme proportions (Forsythe 2012, 101; Nowak 2011), nor is one likely to be established in the foreseeable future. Nor is there an international civil court that would allow individuals to bring legal actions against their own state or other states for violating their human rights (Gibney 2002, 55). It is time to find new ways to call states and their leaders to account at the early stage of state-induced famine, rather than wait until a sufficient number of people has been murdered or starved before turning to the ICC, the only punitive international human rights court that currently exists, and whose jurisdiction is currently limited to genocide, war crimes, and crimes against humanity.

Moreover, even if extreme state food crimes such as occurred in North Korea can be referred to the ICC as crimes against humanity, that institution has a mandate only to punish individuals for human rights violations. Indictment of individual leaders does not address the real problem, the existence of entire regimes that persecute significant sections of their own populations, as in North Korea, Zimbabwe, and Venezuela, or of people under their control, as in Israel. It is a paradox of international law that states are considered responsible for promoting, protecting, and fulfilling human rights, but only individuals are held accountable for their violation. As Baehr noted, "The strength of international criminal tribunals is that they help to serve to individualize guilt. However, one may pause to wonder to what extent this is indeed an advantage" (Baehr 2001, 107–08). Should the world community do more than indict individuals for systemic crimes in which entire political regimes, their armies, and many civilians are implicated? How, if at all, is it possible to punish an entire political regime, rather than only individual actors within it?

Are Human Rights Treaties Effective?

A treaty on the right to food would not be able to solve the problem that it is entire regimes, not only individuals, who are responsible for state food crimes. Moreover, a treaty on the right to food would probably have no influence at all on a country such as North Korea, which is a totalitarian state. There is no evidence that dictators are deterred from gross violations of human rights by the threat of punitive international action, especially given international human rights law's lack of enforcement powers. The importance of such a treaty, rather, lies in its bringing together all aspects of international law pertaining to the right to food and its possible effect on a range of countries, most of which are not totalitarian. Human rights treaties have an educative effect; they may be able to influence the behavior of some states some of the time in a positive direction, and they provide a guide and touchstone for civil society organizations. States and their elites, moreover, sometime try to improve their human rights records for reasons of prestige, to be accepted as legitimate members of the international family of nations (Simmons 2009, 13). The international community is collectively engaged in a long-term project to inscribe human rights in the consciences and policies of all human rights actors, politicians as well as activists.

The evidence regarding the efficacy of human rights laws is mixed; indeed, it could be argued that although the human rights legal regime is extensive, it has not had much, if any, real positive effect since 1945. Some scholars argue that there is no evidence that when a state signs a human rights treaty its actual human rights performance improves (Keith 1999). It seems that states sign treaties and take part in the ritual of United Nations human rights monitoring to gain international and internal legitimacy, rather than to improve their domestic human rights performance (Hathaway 2002, 2013–14). On the other hand, some states are acculturated by international norms to improve their own human rights performance (Stacy 2009, 124), and states that are criticized by UN monitoring bodies for poor protection of human rights after signing the International Covenant on Civil and Political Rights (ICCPR) and the Convention against Torture sometimes improve their performance (Clark 2009). Most of this evidence, however, pertains to civil and political rights such as the right not to be tortured, not to the right to food. Nevertheless, as both the case studies in Part II and the analysis throughout show, without civil and political rights it is unlikely that the right to food will be realized.

In a review of statistical research on correlations between states' accessions to human rights treaties and their actual human rights performance, Hafner-Burton concludes that democratic and newly democratizing states are most likely to improve their human rights performance after signing human rights treaties (Hafner-Burton 2013, 71). Earlier work by Hathaway and Landman came to similar conclusions (Hathaway 2002, 2019; Landman 2005, 6–7). Confirming my own analysis in Chapters 10 and 11, both Landman and Hafner-Burton suggest that large-scale social changes such as economic development and establishment of the rule of law and democratic institutions are much more important for the protection of human rights than formal adherence to international human rights treaties (Landman 2005, 9; Hafner-Burton 2013, 85).

Against this rather pessimistic view, some scholars theorize that some governments undergo "norm socialization" (Risse and Sikkink 1999, 5); that is, they are socialized to accept human rights norms and implement them domestically. In this pattern of norm socialization, moral persuasion is particularly important. Domestic opposition and international pressure by other states and by international organizations may influence states to sign human rights treaties and then implement their provisions. These factors are particularly effective if the regime in question seeks international legitimacy. Unfortunately, they seem to have had little effect in the four contemporary cases discussed in Part II.

In North Korea, little to no domestic opposition existed, with the possible exception of periodic (and quickly suppressed) local rebellions and internal faction-building. International pressure until 2015 was confined mainly to North Korea's nuclear threat, not to its policies regarding food. Nor was North Korea much interested in international legitimacy. Zimbabwe was subjected to international pressure from the West but enjoyed a high degree of legitimacy within Africa; Mugabe did not seem to care about wider international legitimacy. Domestic opposition did exist, but judicious – and sometimes extreme, as immediately before and after the 2008 elections – use of violence resulted in the opposition's trying to cooperate with the regime to avoid further punishments.

In Venezuela, politics became a conflict over the Chávez and Maduro food policies. The response of the government to opposition demands was repression of political rights, in the worst cases by imprisonment, torture, and even assassinations. Domestic opposition in Venezuela combined with weak, but growing, international pressure, but the Maduro government was uninterested in international legitimacy, except among a small group of leftist states such as Cuba and Iran. Within Israel, an active and strong domestic opposition to policies in the West Bank and Gaza (WBG) existed. International pressure on Israel was also very strong; however, it was balanced by almost uncritical support of Israel by the US. And Israeli governments, especially the hard-right ethno-nationalists who dominated Israel at the end of the period under study, were increasingly uninterested in international legitimacy, as they viewed their domination of WBG as a zero-sum game in which the actual existence of Israel (and by implication, of the Jewish people as a whole) was at stake.

This suggests that for these four countries, a treaty on the right to food might be little more than a piece of paper, even if for reasons of government prestige or international legitimacy their leaders decided to sign it. Hafner-Burton notes that "laws generally don't relate well to protections for human rights in settings where rights are most in jeopardy" (Hafner-Burton 2013, 73). We have seen in this volume that this is the case for North Korea, a totalitarian state since its inception, and for Zimbabwe, which turned increasingly to anti-democratic politics during the twenty-first century, undermining the rule of law, manipulating elections, and repressing its opposition.

While North Korea and Zimbabwe seem effectively beyond the reach of international human rights law, Venezuela might be susceptible to naming and shaming by international organizations for the threats its policies pose to the right to food. Simmons concludes from a large quantitative study that while democracies sign human rights treaties when they are already committed to their principles, and human rights treaties have no effect on autocratic countries, countries with unstable political institutions exhibit quite high positive (for human rights) effects after signing the treaties (Simmons 2009, 16, 108). This suggests that were it to sign a hypothetical treaty on the right to food, Venezuela might be more inclined to guarantee that right than it was in the early twenty-first century. And countries such as Israel and Canada, which are and were colonial settler states but are also political democracies, might be shamed by the existence of a new treaty on the right to food into paying more attention to the food rights of the populations they have colonized.

In Canada, Israel, Venezuela, and even possibly Zimbabwe, an international treaty on the right to food would give civil society organizations one more resource to shame their own governments into policy changes, one more way to "speak rights to power" (Brysk 2013). Even if states do not improve their human rights performance after signing human rights treaties, those treaties become a resource that domestic human rights activists can use. "[T]reaties are more than scraps of paper. They can become powerful instruments in the hands of rights claimants to hold governments to their promised behavior" (Simmons 2009, 111). One should not conclude from the apparent hopelessness of autocratic – indeed totalitarian – states such as North Korea that human rights treaties are ineffective everywhere.

The Right to Food as an Aspect of Fundamental Human Decency

One might argue that whether or not the international human rights regime exists, human rights are a mere fictional construct. Unless they are enacted into effective national positive law, they have little or no meaning. And it seems that they are only enacted into effective law once a country has become so wealthy and democratic that it is likely to respect human rights regardless of whether it signs international treaties. While some countries may be more likely to respect human rights after having signed international human rights Covenants, others only sign when human rights have already been entrenched. To discuss human rights gaps in totalitarian or authoritarian countries, or countries under occupation, may be putting the cart before the horse. Economic development and political change may be the real keys to rights protection, not the articulation of human rights principles.

I agree that human rights are a social construction. They represent an international consensus on what the rules should be to provide fair and just societies in which, as the preamble to the Universal Declaration of Human Rights proclaims, "the dignity and worth of the human person" is always and everywhere protected (United Nations General Assembly 1948, preamble, par. 5). Human rights are what decent people think human beings need in order to live decent lives. Among these is the fundamental right to life, protecting individuals not only against arbitrary execution by the state but also against arbitrary deprivation of food. As there is some evidence that international human rights treaties do have some positive effect some of the time, it is worth articulating the principles of the right to food in a separate treaty. This treaty could provide support to domestic and international civil society organizations to pressure states not to institute or implement faminogenic policies, and to remedy malnutrition, whether intentionally, recklessly, or incompetently created.

The right to food is a core human right. It deserves its own treaty, even if, like all other international human rights treaties, a treaty on the right to food is ultimately unenforceable.

Bibliography

Aaronson, S. and I. Higham (2013). " 'Re-Righting Business': John Ruggie and the Struggle to Develop International Human Rights Standards for Transnational Firms." *Human Rights Quarterly* 35(2): 333–64.

Abdelaziz, K. (2014, December 14). "Sudan's President Omar al-Bashir Claims Victory over ICC after It Drops Darfur War Crimes Investigation." The Independent.

Abouharb, M. R. and D. Cingranelli (2007). *Human Rights and Structural Adjustment*. New York, Cambridge University Press.

Abraham, M., C. deAlbuquerque, et al. (2011). *Maastricht Principles on Extraterritorial Obligations of States in the Area of Economic, Social and Cultural Rights*. Maastricht, Maastricht University.

Affonço, D. (2007). *To the End of Hell: One Woman's Struggle to Survive Cambodia's Khmer Rouge*. London, Reportage Press.

Africa Research Bulletin (2008, July 1–31). "Zimbabwe: The Road to Talks." Africa Research Bulletin.

African Union (2000). Constitutive Act of the African Union, African Union.

(2008, July 1). African Union Summit Resolution on Zimbabwe. Sharm el-Sheikh. 11th Ordinary Session.

(2009). African Union Convention for the Protection and Assistance of Internally Displaced Persons in Africa. Kampala.

Agence France-Presse (2010, October 5). Botswana Urges End to Zimbabwe Sanctions. Agence France-Presse.

Agricultural Guiding and Awareness Society et al (2013). Farming Injustice: International Trade with Israeli Agricultural Companies and the Destruction of Palestinian Farming, Palestinian Farming and Civil Society Organisations.

AIDS-Free World (2009). Electing to Rape: Sexual Terror in Mugabe's Zimbabwe. New York.

Al Husseini, J. (2010). "UNRWA and the Refugees: A Difficult but Lasting Marriage." *Journal of Palestine Studies* 11(1): 6–26.

Al Jazeera (2015, January 30). Mugabe Appointed African Union Chairman. Al Jazeera.

Alexander, J. (2009, March 21). "Death and disease in Zimbabwe's prisons." *The Lancet* 373(9668): 995–96.

Allen, K. (1998). "Sharing Scarcity: Bread Rationing and the First World War in Berlin, 1914–1923." *Journal of Social History* 32(2): 371–93.

Allen, L. (2006). "Social Security: How Palestinians Survive a Humanitarian Crisis." *Middle East Report* 240: 12–19.

Almog, D. (2004). "Tunnel-Vision in Gaza." *The Middle East Quarterly* (summer): 3–11.

Alsheh, Y. (2011). The Intellectual and Political Origins of the United Nations' Convention on the Prevention and Punishment of the Crime of Genocide 1933–1948. Department of History. Tel-Aviv, Tel-Aviv University. Ph.D.

(2016). The Self-Congratulatory Narrative Concerning the Boycotts and Sanctions Campaign on Apartheid South Africa. *Boycotts Past and Present*. D. Feldman, M. L. Miller and S. Uri (ed.). London, Palgrave in press.

Alston, P. (1984). International Law and the Right to Food. *Food as a Human Rights*. Asbjorn Eide et al. (ed.). Tokyo, United Nations University.

Alvarez Herrera, B. (2006). "A Benign Revolution: In Defense of Hugo Chavez." *Foreign Affairs* 85(4): 195–98.

Amnesty International (2009). *Troubled Waters-Palestinians Denied Fair Access to Water: Israeli-Occupied Palestinian Territories*. London, Amnesty International.

(2010, July 15). *Starving North Koreans Forced to Survive on Diet of Grass and Tree Bark*. London, Amnesty International.

(2011). *Israel and the Occupied Palestinian Territories*. London, Amnesty International.

(2012a). *Annual Report 2012: Zimbabwe*. London, Amnesty International.

(2012b). *Annual Report: The State of the World's Human Rights: Venezuela*. London, Amnesty International.

(2012c). *Israel and the Occupied Palestinian Territories*. London, Amnesty International.

(2013). "Changing the Soup but not the Medicine?" *Abolishing Re-Education through Labour in China*. London, Amnesty International.

Anaya, J. (2013, October 15). Statement Upon Conclusion of the Visit to Canada, United Nations Human Rights Council.

Anderson, J. (2013, April 10). *In Venezuelan Election, Food Is a Voting Issue*. Associated Press.

Annan, K. (2005). *In Larger Freedom: Towards Development, Security and Human Rights for All*. New York, United Nations.

Anonymous (2009). "Statistical Indicators on the Eve of Operation Cast Lead." *Journal of Palestine Studies* 38(3): 169–71.

Apodaca, C. (2014). The Right to Food. *Handbook of Human Rights*. T. Cushman (ed.). New York, Routledge: 349–58.

Applebaum, A. (2003). *Gulag: A History*. New York, Anchor Books.

Article 19 (1990). *Starving in Silence: A Report on Famine and Censorship*. London, Article 19.

Associated Press (2007, March 14). African Union Chairman Calls Situation in Zimbabwe 'Embarrassing'.

(2011, October 30). Hugo Chavez Orders Seizure of British Company's Land for Venezuelan State. The Guardian.

(2012, February 2). Venezuela's Oil Exports to US Decline, Reflecting Downward Trend during Chavez Government.

(2013, June 9). Finding Scarce Food and Toilet Paper in Venezuela – Now There's a Free Mobile App For That.

(2014, March 11). Students, University Attacked in Central Venezuela. *The New York* Times.

(2014, May 31). Israel's Desalination Program Averts Future Water Crises. Haaretz.com.

Azieri, M. (2009). "The Castro-Chavez Alliance." *Latin American Perspectives* 36(1): 99–110.

B'Tselem (2005, February 17). B'Tselem to IDF Chief of Staff Ya'alon: Adopt the Recommendation to Stop House Demolitions.

(2009, December 27). One and a Half Million People Imprisoned.

(2010, July). By Hook and By Crook: Israeli Settlement Policy in the West Bank.

(2011, May). Dispossession and Exploitation: Israel's Policy in the Jordan Valley and Northern Dead Sea.

(2012, July 16). The Separation Barrier-Statistics.

(2012, October). Arrested Development: The Long Term Impact of the Separation Barrier.

(2012, October 11). Press Release: Five Attacks on Olive Harvesters and Damaged Olive Groves in Four Days.

(2013, December 25). Settler Violence: Lack of Accountability.

(2013, January 1). Israel's Control of the Airspace and the Territorial Waters of the Gaza Strip.

(2013, May 31). Israelis and Palestinians Killed in the Current Violence.

(2014, February 9). Gaza Strip: Over 90% of Water in Gaza Strip Unfit For Drinking.

(2014, July 24). Firing of Rockets and Other Projectiles into Israel [in Hebrew: transl. Yehonatan Alsheh].

Baehr, P. R. (1990). Human Rights and Peoples' Rights. *Human Rights in a Pluralist World: Individuals and Collectivities.* J. Berting, P. R. Baehr, J. H. Burgers et al. (eds.). Westport, CT, Meckler: 99–107.

(2001). *Human Rights: Universality in Practice.* New York, Palgrave.

Baer, M. (2015). The Palestinian People: Ambiguities of Citizenship. *The Human Right to Citizenship: A Slippery Concept.* R. E. Howard-Hassmann and M. Walton-Roberts (eds.). Philadelphia, University of Pennsylvania Press: 45–61.

Bajoria, J. (2012, February 29). The Six-Party Talks on North Korea's Nuclear Program. Council on Foreign Relations. New York.

Bakan, A. B. and Y. Abu-Laban (2009). "Palestinian Resistance and International Solidarity: The BDS Campaign." *Race & Class* 51(1): 29–54.

(2010). "Israel/Palestine, South Africa and the 'One-State Solution': The Case for an Apartheid Analysis." *Politikon* 37(2–3): 331–51.

Banya, N. (2012, February 3). Zimbabwe Bars Unregistered Foreign Newspapers. Reuters.

Banya, N. and M. Dzirutwe (2011, September 14). Zimbabwe Softens Tone With Foreign Miners. Mail and Guardian Online.

Barnette, J. (2010). "The Goldstone Report: Challenging Israeli Impunity in the International Legal System?" *Global Jurist* 10(3): 1–28.

Bazian, H. (2009). Palestine. *Encyclopedia of Human Rights.* D. P. Forsythe (ed.). New York, Oxford University Press 4: 175–86.

BBC News (2005, June 24). Africa Rejects Action on Zimbabwe.

(2008, July 7). Fury as Zimbabwe Sanctions Vetoed.

(2012, May 25). Zimbabwe's Mugabe: Lift Sanctions, UN's Navi Pillay urges.

Beaumont, P. (2014, December 25). Corruption Hampers Effort to Rebuiild Gaza after Summer Conflict. The Guardian.

(2014, December 31). Palestinian President Signs up to Join International Criminal Court. The Guardian.

(2015, January 16). ICC May Investigate Possible War Crimes in Palestinian Territories. The Guardian.

Becker, J. (2005). *Rogue Regime: Kim Jong Il and the Looming Threat of North Korea.* New York, Oxford University Press.

Beetham, D. (1995). "What Future for Economic and Social Rights?" *Political Studies* 53: 41–60.

Bell, A. (2010, December 2). Zuma, Banda Stand by Mugabe on Sanctions. SW Radio Africa News.

(2010, July 2). SA Farmer Arrested & Evicted from Chipinge Farm. SW Radio Africa News.

(2010, September 1). Mugabe Vows no Reversal of Land Grab. The Zimbabwean.

(2011, May 30). AU Credibility Questioned as Zim Set to Chair Peace Organ. SW Radio Africa News.

(2011, June 3). Top Lawyers Say SADC Turning its Back on Human Rights. SW Radio Africa News.

(2012, February 16). Zimbabwe: Top African Court Urged to Tackle SADC Breach of Human Rights. SW Radio Africa News.

(2014, March 5). Top African Court 'Powerless' to Reinstate SADC Tribunal. Zimbabwe Situation.

Bellamy, A. J. (2015). "A Chronic Protection Problem: The DPRK and the Responsibility to Protect." *International Affairs* 91(2): 225–44.

Belton, K. (2015). Statelessness: A Matter of Human Rights. *The Human Right to Citizenship: A Slippery Concept.* R. E. Howard-Hassmann and M. Walton-Roberts (eds.). Philadelphia, University of Pennsylvania Press: 31–42.

Ben-Eliezer, U. and Y. Feinstein (2007). "The Battle over Our Homes: Reconstructing/Deconstructing Sovereign Practices around Israel's Separation Barrier on the West Bank." *Israel Studies* 12(1): 171–92.

Benvenisti, E. (2004). *The International Law on Occupation.* Princeton, Princeton University Press.

Berger, T. R. (1981). *Fragile Freedoms: Human Rights and Dissent in Canada.* Toronto, Clarke, Irwin and Co.

Bernstein, R. (2007, March 1). "How Not to Deal with North Korea." *New York Review of Books* 54(3): 37–39.

Bernstein, T. P. (2006). "Mao Zedong and the Famine of 1959–60: A Study in Wilfulness." *The China Quarterly* 186: 421–55.

Besada, H. and N. Moyo (2008a). Zimbabwe in Crisis: Mugabe's Policies and Failures. Waterloo, Canada, Centre for International Governance Innovation.

(2008b). Picking Up the Pieces of Zimbabwe's Economy. Waterloo, Canada, Centre for International Governance Innovation.

Bhebhe, N. (2011, September 8). Zimbabwe: Anti-Corruption Commission has Mammoth Task. Zimbabwe Independent.

Bhebhe, V. (2010, August 28). Mugabe Sets up Military State. The Zimbabwean.

Bickerton, I. J. (2012). *The Arab-Israel Conflict: A Guide for the Perplexed*. New York, Continuum.

Blaire, D. (2002). *Degrees in Violence: Robert Mugabe and the Struggle for Power in Zimbabwe*. New York, Continuum.

Blanchard, B. (2012, August 9). North Korean Famine Not Imminent but Flood Impact Not Yet Clear: U.N. The New York Times.

Blecher, R. (2009). "Operation Cast Lead in the West Bank." *Journal of Palestine Studies* 38(3): 64–71.

Bloch, A. (2010). "The Right to Rights?: Undocumented Migrants from Zimbabwe Living in South Africa." *Sociology* 44(2): 233–50.

Bluth, C. (2008). *Korea*. Cambridge, UK, Polity.

Bolivarian Republic of Venezuela (1999). Constitution of Venezuela.

Bourdillon, M. F. C. (2008). Zimbabwe: Society and Cultures. *New Encyclopedia of Africa*. J. Middleton and J. C. Miller (eds.). New York, Thomson Gale 5: 333–36.

Bowcott, O. (2014, December 5). ICC Drops Murder and Rape Charges against Kenyan President. The Guardian.

Bratton, M. and E. Masunungure (2006). "Popular Reactions to State Repression: Murambatsvina in Zimbabwe." *African Affairs* 106(422): 21–45.

Brewer-Carias, A. R. (2010). *Dismantling Democracy in Venezuela: The Chavez Authoritarian Experiment*. New York, Cambridge University Press.

Briceno-Leon, R. (2005). "Petroleum and Democracy in Venezuela." *Social Forces* 84(1): 1–23.

British Library. (undated). "The 1832 Reform Act."

Brysk, A. (2013). *Speaking Rights to Power: Constructing Political Will*. New York, Oxford University Press.

Buchan, R. (2012). "The Palmer Report and the Legality of Israel's Naval Blockade of Gaza." *International and Comparative Law Quarterly* 61(1): 264–73.

Burke, R. (2010). *Decolonization and the Evolution of International Human Rights*. Philadelphia, University of Pennsylvania Press.

Bush, G. W. (2002, January 29). Text of President Bush's 2002 State of the Union Address. The Washington Post.

Butterfield, D., J. Isaac, et al. (2000). Impacts of Water and Export Market Restrictions on Palestinian Agriculture. Hamilton, Ontario, McMaster University and Econometric Research Limited and Applied Research Institute of Jerusalem (ARIJ).

Butterly, J. R. and J. Shepherd (2010). *Hunger: The Biology and Politics of Starvation*. Hanover, NH, University Press of New England.

Byers, M. (2005). *War Law*. Vancouver/Toronto, Douglas & McIntyre.

Byom, K. (2013, July 24). Zimbabwe by the Numbers. Washington, D.C., Freedom House.

Calderisi, R. (2006). *The Trouble with Africa: Why Foreign Aid Isn't Working*. New York, NY, Palgrave Macmillan.

Carens, J. H. (1995). Aliens and Citizens: The Case for Open Borders. *Theorizing Citizenship*. R. Beiner (ed.). Albany, State University of New York Press: 229–53.

Carey, S. C., M. Gibney, et al. (2010). *The Politics of Human Rights: The Quest for Dignity*. New York, Cambridge University Press.

Carter, J. (2006). *Palestine: Peace Not Apartheid*. New York, Simon and Schuster.

Caryl, C. (2008). "The Other North Korea." *New York Review of Books* 55 (13): 25–27.

(2010). "North Korea: The Crisis of Faith." *New York Review of Books* 57 (12): 29–31.

Castaneda, J. G. (2006). "Latin America's Left Turn." *Foreign Affairs* 85 (3): 28–43.

Cawthorne, A. (2012, September 10). Venezuela's Chavez Woos Rich, Warns of "Civil War". Reuters.

(2014, April 26). 16 People Arrested in Venezuela for Raising Prices on Food More than the Government Allows. Reuters.

Central Intelligence Agency (2008). The World Factbook.

(2013a). The World Factbook: Middle East: Gaza Strip.

(2013b). The World Factbook: Middle East: West Bank.

(2013c). The World Factbook: Middle East: Israel.

(2015). World Factbook: Zimbabwe.

CEPAL (2014). Panorama Social de America Latina Comision Economica para America Latina y el Caribe (Economic Commission for Latin America and the Caribbean).

Chadenga, S. (2013, July 26). Mugabe Takes a Swipe at White People. Canada Free Press.

Chalk, F. and K. Jonassohn (1990). *The History and Sociology of Genocide: Analyses and Case Studies*. New Haven, Yale University Press.

Chan, E. and A. Schloenhardt (2007). "North Korean Refugees and International Refugee Law." *International Journal of Refugee Law* 19(2): 215–45.

Chang, J. (1991). *Wild Swans: Three Daughters of China*. New York, Simon and Schuster.

Chang, J. and J. Halliday (2005). *Mao: The Unknown Story*. New York, Alfred A. Knopf.

Charbonneau, L. (2012, November 29). Palestinians Win Implicit U.N. Recognition of Sovereign State. Reuters.

Chen, Y. and L.-A. Zhou (2007). "The Long-term Health and Economic Consequences of the 1959–61 Famine in China." *Journal of Health Economics* 26: 659–81.

Chiefs' Assembly on Education (2012, October 1–3). Federal Funding for First Nations Schools. Palais des Congres de Gatineau, Gatineau, Quebec.

Chikanda, A. (2010). Nursing the Health System: The Migration of Health Professionals from Zimbabwe. *Zimbabwe's Exodus: Crisis, Migration, Survival*. J. Crush and D. Tevara (eds.). Cape Town and Ottawa, Southern African Migration Programme and International Development Research Centre.

China Post. (2010, July 7). Aid Group: NKorea Jailed Kin of Currency Reformer. China Post.

Chinaka, C. (2012, June 14). "Illegal" Hiring Leaves Zimbabwe Army Hungry. Reuters.

Chivara, I. (2013, May 3). Zimbabwe: The Land Issue Revisited. Mail and Guardian.

Choe, S.-H. and D. E. Sanger (2013, December 23). Korea Execution is Tied to Clash Over Businesses. The New York Times.

Clapham, A. (2006). *Human Rights Obligations of Non-State Actors*. New York, Oxford University Press.

Clapp, J. (2012). *Food*. Malden, MA, Polity.

Clark, A. M. (2009). International Sources of Human Rights Change. West Lafayette, IND, Purdue University.

Cliffe, L., J. Alexander, et al. (2011). "An Overview of Fast Track Land Reform in Zimbabwe: Editorial Introduction." *Journal of Peasant Studies* 38(5): 907–38.

Cohen, R. (2010, September 14). Legal Grounds for Protection of North Korean Refugees. Washington, D.C., Brookings Institution.

(2013). World Food Day: The Challenge of North Korea. *Brookings East Asia Commentary No. 71*. Washington, D.C., Brookings Institution.

Cohen, S. E. (2006). "Israel's West Bank Barrier: An Impediment to Peace?" *Geographical Review* 96(4): 682–95.

COI: United Nations General Assembly (2014, February 7). Report of the Detailed Findings of the Commission of Inquiry on Human Rights in the Democratic People's Republic of Korea, Human Rights Council. A/HRC/25/CRP.1.

Coleman-Jensen, A., C. Gregory, et al. (2014). Household Food Security in the United States in 2013: Statistical Supplement. Washington, D.C., United States Department of Agriculture.

Committee on Economic Social and Cultural Rights (1999). General Comment No. 12: The Right to Adequate Food. Geneva, Economic and Social Council, United Nations.

(2002). General Comment No. 15: The Right to Water (arts. 11 and 12 of the International Covenant on Economic, Social and Cultural Rights). Geneva, Economic and Social Council. United Nations.

Conquest, R. (1986). *The Harvest of Sorrow: Soviet Collectivization and the Terror-Famine*. Edmonton, University of Alberta Press.

Cook, J. (2012, October 24). Israel's Starvation Diet Formula in Gaza and the Expansion of the 'Dahiya doctrine'. Mondoweiss.net.

Corcoran, B. (2012, February 2). Mugabe's Poor Health behind Drive by Zanu-PF for Elections, says MDC. Irish Times.

Cordova Cazar, A. L. and F. Lopez-Bermudez (2009). Latin American Populism. *Encyclopedia of Human Rights*. D. P. Forsythe (ed.). New York, Oxford University Press. 3: 400–411.

Corrales, J. (2006). "Hugo Boss." *Foreign Policy* 152: 32–40.

(2011). "A Setback for Chavez." *Journal of Democracy* 22(1): 122–36.

(2013). Explaining Chavismo: The Unexpected Alliance of Radical Leftists and the Military in Venezuela since the late 1990s. *Venezuela Before Chavez: Anatomy of a Collapse*. R. Hausmann and F. Rodriguez (eds.). University Park, PA, Penn State University Press.

(2013, March 14). Comments on Earlier Draft of chapter on Venezuela. R. E. Howard-Hassmann.

(2013, March 7). The House That Chavez Built. Foreign Policy.com.

Corrales, J. and M. Penfold (2011). *Dragon in the Tropics: Hugo Chavez and the Political Economy of Revolution in Venezuela*. Washington, D.C., Brookings Institution Press.

Criddle, J. D. and T. B. Mam (1996). To Destroy You is No Loss: The Odyssey of a Cambodian Family. *From the Gulag to the Killing Fields*. P. Hollander (ed.). Wilmington, DE, ISI Books.

Crush, J. and D. Tevera (2010). Exiting Zimbabwe. *Zimbabwe's Exodus: Crisis, Migration, Survival*. J. Crush and D. Tevera (eds.). Kingston and Cape Town, Southern African Migration Program and International Development Research Centre: 1–49.

Cumings, B. (2005). *Korea's Place in the Sun: A Modern History*. New York, W.W. Norton.

Daguerre, A. (2011). "Antipoverty Programmes in Venezuela." *Journal of Social Policy* 40(4): 835–52.

Daniel, F. J. (2008, April 30). "Stumbling Toward Food Security: Hobbled by Poor Planning, Venezuela Confronts Shortages." International Herald Tribune 15.

(2010, May 16). Chavez Signs New Currency Law against Speculation. Reuters.

Daschuk, J. (2013). *Clearing the Plains: Disease, Politics of Starvation, and the Loss of Aboriginal Life*. Regina, University of Regina Press.

Dashwood, H. (2004). Zimbabwe and Sustainable Peacebuilding. *Durable Peace: Challenges for Peacebuilding in Africa*. T. M. Ali and R. O. Matthews (eds.). Toronto, University of Toronto Press: 219–50.

Dashwood, H. and C. Pratt (1999). Leadership, Participation and Conflict Management: Zimbabwe and Tanzania. *Civil Wars in Africa: Roots and Resolution*. T. M. Ali and R. O. Matthews (eds.). Montreal, McGill-Queen's University Press: 223–54.

Dauvergne, M. (2012). Adult Correctional Statistics in Canada, 2010/2011. Ottawa, Statistics Canada.

Davies, R. W. and S. G. Wheatcroft (2006). "Stalin and the Soviet Famine of 1932–33: A Reply to Ellman." *Europe-Asia Studies* 58(4): 625–33.

Davis, M. (2002). *Late Victorian Holocausts: El Nino Famines and the Making of the Third World*. New York, Verso.

De Nie, M. (1998). "The Famine, Irish Identity, and the British Press." *Irish Studies Review* 6(1): 27–35.

De Schutter, O. (2012). Visit to Canada from 6 to 16 May 2012, Office of the United Nations High Commissioner for Human Rights.

de Waal, A. (1991). "Famine and Human Rights." *Development in Practice* 1(2): 77–83.

de Waal, A. and A. Whiteside (2003). "New Variant Famine: AIDS and Food Crisis in Southern Africa." *Lancet* 362: 1234–37.

DeFalco, R. C. (2009). "The Right to Food in Gaza: Israel's Obligations under International Law." *Rutgers Law Record* 35: 11–22.

Delgado, A. M. (2013, March 27). Venezuela Interim President Maduro Takes on Currency Exchange Website. El Nuevo Herald.

Demick, B. (2009). *Nothing to Envy: Ordinary Lives in North Korea.* New York, Spiegel and Grau.

(2012, October 14). North Korea's Progress Seems to be More Style than Substance. Los Angeles Times.

Democratic People's Republic of Korea, trans. Steve S. Sin, (2009). North Korea Constitution. Pyongyang.

Dershowitz, A. (2010). The Case against the Goldstone Report: A Study in Evidentiary Bias. Accessed at https://dash.harvard.edu/handle/1/3593975.

Deutsche Presse-Agentur (2007, September 4). Zimbabwe Chair of UN Green Commission 'Destroyed Seized Farm'.

Devereux, C. (2012, September 4). Venezuelan Inflation Slows Further as Chavez Eyes Votes. Business Week.

Devereux, S. (2007a). Introduction: From 'old famines' to 'new famines'. *The New Famines: Why Famines Persist in an Era of Globalization.* S. Devereux (ed.). New York, Routledge: 1–26.

(2007b). Sen's Entitlement Approach: Critiques and Counter-critiques. *The New Famines: Why Famines Persist in an Era of Globalization.* S. Devereux (ed.). New York, Routledge: 66–89.

Dickinson, H. and T. Wotherspoon (1992). From Assimilation to Self-Government: Towards a Political Economy of Canada's Aboriginal Policies. *Deconstructing a Nation: Immigration, Multiculturalism & Racism in '90s Canada.* V. Satzewich (ed.). Halifax, Fernwood Publishing: 405–21.

Dicklitch, S. and R. E. Howard-Hassmann (2007). Public Policy and Economic Rights in Ghana and Uganda. *Economic Rights: Conceptual, Measurement, and Policy Issues.* S. Hertel and L. Minkler (eds.). New York, Cambridge University Press: 325–44.

Dietrich, D. J. (1981). "Holocaust as Public Policy: The Third Reich." *Human Relations* 34(6): 445–62.

Dikötter, F. (2010). *Mao's Great Famine: The History of China's Most Devastating Catastrophe, 1958–1962.* New York, Walker & Co.

Donath, M. (2014, November 18). U.N. Panel Calls for North Korea Referral to International Court. Reuters.

Donnelly, J. (2003). *Universal Human Rights in Theory and Practice,* 2nd edition. Ithaca, NY, Cornell University Press.

(2007). The West and Economic Rights. *Economic Rights: Conceptual, Measurement, and Policy Issues.* S. Hertel and L. Minkler (eds.). New York, Cambridge University Press: 37–55.

Dore, D. (2012, May 4). The Nationalist Narrative and Land Policy in Zimbabwe. Sokwanele.

(2012, November 13). Myths, Reality and the Inconvenient Truth about Zimbabwe's Land Resettlement Programme. Sokwanele.

Dowty, A. (2012). *Israel/Palestine,* 3rd edition. Cambridge, UK, Polity.

D'Souza, F. (1990). Preface. *Starving in Silence: A Report on Famine and Censorship.* London, Article 19.

Duarte Villa, R. (2007). "Venezuela: Political Changes in the Chavez Era." *Estudos Avancados* 21(55): 153–72.

Dube, G. (2011, June 2). Zimbabwe Government, Civil Service Representatives, Deadlock on Wages. VoANews.com.

(2012, May 8). Hunger-Stricken Zimbabwe Villagers Trade Off Livestock at Low Prices. VoANews.com.

Dugger, C. W. (2008, October 12). Mugabe Claims Security Ministries, Jeopardizing Deal. The New York Times.

DVA Group and Selinger Group (2013, January 15). *Venezuelan Daily Brief.* Online.

(2013, January 18). *Venezuelan Daily Brief.* Online.

(2013, January 22). *Venezuelan Daily Brief.* Online.

(2013, January 25). *Venezuelan Daily Brief.* Online.

The Economist (2001, April 26). Back to the Soil.

(2008, May 10). North Korea: Let Them Eat Juche. 1.

(2008, September 27). The Odd Couple: A Special Report on the Koreas. 1–19.

(2009, January 3). Socialism with Cheap Oil: Venezuela. 26.

(2009, February 21). Chavez For ever? Venezuela's Term-limits Referendum. 39.

(2009, March 7). Whose Land? 57–58.

(2009, March 12). Socialism in Venezuela: Feeding Frenzy. 40.

(2009, May 9). Socialism v. Labour: Trade Unions in Venezuela. 39.

(2009, June 6). An (iron) Fistful of Help: Development Aid from Authoritarian Regimes. 59.

(2009, September 10). "Robert Mugabe off the hook as usual." 52–53.

(2009, October 24). Hell on Earth. 56.

(2009, December 12). Fall of the Boligarchs: Banking in Venezuela. 40.

(2010, January 16). Mad, Bad and Dangerous to Know. 45.

(2010, January 30). Venezuela's Drift to Authoritarianism: Wolf Sheds Fleece. 44–46.

(2010, April 24). Foreigners and Local Whites Out. 48.

(2010, May 29). Not Waving. Perhaps Drowning. 23–25.

(2010, June 12). Venezuelan Socialism: Food Fight. 43.

(2011, January 1). Hugo Chavez's Venezuela: A Coup against the Constitution. 31.

(2011, February 26). Venezuela's Economy: Oil Leak. 43.

(2011, June 25). A New Road Map for Zimbabwe? 57.

(2011, September 17). Deprive and Rule. 42.

(2012, February 11). Mano a Mano. 39.

(2012, August 11). Venezuela's Army: The Vote that Counts. 32.

(2012, September 1). Venezuela's Refinery Disaster: A Tragedy Foretold. 39.

(2012, September 29). Venezuela's Presidential Election: Henrique and Hugoliath.

(2013, February 9). Venezuela's Economy: Out of Stock. 40.

(2013, February 23). Robert Mugabe's Last Throw? 45–46.

(2013, May 4). Squeeze Them Out. 50–51.

(2013, May 11). Park's Progress. 58.

(2013, August 10). Stealing the Vim from Zim. 41.

(2013, December 14). Crying Uncle: Kim Jong Un has Managed the Improbable Feat of Making North Korea even Scarier. 52.

(2014, February 1). Venezuela and Argentina: The Party is Over. 27–29.

(2014, February 22). Protests in Venezuela: A Tale of Two Prisoners. 30–31.

(2014, March 8). North Korea: Better Tomorrow? 42–43.

(2014, May 17). Venezuela's Unrest: Stumbling Towards Chaos. 36.

(2014, August 30). Long May it Hold. 43.

(2014, October 4). A Sea of Despair. 56.

(2014, December 6). The Cuban Question. 40.

(2015, February 28). North Korea's Economy; Spring Release. 32–34.

(2015, April 4). Venezuela: Maduro's Muzzle. 32–33.

(2015, April 25). Blood at the End of the Rainbow: Xenophobia in South Africa. 44.

(2015, May 2). Netanyahu v the Supreme Court. 39.

(2015, June 20). Food and Venezuela: Let Them Eat Chavismo. 36.

Ecumenical Zimbabwe Network (2008, June 25). Call for International Intervention in Zimbabwe. Pambuzuka News.

Edelman, M. and C. James (2011). "Peasants' Rights and the UN System: Quixotic Struggle? Or Emancipatory Idea Whose Time Has Come?" *Journal of Peasant Studies* 38(1): 81–108.

Editors (2012, March 22). Don't Punish Kim Jong Un's People for his Missile Madness. Bloomberg News.

Edkins, J. (2007). The Criminalization of Mass Starvations: From Natural Disaster to Crime against Humanity. *The New Famines: Why Famines Persist in a Era of Globalization*. S. Devereux (ed.). New York, Routledge: 50–65.

Egeland, G. M., A. Pacey, et al. (2010). "Food Insecurity Among Inuit Preschoolers: Nunavut Inuit Child Health Survey, 2007–2008." *Canadian Medical Association Journal* 182 (3): 243–48.

Egeland, G. M., L. Johnson-Down, et al. (2011). "Food Insecurity and Nutrition Transition Combine to Affect Nutrient Intakes in Canadian Arctic Communities." *The Journal of Nutrition* 141: 1746–53.

Eide, A. (1989). "Realization of Social and Economic Rights and the Minimum Threshold Approach." *Human Rights Law Journal* 10(1–2): 35–51.

(2006). Economic, Social, and Cultural Rights as Human Rights. *Human Rights in the World Community: Issues and Action*, 3rd edition. R. P. Claude and B. H. Weston (eds.). Philadelphia, University of Pennsylvania Press: 170–79.

El Amrani, I. (2013, February 20). Tunnel Vision. The New York Times.

El Universal (2012, November 1). Imports Feed Consumption in Venezuela.

(2013, June 12). Maduro Estimates Overconsumption at 30%.

(2013, September 19). Cargo Ships with 353 Tons of Food Stuck in Puerto Cabello, Venezuela.

(2013, November 18). Industrias estatizadas registran perdidas: Control estatal en empresas ha impactado su salud financiera.

Elizur, Y. (2014, January 24). Over and Drought: Why the End of Israel's Water Shortage is a Secret. Haaretz.com.

Elliott, J. (2009, September 29). Zimbabwe: Hold the Line. Huffington Post.

Ellman, M. (2005). "The Role of Leadership Perceptions and of Intent in the Soviet Famine of 1931–34." *Europe-Asia Studies* 57(6): 823–41.

Ellner, S. (2007). "Toward a 'Multipolar World': Using Oil Diplomacy to Sever Venezuela's Dependence." *NACLA Report on the Americas* 40(5): 15–43.

Ellsworth, B. (2009, March 7). Chavez Takes on Venezuela's Food Sector: Showdowns with Industry Have Cut Country's GDP. Reuters.

Engels, F. (1969 [first English edition 1892: first German edition 1845]). *The Condition of the Working Class in England*. London, Panther Books.

Epstein, E. (2013, February 21). Economic Conflict Boils on the Chinese-North Korean Border. MSN News.

Evans, G. (2008). *The Responsibility to Protect: Ending Mass Atrocity Crimes Once and for All*. Washington, DC, Brookings Institution Press.

Evans, S. (2015, January 14). A Quiet Revolution in North Korea. BBC News.

Fajardo, T. (accessed December 3, 2014). Soft Law. Oxford Bibliographies. *web*.

Falk, R. A. (2005). "Toward Authoritativeness: The ICJ Ruling on Israel's Security Wall." *American Journal of International Law* 99(1): 42–52.

FAO/WFP (2011, November 25). FAO/WFP Crop and Food Security Assessment Mission to the Democratic People's Republic of Korea. Rome, Food and Agriculture Organization and World Food Programme.

FAOSTAT Zimbabwe: Country Profile. Rome, Food and Agriculture Organization.

Farer, T. (1991). "Israel's Unlawful Occupation." *Foreign Policy* 82: 37–58.

Farsakh, L. (2000). "Under Siege: Closure, Separation and the Palestinian Economy." *Middle East Research and Information Project* 217: 22–25.

Feffer, J. (2006). North Korea and the Politics of Famine. *FPIF Special Report*. Washington, DC, Foreign Policy in Focus.

Feierstein, D. (2006). "Political Violence in Argentina and its Genocidal Characteristics." *Journal of Genocide Research* 8(2): 149–68.

Fein, H. (1979). *Accounting for Genocide: National Responses and Jewish Victimization during the Holocaust*. Chicago, IL, University of Chicago Press.

(1990). "Genocide: A Sociological Perspective." *Current Sociology* 38(1): 1–126.

(1993). "Genocide by Attrition 1939–1993: The Warsaw Ghetto, Cambodia and Sudan." *Health and Human Rights* 2(2): 11–45.

Feldman, I. (2009). "Gaza's Humanitarianism Problem." *Journal of Palestine Studies* 38(3): 22–37.

Felice, W. F. (1996). *Taking Suffering Seriously: The Importance of Collective Human Rights*. Albany, NY, State University of New York Press.

Feunteun, T. (2015). "Cartels and the Right to Food: An Analysis of States' Duties and Options." *Journal of International Economic Law* 18: 341–82.

Fields, J. (2013, April 18). Zimbabwe's Last White Ruler Struck Off Voter Role. Scotsman.

Figes, O. (2007). *The Whisperers: Private Life in Stalin's Russia*. New York, Picador.

Food and Agriculture Organization (2005). Voluntary Guidelines to Support the Progressive Realization of the Right to Adequate Food in the Context of National Food Security. Rome, Food and Agriculture Organization.

(2013). Food Security Indicators, Food and Agriculture Organization.

Food and Agriculture Organization and Office for the Coordination of Humanitarian Affairs (2010, May). Farming without Land, Fishing without Water: Gaza Agriculture Section Struggles to Survive, United Nations.

Food Banks Canada (2012). Hunger Count 2012: A Comprehensive Report on Hunger and Food Bank Use in Canada, and Recommendations for Change. Mississauga, Ontario, Food Banks Canada.

Forsythe, D. P. (2012). *Human Rights in International Relations*, 3rd edition. New York, Cambridge University Press.

Fox News (2013, March 25). Administration Moves $500m in Palestinian Aid, as Agencies Scramble to Delay Furloughs. Fox News.

Fox News Latino (2011, June 24). Thousands of Venezuelans Have Gotten Political Asylum in the U.S. Fox News.

Fraunces, M. G. (1992). "The International Law of Blockade: New Guiding Principles in Contemporary State Practice." *The Yale Law Journal* 101(4): 893–918.

French, P. (2007). *North Korea, the Paranoid Peninsula: A Modern History*, 2nd edition. New York, Zed.

Frideres, J. S. (1988). *Native Peoples in Canada: Contemporary Conflicts*, 3rd edition. Scarborough, ON, Prentice-Hall.

Frisch, H. and M. Hofnung (2007). "Power or Justice? Rule and Law in the Palestinian Authority." *Journal of Peace Research* 44(3): 331–48.

G8 Leaders (2008, July 8). Statement on Zimbabwe. Hokkaido Toyako Summit, G8.

Galloway, G. (2013, October 4). Atleo Hopes UN Visit will 'hold a mirror' to Gap between Canada and First Nations. Globe and Mail.

Gasser, H.-P. (2009). Humanitarian Law. *Encyclopedia of Human Rights*. D. P. Forsythe (ed.). New York, Oxford University Press. 2: 462–72.

Gause, K. E. (2011). *North Korea under Kim Chong-il: Power, Politics, and Prospects for Change*. Santa Barbara, CA, Praeger.

Gavaghan, J. (2009, April 2). Life in Mugabe's Hell Hole: Zimbabwe Jail Exposed in Secret Film that Shows Inmates Starving to Death. Mail Online.

Geneva Convention (1949). Convention (IV) Relative to the Protection of Civilian Persons in Time of War, Geneva.

Genocide Scholars and Professionals (2009, February 24). Declaration of Genocide Scholars and Professionals on Israel and Palestine.

Gibbs, T. (2006). "Business as Unusual: What the Chavez Era Tells Us about Democracy under Globalisation." *Third World Quarterly* 27(2): 265–79.

Gibney, M. (2002). "On the Need for an International Civil Court." *Fletcher Forum on World Affairs* 26: 47–56.

(2008). *International Human Rights Law: Returning to Universal Principles*. Lanham, MD, Rowman and Littlefield.

(2015). *International Human Rights Law: Returning to Universal Principles*, 2nd edition. New York, Rowman and Littlefield.

Girling, R. (2006, July 2). Defence of the Realm. Sunday Times Features.

Gisha (2008, December). Gaza Closure Defined: Collective Punishment. Legal Center for Freedom of Movement.

(2012, October 17). "Red Lines" Presentation Released after 3.5-year Legal Battle: Israel Calculated the Number of Calories It Would Allow Gaza Residents to Consume. Legal Center for Freedom of Movement.

Global Centre for the Responsibility to Protect (2009, January 30). Zimbabwe: What Can be Done, Who Must Act? New York, Ralph Bunche Institute for International Studies, CUNY Graduate Center.

Glover, J. (2001). *Humanity: A Moral History of the Twentieth Century*. London, Pimlico.

Godwin, P. (2010). *The Fear: Robert Mugabe and the Martyrdom of Zimbabwe*. New York, Little, Brown and Company.

Goedde, P. (2010). "Legal Mobilization for Human Rights Protection in North Korea: Furthering Discourse or Discord?" *Human Rights Quarterly* 32 (3): 530–74.

Goldstone, R. (2009). Human Rights in Palestine and Other Occupied Arab Territories: Report of the United Nations Fact-Finding Mission on the Gaza Conflict. Human Rights Council. New York, United Nations General Assembly.

Gonda, V. and B. Zulu (2012, February 8). Zimbabwe President, PM Said to Agree Acting Status for Police Chief Chihuri. VoANews.com.

Good Friends: Research Institute for North Korean Society (2012, May 23). North Korea Today No. 456: Three Major Steel Mills Experiencing Severe Food Shortage.

Goodkind, D. and L. West (2001). "The North Korean Famine and its Demographic Impact." *Population and Development Review* 27(2): 219–38.

Gordon, N. (2008). *Israel's Occupation*. Berkeley, University of California Press.

(2014, April 21). Personal Communication. R. E. Howard-Hassmann.

Gordon, N. and Y. Cohen (2012). "Western Interests, Israeli Unilateralism, and the Two-State Solution." *Journal of Palestine Studies* 61(3): 6–18.

Gordon, N. and D. Filc (2005). "Hamas and the Destruction of Risk Society." *Constellations* 12(4): 542–60.

Gott, R. (2011). *Hugo Chavez and the Bolivarian Revolution*. New York, Verso.

Government of Canada (1982). Canadian Charter of Rights and Freedoms Ottawa, Government of Canada.

Government of the United Kingdom (1914). Defence of the Realm Consolidation Act, 27 November 1914. London.

Government of Venezuela (2015, January 27). Gaceta Oficial de la Republica Bolivariana de Venezuela, no. 40.589 (trans. Antulio Rosales), Ministry of Defense.

Government of Zimbabwe (2007). Indigenisation and Economic Empowerment Act, 2007. Harare, Government of Zimbabwe.

(2013). Constitution of Zimbabwe. Harare, Government of Zimbabwe.

Grant, W. (2010, November 15). Why Venezuela's Government is Taking Over Apartments. BBC News.

Greenberg, J. (2011, July 22). Israeli Anti-boycott Law Stirs Debate on Settlement Products. Washington Post.

Greenslade Blog (2010, November 22). Exiled Zimbabwe Editor Faces Arrest. Greenslade Blog, Guardian.co.uk.

Grundy, T. (2006, October 2). Whatever Happened to Didymus Mutasa? London, Institute for War Reporting.

Gubbay, A. R. (1997). "The Protection and Enforcement of Fundamental Human Rights: The Zimbabwean Experience." *Human Rights Quarterly* 19(2): 227–54.

Gupta, G. (2014, January 23). Venezuela: The 'Cheapest' Country in the World. World.Time.Com.

Gutierrez, A. (2013a). *El Sistema Alimentario Venezolano A Comienzos Del Siglo XXI: Evolucion, Balance y Desafios.* Merida, Venezuela, Consejo de Publicaciones-FACES ULA.

(2013b). Telephone Conversation with Antulio Rosales on Venezuelan Food Statistics. A. Rosales. Waterloo, Ontario.

Hafner-Burton, E. M. (2013). *Making Human Rights a Reality.* Princeton, Princeton University Press.

Haggard, S. and M. Noland (2007). *Famine in North Korea: Markets, Aid, and Reform.* New York, Columbia University Press.

(2009). Repression and Punishment in North Korea: Survey Evidence of Prison Camp Experiences. Honolulu, East-West Center.

(2011). *Witness to Transformation: Refugee Insights into North Korea.* Washington, DC, Peterson Institute for International Economics.

Haig-Brown, C. (1988). *Resistance and Renewal: Surviving the Indian Residential School.* Vancouver, Tillacum Library.

Halbertal, M. (2009, November 6). The Goldstone Illusion. *New Republic.*

Hammer, J. (2008a, June 26). "The Reign of Thuggery." *New York Review of Books* 55(11): 26–29.

(2008b, August 14). "Scandal in Africa." *New York Review of Books* 55(13): 4.

(2009a, February 12). "Will He Rule South Africa?" *New York Review of Books* 56(2): 28–31.

(2009b, October 25). "Dictator Mugabe Makes a Comeback." *New York Review of Books* 56(16): 48–49.

Hanke, S. H. (2009). R.I.P. Zimbabwe Dollar. Johns Hopkins University, Cato Institute.

(2013, June 22). Why the World Should be Rallying for the 'Yuan-ization' of North Korea. Business Insider.

Hanlon, J., J. Manjengwa, et al. (2013). *Zimbabwe Takes Back Its Land.* Sterling, Virginia, Kumarian Press.

Harff, B. and T. R. Gurr (1988). "Toward Empirical Theory of Genocides and Politicides: Identification and Measurement of Cases since 1945." *International Studies Quarterly* 32(3): 359–71.

Hassig, R. and K. Oh (2009). *The Hidden People of North Korea: Everyday Life in the Hermit Kingdom.* New York, Rowman and Littlefield.

Hathaway, J. C. (2014). "Food Deprivation: A Basis for Refugee Status?" *Social Research* 81(2): 327–39.

Hathaway, O. (2002). "Do Human Rights Treaties Make a Difference?" *The Yale Law Journal* 111(8): 1935–2042.

Haugen, H. M. (2009). "Food Sovereignty–An Appropriate Approach to Ensure the Right to Food?" *Nordic Journal of International Law* 78: 263–93.

Hawk, D. (2003). The Hidden Gulag: Exposing North Korea's Prison Camps. Washington, D.C., U.S. Committee for Human Rights in North Korea.

Hawkins, T. (2009). The Mining Sector in Zimbabwe and its Potential Contribution to Recovery, United Nations Development Programme.

(2013, June 5). Inconvenient Truths about Land Resettlement in Zimbabwe. Nehanda Radio: Zimbabwe News and Internet Radio Station.

Helfont, T. (2010). "Egypt's Wall with Gaza & the Emergence of a New Middle East Alignment." *Orbis: A Journal of World Affairs*, 54(3): 426–40.

Hellinger, D. (2011). "Obama and the Bolivarian Agenda for the Americas." *Latin American Perspectives* 38(4): 46–62.

Hellum, A. and B. Derman (2004). "Land Reform and Human Rights in Contemporary Zimbabwe: Balancing Individual and Social Justice through an Integrated Human Rights Framework." *World Development* 32(10): 1785–805.

Hidalgo, M. (2009). "Hugo Chavez's 'Petro-socialism.' " *Journal of Democracy* 20 (2): 78–92.

Hill, G. (2005). *What Happens after Mugabe? Can Zimbabwe Rise from the Ashes?* Cape Town, Zebra Press.

HM Treasury (2014, February 25). Financial Sanctions Notice: Zimbabwe, United Kingdom.

Hogan, E. N. (2012). "Fieldnotes from Jerusalem and Gaza, 2009–11." *Journal of Palestine Studies* 41(2): 99–114.

Howard, G. and J. Bartram (2003). Domestic Water Quantity, Service Level and Health. Geneva, World Health Organization.

Howard, N. P. (1993). "The Social and Political Consequences of the Allied Food Blockade of Germany." *German History* 11(2): 161–88.

Howard, R. (1983). "The Full-Belly Thesis: Should Economic Rights take Priority over Civil and Political Rights? Evidence from Sub-Saharan Africa." *Human Rights Quarterly* 5(4): 467–90.

(1986). *Human Rights in Commonwealth Africa.* Totowa, NJ, Rowman and Littlefield.

(1995). *Human Rights and the Search for Community.* Boulder, CO, Westview.

Howard-Hassmann, R. E. (2003). *Compassionate Canadians: Civic Leaders Discuss Human Rights.* Toronto, University of Toronto Press.

(2010). *Can Globalization Promote Human Rights?* University Park, Pennsylvania, Pennsylvania State University Press.

(2012a). "Human Security: Undermining Human Rights?" *Human Rights Quarterly* 34(1): 88–112.

(2012b). "The Skeptical Forsythe: Peace, Human Rights, and Realpolitik." *Journal of Human Rights* 11(3): 356–59.

(2013). "Reconsidering the Right to Own Property." *Journal of Human Rights* 12(2): 180–97.

(2016 in press). State Enslavement in North Korea. *Contemporary Slavery and Human Rights*. J. Quirk and A. Bunting (eds.). Vancouver, University of British Columbia Press.

Howard-Hassmann, R. E. and C. E. Welch, eds. (2006). *Economic Rights in Canada and the United States*. Philadelphia, University of Pennsylvania Press.

Howe, P. (2002). "Reconsidering 'Famine'". *IDS (Institute of Development Studies) Bulletin* 33(4): 19–27.

(2007). Priority Regimes and Famine. *The New Famines: Why Famines Persist in an Era of Globalization*. S. Devereux (ed.). New York, Routledge: 336–62.

Human Rights Council (2010, September 24). Human Rights and Access to Safe Drinking Water and Sanitation. New York, United Nations.

Human Rights Watch (2002). Fast Track Land Reform in Zimbabwe. New York.

(2003a). Zimbabwe: Food Used as Political Weapon. New York.

(2003b). Zimbabwe: Not Eligible: The Politicization of Food in Zimbabwe. New York.

(2006a). A Matter of Survival: The North Korean Government's Control of Food and the Risk of Hunger. New York.

(2006b). World Report 2006: Events of 2005: Zimbabwe. New York.

(2007, March). North Korea: Harsher Policies against Border-Crossers. New York.

(2008a). A Decade under Chavez: Political Intolerance and Lost Opportunities for Advancing Human Rights in Venezuela. New York.

(2008b). Zimbabwe: Reverse Ban on Food Aid to Rural Areas. New York.

(2009a). Crisis without Limits: Human Rights and Humanitarian Consequences of Political Repression in Zimbabwe. New York.

(2009b). False Dawn: The Zimbabwe Power-Sharing Government's Failure to Deliver Human Rights Improvements. New York.

(2009c). Diamonds in the Rough: Human Rights Abuses in the Marange Diamond Fields of Zimbabwe. New York.

(2010a). Deliberate Chaos: Ongoing Human Rights Abuses in the Marange Diamond Fields of Zimbabwe. New York.

(2010b). World Report: Events of 2009. New York.

(2010, December 19). Israel/West Bank: Separate and Unequal. New York.

(2011). World Report: Events of 2010. New York.

(2012, October 3). Gaza: Arbitrary Arrests, Torture, Unfair Trials. New York.

(2013, April 4). Gaza: 'Collaborator' Murders Go Unpunished. New York.

(2013, July 28). Gaza: Let Media Offices Open. New York.

(2013, July 30). Palestine: Palestinian Authority Police Beat Protestors. New York.

Hummel, S. (2013, June 17). Venezuela: Eagerly Awaiting Food Aid from "Allied Countries". The Argentina Independent.

Hwang, K. M. (2010). *A History of Korea: An Episodic Narrative*. New York, Palgrave Macmillan.

Ide, W. (2012, February 29). North Korea to End Nuclear Tests for Food Aid. VoANews.Com.

(2012, March 28). US Suspends Food Assistance to North Korea. VoANewsCom.

Indian and Northern Affairs Canada (2008). Measuring the Well-Being of Aboriginal Peoples in Canada: The Registered Indian and Inuit Human Development Index and Community-Well-Being Index. Ottawa.

Inter-American Commission on Human Rights (2009, December 30). Democracy and Human Rights in Venezuela, Organization of American States.

Internal Displacement Monitoring Centre (2008, August). The Many Faces of Displacement: IDPs in Zimbabwe. Geneva.

International Bar Association Human Rights Institute (2007). Venezuela: Justice under Threat, International Bar Association.

International Commission on Intervention and State Sovereignty (2001). The Responsibility to Protect. Ottawa, International Development Research Centre.

International Court of Justice (2004, July 9). Press Release 2004/28: Legal Consequences of the Construction of a Wall in the Occupied Palestinian Territory. 2004/28. International Court of Justice.

International Criminal Court (1998). Rome Statute of the International Criminal Court.

(2009). ICC Issues a Warrant of Arrest for Omar Al Bashir, President of Sudan.

(2014, June). Situation of the Republic of Korea: Article 5 Report. The Hague, Office of the Prosecutor.

International Crisis Group (2004). Blood and Soil: Land, Politics and Conflict Prevention in Zimbabwe and South Africa. Brussels.

(2005). Post-election Zimbabwe: What Next? Brussels. Africa Briefing No. 93.

(2008, December 16). Ending Zimbabwe's Nightmare: A Possible Way Forward. Pretoria/Brussels. Africa Briefing No. 56.

(2012, February 6). Zimbabwe's Sanctions Standoff. Africa Briefing No. 86.

International Institute for Strategic Studies (2011). The Military Balance 2010. London.

International Justice Resource Center (accessed December 19, 2014). Universal Jurisdiction. San Francisco.

International Monetary Fund (2014, September 12). West Bank and Gaza: Report to the Ad Hoc Liaison Committee.

Investor's Business Daily (2015, January 16). Shortages Undermine Venezuela's Teetering Socialism. Investor's Business Daily.

IRIN Humanitarian News and Analysis (2006, July 8). AU Suspends Report on Zimbabwe Rights Abuses, UN Office for the Coordination of Humanitarian Affairs.

(2011, March 16). Zimbabwe: UN Agencies Barred from Food Assessment for 'political reasons', UN Office for the Coordination of Humanitarian Affairs.

(2012, February 17). Zimbabwe: More NGO Bannings Feared, UN Office for the Coordination of Humanitarian Affairs.

(2012, May 21). Zimbabwe: Small Grains are Tough Sell, UN Office for the Coordination of Humanitarian Affairs.

Jackson, A. (1996). Germany, The Home Front (2): Blockade, Government and Revolution. *Facing Armageddon: The First World War Experienced.* H. Cecil and P. Liddle (eds.). London, Leo Cooper.

Jacobs, D. (2010, February 17). Moving Past the Genocide Debate: Mass Atrocities and the International Community. *Conference on Theory vs. Policy? Connecting Scholars and Practitioners.* New Orleans.

James, I. (2010, August 31). Farmer-turned-hunger Striker Dies in Venezuela. Associated Press.

Jappah, J. V. and D. T. Smith (2012). "State Sponsored Famine: Conceptualizing Politically Induced Famine as a Crime against Humanity." *Journal of International and Global Studies* 4(1).

Jayne, T. S., M. Chisvo, et al. (2006). Zimbabwe's Food Insecurity Paradox: Hunger Amid Potential. *Zimbabwe's Agricultural Revolution Revisited.* M. Rukini, P. Tawonezvi, and C. Eicher (eds.). Harare, University of Zimbabwe Publications: 525–41.

Jerusalem Post (2014, July 20). The Corruption at the Head of Hamas.

Jonassohn, K. (1991). Hunger as a Low Technology Weapon: Wth Special Reference to Genocide. Occasional Papers. Concordia University, Montreal, Montreal Institute for Genocide Studies.

(1992). The Tragic Circle of Famine, Genocide and Refugees. Occasional Papers. Concordia University, Montreal, Montreal Institute for Genocide and Human Rights Studies.

Jones, A. (2006). *Genocide, a Comprehensive Introduction,* 2nd edition. New York, Routledge.

Jones, B. (2007). *Hugo! The Hugo Chavez Story from Mud Hut to Perpetual Revolution.* Hanover, New Hampshire, Steerforth Press.

Kang, Chol-Hwan (2006). The Aquariums of Pyongyang. *From the Gulag to the Killing Fields: Personal Accounts of Political Violence and Repression in Communist States.* P. Hollander (ed.). Wilmington, DE, ISI Books: 683–97

Kang, G. M. (2006). "A Case for the Prosecution of Kim Jong Il for Crimes against Humanity, Genocide, and War Crimes." *Columbia Human Rights Law Review* 38: 50–113.

Karimakwenda, T. (2012, August 23). Zimbabwe: Land Reform Chaos Continues in Zimbabwe. SW Radio Africa.

(2012, October 4). Zimbabwe: Zanu-PF Forcing Resettled Farmers to Join Party Structures. SW Radio Africa.

Keith, L. C. (1999). "The United Nations International Covenant on Civil and Political Rights: Does It Make a Difference in Human Rights Behavior?" *Journal of Peace Research* 36(1): 95–118.

Kelly, J. (2012). *The Graves Are Walking: The Great Famine and the Saga of the Irish People.* New York, Henry Holt.

Kelly, J. and P. A. Palma (2004). The Syndrome of Economic Decline and the Quest for Change. *The Unraveling of Representative Democracy in Venezuela.* J. L. McCoy and D. J. Myers (eds.). Baltimore, MD, Johns Hopkins University Press: 202–30.

Kent, G. (2005a). *Freedom from Want: The Human Right to Adequate Food.* Washington, D.C., Georgetown University Press.

(2005b). The Human Rights Obligations of Intergovernmental Organizations. UN Chronicle, *online edition* (42, 3).

(2009). Right to Food and Adequate Standard of Living. *Encyclopedia of Human Rights*. D. P. Forsythe (ed.). New York, Oxford. 2: 225–36.

Kestler-D'Amours, J. (2013, February 28). Aid Hurting Palestinians. Inter Press Service.

Khan, I. (2009). *The Unheard Truth: Poverty and Human Rights*. New York, W.W.Norton.

Khen, H. M.-E. (2011). "Having It Both Ways: The Question of Legal Regimes in Gaza and the West Bank." *Israel Studies* 16(2): 55–80.

Khoury, J. (2015, March 4). Israel to Double Amount of Water Supplied to Gaza. Ha'aretz.

Kiernan, B. (1997). The Cambodian Genocide–1975–1979. *Century of Genocide: Eyewitness Accounts and Critical Views*. S. Totten, W. S. Parsons, and I. W. Charny (eds.). New York, Garland Publishing.

Kim, M. (2008). *Escaping North Korea: Defiance and Hope in the World's Most Repressive Country*. New York, Rowman and Littlefield.

Kim, Y. (2011). *North Korean Foreign Policy: Security Dilemma and Succession*. Lanham, MD, Lexington Books.

King-Irani, L. (2003). "Does International Justice have a Local Address? Lessons from the Belgian Experiment." *Middle East Report* 229: 20–25.

Kinley, D. (2009). *Civilising Globalisation: Human Rights and the Global Economy*. New York, Cambridge University Press.

Kinzer, S. (2008, June 12). "Life Under the Ortegas." *New York Review of Books* 55(10): 60–63.

Kornblith, M. (2006). Sowing Democracy in Venezuela: Advances and Challenges in a Time of Change. *State and Society in Conflict: Comparative Perspectives on Andean Crises*. P. W. Drake and E. Hershberg (eds.). Pittsburgh, University of Pittsburgh Press: 288–314.

(2013). "Chavismo after Chavez?" *Journal of Democracy* 24(3): 47–61.

Kretzmer, D. (2009). West Bank and Gaza. *Encyclopedia of Human Rights*. D. P. Forsythe (ed.). New York, Oxford. 5: 311–22.

Kriger, N. (2005). "ZANU (PF) Strategies in General Elections, 1980–2000: Discourse and Coercion." *African Affairs* 104(414): 1–34.

Kulchyski, P. (2013). *Aboriginal Rights Are Not Human Rights: In Defence of Indigenous Struggles*. Winnipeg, ARP Books.

Kuper, L. (1981). *Genocide: Its Political Use in the Twentieth Century*. New York, Penguin.

Kurmanaev, A. and A. Willis (2014, January 8). Hunt for Food Sends Venezuelans to Colombian Border Towns. Bloomberg News.

Kuwali, D. (2009, March). The African Union and the Challenges of Implementing the "Responsibility to Protect". *Policy Notes*, 2009/4. Uppsala, Sweden, Nordiska Afrikainstitutet.

Kwaak, J. S. (2013, April 22). North Korea Asks Mongolia for Food Aid. Wall Street Journal.

Laing, A. (2013, May 6). Mugabe's Party 'Using Food Aid to Buy Political Support'. The Independent.

Lamb, C. (2006). *House of Stone: The True Story of a Family Divided in War-Torn Zimbabwe*. London, Harper Press.

Landes, R. (2009a). Goldstone's Gaza Report: Part One: A Failure of Intelligence. Accessed at http://spme.org/spme-research/analysis/richard-landes-goldstones-gaza-report-part-one-a-failure-of-intelligence/7868/

(2009b). Goldstone's Gaza Report: Part Two: A Miscarriage of Human Rights. Accessed at http://rubincenter.org/2009/12/landes2-2009-12-02/

Landler, M. (2010, August 30). New U.S. Sanctions Aim at North Korean Elite. New York Times.

Landman, T. (2005). *Protecting Human Rights: A Comparative Study.* Washington, D.C., Georgetown University Press.

(2013). *Human Rights and Democracy: The Precarious Triumph of Ideals.* London, Bloomsbury.

Lankov, A. (2009). "Changing North Korea: An Information Campaign Can Beat the Regime." *Foreign Affairs* 88(6): 95–105.

(2013). *The Real North Korea: Life and Politics in the Failed Stalinist Utopia.* New York, Oxford University Press.

Lapper, R. (2006). Living with Hugo: U.S. Policy Toward Hugo Chavez's Venezuela. New York, Council on Foreign Relations.

Laurence, J. and J. Kim (2012, January 16). Transition of Power Going 'Relatively Smoothly' in North Korea: South Minister. National Post.

Lebovic, J. H. and E. Voeten (2006). "The Politics of Shame: The Condemnation of Country Human Rights Practices in the UNCHR." *International Studies Quarterly* 50: 861–88.

Lee, S. (2005). The DPRK Famine of 1994–2000: Existence and Impact. Seoul, Korea Institute for National Unification.

Leitenberg, M. (2012). "North Korean Genocide, Nuclear Weapons and Food Assistance." *The ISG [Institute for the Study of Genocide] Newsletter* 47: 1–2.

Lessing, D. (2003). "The Jewel of Africa." *New York Review of Books.* 50: 6–10.

Li, W. and D. T. Yang (2005). "The Great Leap Forward: Anatomy of a Central Planning Disaster." *Journal of Political Economy* 113(4): 840–77.

Liang-Fenton, D. (2007). "Failing to Protect: Food Shortages and Prison Camps in North Korea." *Asian Perspective* 31(2): 47–74.

Lim, B. K. (2012, May 17). Exclusive: China Pushes North Korea to Drop Nuclear Test Plan: Sources. Reuters.

Lindsay, J. G. (2012, Fall). "Reforming UNRWA." *Middle East Quarterly*: 85–91.

Lodish, E. (2011, June 24). Cannibalism in North Korea. Minnpost.com.

Loewenberg, P. (1971). "The Psychohistorical Origins of the Nazi Youth Cohort." *American Historical Review* 76(5): 1457–502.

(1996). Germany, the Home Front (I): The Physical and Psychological Consequences of Home Front Hardship. *Facing Armageddon: The First World War Experienced.* H. Cecil and P. Liddle (eds.). London, Leo Cooper: 554–62.

Lofaro, J. (2013, March 4). Health Minister Leona Aglukkaq Slams UN Right-to-food Report. Metro News.

Loucaides, L. G. (2004). "The Protection of the Right to Property in Occupied Territories." *International Comparative Law Quarterly* 53: 677–90.

Lourens, C. (2011, September 1). Impala Platinum in Talks with Zimbabwe as Deadline Expires. Bloomberg News.

Lupu, N. (2010). "Who Votes for Chavismo? Class Voting in Hugo Chavez's Venezuela." *Latin American Research Review* 45(1): 7–32.

Lustick, I. S. and A. M. Lesch (2005). The Failure of Oslo and the Abiding Question of the Refugees. *Exile and Return: Predicaments of Palestinians and Jews.* A. M. Lesch and I. S. Lustick (eds.). Philadelphia, University of Pennsylvania Press: 3–16.

Ma'an News Agency (2011, February 19). Demolitions, Drought and Displacement in the West Bank.

Mace, J. E. (1997). Soviet Man-Made Famine in Ukraine. *Century of Genocide: Eyewitness Accounts and Critical Views.* S. Totten, W. S. Parsons, and I. W. Charny (eds.). New York, Garland: 78–90.

Madongo, I. (2011, June 27). ZANU PF Youth Terrorise Harare Residents Meeting. swradioafrica.com.

Magliveras, K. D. and G. J. Naldi (2013). "The International Criminal Court's Involvement with Africa: Evaluation of a Fractious Relationship." *Nordic Journal of International Law* 82: 417–46.

Maguwu, F. (2008). "Land Reform, Famine and Environmental Degradation in Zimbabwe." *Journal of Human Security* 3(2): 32–46.

Mail and Guardian Online (2011, June 21). Zimbabwe Defiant over Right to Export Gems.

Majaji, T. (2014, September 11). Mugabe's Anti-white Ranting A Diversionary Tactic to Mask Failures. New Zimbabwe.

Makadho, J. (2006). Land Redistribution Experiences in Zimbabwe 1998–2004. *Zimbabwe's Agricultural Revolution Revisited.* M. Rukini, P. Tawonezvi, and C. Eicher (eds.). Harare, University of Zimbabwe Publications: 165–88.

Makasure, O. (2014, December 7). Comments on Draft Chapter 5. R. E. Howard-Hassmann. Brantford, Ontario.

Mangudhla, T. (2013, May 24). Zimbabwe: Zim Faces Food Crisis. Zimbabwe Independent.

Manna', A. (2013). "The Palestinian Nakba and its Continuous Repercussions." *Israel Studies* 18(2): 86–99.

Maodza, T. (2012, December 7). Zimbabwe: 210 White Farmers Refuse to Vacate Gazetted Land. The Herald.

Maphosa, F. (2007). "Remittances and Development: The Impact of Migration to South Africa on Rural Livelihoods in Southern Zimbabwe." *Development Southern Africa* 24(1): 123–35.

Marcano, C. and A. Barrera Tyszka (2006). *Hugo Chavez.* New York, Random House.

Marchak, P. (2008). *No Easy Fix: Global Responses to Internal Wars and Crimes against Humanity.* Montreal, McGill-Queen's University Press.

Marcus, D. (2003). "Famine Crimes in International Law." *American Journal of International Law* 97(2): 245–81.

Margolin, J.-L. (1999a). Cambodia: The Country of Disconcerting Crimes. *The Black Book of Communism: Crimes, Terror, Repression.* S. Courtois, N.

Werth, J.-L. Panne, et al. (eds.). Cambridge, MA, Harvard University Press: 577–635.

(1999b). China: A Long March into Night. *The Black Book of Communism: Crimes, Terror, Repression.* S. Courtois, N. Werth, J.-L. Panne, et al. (eds.). Cambridge, MA, Harvard University Press: 463–546.

Martel, F. (2015, April 13). Venezuela's President Maduro Reneges on Anti-Obama Petition Pledge. Breitbart News Network.

Martin, R. (2006). "The Rule of Law in Zimbabwe." *The Round Table* 95(384): 239–53.

Martin, S. (2015, April 24). Basic Food Items out of Reach for Four in Five Venezuelans. Panama Post.

Mashingaidze, T. M. (2011). What Blacks, Which Africans and in Whose Zimbabwe? Pan-Africanism, Race and the Politics of Belonging in Postcolonial Zimbabwe *Redemptive or Grotesque Nationalism? Rethinking Contemporary Politics in Zimbabwe.* S. J. Ndlovu-Gatsheni and J. Muzondidya (eds.). Oxford, Peter Lang: 261–88.

Mashiri, C. (2010, October 15). Zimbabwe–How Costly is Kleptocracy? The Zimbabwe Telegraph.

Massad, S. G., F. J. Nieto, et al. (2011). "Health-related Quality of Life of Palestinian Preschoolers in the Gaza Strip: A Cross-sectional Study." *BMC Public Health* 11 (253).

Masters, J. (2012, November 27). Hamas, Council on Foreign Relations.

Mathuthu, M. (2014, January 16). Zim Prisoners Facing Starvation. SW Radio Africa.

McDermott, J. (1986). "Total War and the Merchant State: Aspects of British Economic Warfare against Germany, 1914–16." *Canadian Journal of History* 21: 61–76.

McGirk, J. (2008). "Gaza's Humanitarian Crisis Deepens." *The Lancet* 371(9610): 373–74.

Mearsheimer, J. J. and S. M. Walt (2007). *The Israel Lobby and U.S. Foreign Policy.* New York, Farrar, Straus and Giroux.

MercoPress (2011, December 17). *Venezuelan Supreme Court Endorses Land Grabbing Alleging the Right to Food.*

Meredith, M. (2005). *The Fate of Africa: A History of Fifty Years of Independence.* New York, PublicAffairs.

(2007). *Mugabe: Power, Plunder, and the Struggle for Zimbabwe.* New York, PublicAffairs.

Mhofu, S. (2012, August 13). WFP Seeks to Avert Zimbabwe Hunger. VoANews.com.

Middle East Monitor (2011, February 24). The Economic Mirage in the West Bank-Ramallah.

(2014, September 15). Venezuela Sends More Aid Planes to Gaza.

Midlarsky, M. I. (2005). *The Killing Trap: Genocide in the Twentieth Century.* New York, Cambridge University Press.

Migdalovitz, C. (2010, June 23). Israel's Blockade of Gaza, the *Mavi Marmara* Incident, and Its Aftermath. Washington, DC, Congressional Research Service.

Milloy, J. S. (1999). *"A National Crime"*. *The Canadian Government and the Residential School System, 1879 to 1986*. Winnipeg, University of Manitoba Press.

Ministry of Defence (2008, January 27). Food Consumption in the Gaza Strip-Red Lines (unofficial trans. by Gisha), State of Israel.

Moon, K. H. S. (2008). "Beyond Demonization: A New Strategy for Human Rights in North Korea." *Current History* 107(710): 263–68.

Moon, S. (2015, January 14). North Korea Lightens Combat Kit for Soldiers Weakened by Hunger. Radio Free Asia.

Moon, W. J. (2009). "The Origins of the Great North Korean Famine: Its Dynamics and Normative Implications." *North Korean Review* 5(1): 105–22.

Moore, G. J. (2008). "How North Korea Threatens China's Interests: Understanding Chinese 'Duplicity' on the North Korean Nuclear Issue." *International Relations of the Asia-Pacific* 8(1): 1–29.

(2014). Introduction: The Problem with an Operationally Nuclear North Korea. *North Korean Nuclear Operationality: Regional Security and Non-Proliferation*. G. J. Moore (ed.). Baltimore, Johns Hopkins University Press.

Moreu, L. F. (2011). Food Aid: How It Should be Done. *Accounting for Hunger: The Right to Food in the Era of Globalisation*. O. DeSchutter and K. Y. Cordes (eds.). Oxford, Hart: 239–64.

Morgan, E. (2010). "The UN's Book of Judges." *Global Governance* 16(2): 160–72.

Morris, B. (2004). *The Birth of the Palestinian Problem Revisited*. New York, Cambridge University Press.

Morsink, J. (1999). *The Universal Declaration of Human Rights: Origins, Drafting and Intent*. Philadelphia, PA, University of Pennsylvania Press.

Mosby, I. (2013). "Administering Colonial Science: Nutrition Research and Human Biomedical Experimentation in Aboriginal Communities and Residential Schools, 1942–1952." *Histoire Sociale/Social History* 46(91): 145–72.

Mountain, R. (2011, September 22). Humanitarian Aid for Palestinians Shouldn't be Necessary. The Guardian.

Moyo, S. (2006). The Evolution of Zimbabwe's Land Acquisition. *Zimbabwe's Agricultural Revolution Revisited*. M. Rukini, P. Tawonezvi, and C. Eicher (eds.). Harare, University of Zimbabwe Publications.

Mtondoro, F. S., G. Chitereka, et al. (2013). Research Paper on the Power Dimension to Mineral-Related Corruption. Harare, Transparency International Zimbabwe.

Mugabe, R. G. (2009, November 17). Statement by His Excellency the President of the Republic of Zimbabwe, Comrade Robert Gabriel Mugabe, at the United Nations World Food Summit. Rome.

(2011, September 22). Full Text of Robert Mugabe Speech at UN Assembly. Nehanda Radio.

Mugabe, T. (2012, November 2). Zimbabwe: Govt Scoffs at White Former Farmers' Threats. The Herald.

Muico, N. K. (2005). An Absence of Choice: The Sexual Exploitation of North Korean Women in China. London, Anti-Slavery International.

Munoz, S. S. (2013, April 10). Key Issue in Venezuelan Vote: Food. WSJ.com.

Mutenga, T. (2012, August 10). Zimbabwe: Draft Constitution Displeases Displaced Farmers. Financial Gazette.

Myers, B. R. (2010). *The Cleanest Race: How North Koreans See Themselves – And Why It Matters*. Brooklyn, N.Y., Melville House.

Myers, D. J. (2008). Venezuela: Delegative Democracy or Electoral Autocracy? *Constructing Democratic Governance in Latin America*, 3rd edition. J. I. Dominguez and M. Shifter (eds.). Baltimore, MD, Johns Hopkins University Press: 285–320.

Myers, M. (2009). "Negative Impact of Policy on Humanitarian Assistance in Gaza." *Middle East Policy* 16(2): 116–21.

Nading, J. M. (2002). "Property under Siege: The Legality of Land Reform in Zimbabwe." *Emory International Law Review* 16: 737–800.

Naim, M. (2006). Introduction. *Hugo Chavez*. C. Marcano and A. Barrera Tyszka (eds.). New York, Random House.

(2013, January 3). An Economic Crisis of Historic Proportions. The New York Times.

Naimark, N. M. (2010). *Stalin's Genocides*. Princeton, Princeton University Press.

Nathan, L. (2013). "The Disbanding of the SADC Tribunal: A Cautionary Tale." *Human Rights Quarterly* 35(4): 870–92.

Natsios, A. S. (2001). *The Great North Korean Famine: Famine, Politics, and Foreign Policy*. Washington, D.C., United States Institute of Peace Press.

Naval Conference of London (1909). Declaration Concerning the Laws of Naval War C. T. S. 338. Minneapolis, University of Minnesota Human Rights Library.

Navoth, M. (2014, April 6). Israel's Relationship with the UN Human Rights Council; Is There Hope for Change?, Jerusalem Center for Public Affairs.

Newsday (2011, November 10). White Farmers under Siege.

NewsdzeZimbabwe (2012, June 11). Evicted White Farmers Supplying Bulk of Imported Maize.

Ngor, H. (1987). A Cambodian Odyssey. *From the Gulag to the Killing Fields*. P. Hollander (ed.). New York, Macmillan: 439–47.

Niada, L. (2006–2007). "Hunger and International Law: The Far-Reaching Scope of the Human Right to Food." *Connecticut Journal of International Law* 22: 131–201.

Nichols, J. E. (2012). "A Conflict of Diamonds: The Kimberley Process and Zimbabwe's Marange Diamond Fields." *Denver Journal of International Law and Policy* 40: 649–85.

Nkomo, N. (2011, September 15). Zimbabwe AG Tomana Steps Up Legal Challenges to Western Sanctions. Voice of America.

Noland, M. (2007). North Korea as a 'New' Famine. *The New Famines: Why Famines Persist in an Era of Globalization*. S. Devereux (ed.). New York, Routledge: 197–221.

Noland, M., S. Robinson, et al. (2001). "Famine in North Korea: Causes and Cures." *Economic Development and Cultural Change* 49(4): 741–67.

Nossek, H. and K. Rinnawi (2003). "Censorship and Freedom of the Press under Changing Political Regimes: Palestinian Media from Israeli Occupation to the Palestinian Authority." *Gazette* 65(2): 183–202.

Nowak, M. (2011). It's Time for a World Court of Human Rights. *New Challenges for the UN Human Rights Machinery: What Future for the UN Treaty Body System and the Human Rights Council Procedures?* C. Bassiouni and W. A. Schabas (eds.). Antwerp, Intersentia.

Nuclear Threat Institute (2012, August). North Korea: Chemical. Monterey, CA, James Martin Center for Nonproliferation Studies, Monterey Institute of International Studies.

Nyamurundira, R. (2011, December 22). Zimbabwe: US – The Desperate Act of Sanctioning Country's Diamond Companies. The Herald.

NZHerald (2005, July 2). Australia Joins NZ on Push over Zimbabwe.

Obama, B. (2015, March 9). Executive Order–Blocking Property and Suspending Entry of Certain Persons Contributing to the Situation in Venezuela. The White House, Office of the Press Secretary.

Oberleitner, G. (2005). "Human Security: A Challenge to International Law?" *Global Governance* 11(2): 185–203.

Oborne, P. (2003). A Moral Duty to Act There. London, Centre for Policy Studies.

(2012, July 18). We Must Have the Courage to Bring Zimbabwe in from the Cold. The Telegraph.

Offer, A. (1989). *The First World War: An Agrarian Interpretation.* Oxford, The Clarendon Press.

(2000). The Blockade of Germany and the Strategy of Starvation, 1914–1918: An Agency Perspective. *Great War, Total War: Combat and Mobilization on the Western Front, 1914–1918.* R. Chickering and S. Forster (eds.). Cambridge, Cambridge University Press: 169–87.

Office for the Coordination of Humanitarian Affairs (2009, July 15). Zimbabwe; Cholera Update.

(2014, September). Occupied Palestinian Territory. Gaza Crisis Appeal. East Jerusalem, United Nations.

Office of Foreign Assets Control (2013, December 18). Zimbabwe Sanctions Program. Washington, D.C., Department of the Treasury.

Ó Gráda, C. (2009). *Famine: A Short History.* Princeton, Princeton University Press.

O'Malley, P. (2005, March 30). South Africa's Failure in Zimbabwe. The Boston Globe.

Open Society Institute (2009, October 21). Lack of Citizenship Rights a Major Cause of Conflict in Africa.

Organization of African Unity (1969). Organization of African Unity Convention on the Specific Aspects of Refugee Problems in Africa. Addis Ababa.

Organization of American States (2002, April 13). Situation in Venezuela, Permanent Council of the OAS.

Painter, N. I. (2010). *The History of White People.* New York, W.W. Norton.

Palestinian Center for Human Rights (2011, December 27). 3 Years After Operation Cast Lead Justice Has Been Comprehensively Denied: PCHR Release 23 Narratives Documenting the Experiences of Victims. Gaza City.

(2015, March 4). Statistics: Victims of the Israeli Offensive on Gaza since 08 July 2014. Gaza City.

Palmer Report (2011, September). Report of the Secretary-General's Panel of Inquiry on the 31 May 2010 Flotilla Incident. New York, United Nations.

Pan-African Parliament (2008, June 27). Report of the Pan African Parliament Election Observer Mission: Presidential Run-Off Election and House of Assembly By-Elections, Republic of Zimbabwe.

Park, K.-A. (2010). "People's Exit in North Korea: New Threat to Regime Stability?" *Pacific Focus* 25(2): 257–75.

(2011). "Economic Crisis, Women's Changing Economic Roles, and Their Implications for Women's Status in North Korea." *The Pacific Review* 24(2): 159–77.

Park, R. (2011). "North Korea and the Genocide Movement." *ISG [Institute for the Study of Genocide] Newsletter* (46): 11–13.

Park, Young-ho, K. Su-am, et al. (2010). White Paper on Human Rights in North Korea. Seoul, Korea Institute for National Unification.

Patel, R. (2009). "Food Sovereignty." *Journal of Peasant Studies* 36(3): 663–706.

Patel, R. and P. McMichael (2009). "A Political Economy of the Food Riot." *Review, A Journal of the Fernand Braudel Center* 32(1): 9–35.

Paullier, J. (2012, January 2). Lo que se sabe de las expropiaciones de Chavez. *BBC Mundo.*

Pelham, N. (2012). "Gaza's Tunnel Phenomenon: The Unintended Dynamics of Israel's Siege." *Journal of Palestine Studies* 41(4): 6–31.

Penfold-Becerra, M. (2007). "Clientelism and Social Funds: Evidence from Chavez's Missions." *Latin American Politics and Society* 49(4): 63–84.

Petroleos de Venezuela S.A. (2012). Informe de gestion anual [Annual Business Report]. Caracas, Venezuela.

Phimister, I. and B. Raftopoulos (2004). "Mugabe, Mbeki and the Politics of Anti-Imperialism." *Review of African Political Economy* 31(101): 385–400.

Physicians for Human Rights (2009). Health in Ruins: A Man-Made Disaster in Zimbabwe. Cambridge, MA.

Physicians for Human Rights Denmark (2002, May 21). Zimbabwe: Post Presidential Election March to May 2002: "We'll Make Them Run".

(2002, November 20). Voting ZANU for Food: Rural District Council and Insiza Elections. Physicians for Human Rights.

Pillitu, P. A. (2003). "European 'Sanctions' against Zimbabwe's Head of State and Foreign Minister: A Blow to Personal Immunities of Senior State Officials?" *Journal of International Criminal Justice* 1: 453–61.

Pollis, A. and P. Schwab (1980). Human Rights: A Western Construct with Limited Applicability. *Human Rights: Cultural and Ideological Perspectives.* A. Pollis and P. Schwab (eds.). New York, Praeger: 1–18.

Polzer, T. (2008). "Responding to Zimbabwean Migration in South Africa: Evaluating Options." *South African Journal of International Affairs* 15(1): 1–28.

(2010). Silence and Fragmentation: South African Responses to Zimbabwean Migration. *Zimbabwe's Exodus: Crisis, Migration, Survival.* J. Crush and D. Tevera (eds.). Kingston and Cape Town, Southern African Migration Project and International Development Research Centre: 379–99.

Porter, R. (2011). *From Mao to Market: China Reconfigured.* New York, Columbia University Press.

Posner, E. (2014, December 4). The Case against Human Rights. The Guardian.

Potts, D. (2006). "'Restoring Order'? Operation Murambatsvina and the Urban Crisis in Zimbabwe." *Journal of Southern African Studies* 32(2): 273–91.

———. (2010). Internal Migration in Zimbabwe: The Impact of Livelihood Destruction in Rural and Urban Areas. *Zimbabwe's Exodus: Crisis, Migration, Survival.* J. Crush and D. Tevera (eds.). Kingston and Cape Town, Southern African Migration Programme and International Development Research Centre: 79–109.

Powell, K. and S. Baranyi (2005). Delivering on the Responsibility to Protect in Africa. Policy Brief. Ottawa, The North-South Institute.

Power, E. M. (2008). "Conceptualizing Food Security for Aboriginal People in Canada." *Canadian Journal of Public Health* 99(2): 95–97.

Power, S. (2003). "How to Kill a Country." *The Atlantic Monthly* 292(5).

President and Parliament of Zimbabwe (2005). Constitution of Zimbabwe Amendment (No. 17) Act 2005. Harare, Government of Zimbabwe.

PROVEA [National Program of Human Rights Education and Action] (2012). Informe Anual septiembre 2010-octubre 2011. Derecha a la tierra [Annual Report October 2010–September 2011: Right to land].

Pu Ning (2007). Red in Tooth and Claw: Twenty-Six Years in Communist Chinese Prisons. *From the Gulag to the Killing Fields: Personal Accounts of Political Violence and Repression in Communist States.* P. Hollander (ed.). Wilmington, DE, ISI Books: 364–81.

Qarmout, T. and D. Beland (2012). "The Politics of International Aid to the Gaza Strip." *Journal of Palestine Studies* 41(4): 32–47.

Qouta, S. and J. Odeh (2005). "The Impact of Conflict on Children: The Palestinian Experience." *Journal of Ambulatory Care Management* 28(1): 75–79.

Radi, S., T. A. Mourad, et al. (2009). "Nutritional Status of Palestinian Children Attending Primary Health Care Centers in Gaza." *Indian Journal of Pediatrics* 76: 163–66.

Radio VoP (2012, February 16). NGO Ban to Distribute Food to Hungry Villagers Dismissed.

Rangasami, A. (1985). "'Failure of Exchange Entitlements' Theory of Famine: A Response." *Economic and Political Weekly* 20(41, 42): 1747–52, 1797–1801.

Ravallion, M. (1997). "Famines and Economics." *Journal of Economic Literature* 35(3): 1205–42.

Refugee and Immigration Ministries (n.d.). Venezuelan and Colombian Refugees and Internally Displaced, Disciples Home Missions.

Reuters (2011, November 7). Chavez Says Foes Would Harm Slums, See Off Cubans.

Richardson, C. J. (2005). "The Loss of Property Rights and the Collapse of Zimbabwe." *Cato Journal* 25(3): 541–65.

Rigoulot, P. (1999). Crimes, Terror, and Secrecy in North Korea. *The Black Book of Communism: Crimes, Terror, Repression.* S. Courtois, N. Werth, J.-L. Panne, et al. Cambridge, MA, Harvard University Press: 547–64.

Risse, T. and K. Sikkink (1999). The Socialization of International Human Rights Norms into Domestic Practice: Introduction. *The Power of Human Rights: International Norms and Domestic Change.* T. Risse, S. C. Ropp, and K. Sikkink. New York, Cambridge: 1–38.

Riveiro, M. B., L. Rosende, et al. (2013). "Genocide on Trial: Case Note and Extracts of "Circuito Camps" Judgment." *Genocide Studies and Prevention* 8(1): 57–65.

Roberts, A. (1990). "Prolonged Military Occupation: The Israeli-Occupied Territories Since 1967." *American Journal of International Law* 84(1): 44–103.

Robertson, E. (2014, January 13). Venezuelan Government to Continue Pace of Land Expropriations for "Agrarian Socialism". venezuelanalysis.com.

Robertson, R. E. (1990). The Right to Food-Canada's Broken Covenant. *Canadian Human Rights Yearbook, 1989–90.* Ottawa, University of Ottawa, Human Rights Research and Education Centre.

Rodriguez, F. (2008). "An Empty Revolution: The Unfulfilled Promises of Hugo Chavez." *Foreign Affairs* 87(2): 49–62.

Rodriguez Pons, C. and D. Cancel (2011, February 21). Chavez's Currency Market Takeover Spurs Lines for Dollars. Bloomberg.

Rodriguez Rojas, J. E. (2009). "Evolucion de la dependencia externa proteinica y sus determinantes macroeconomicos en el periodo 1989–2006 [Evolution of Dependence on External Proteins and its Macroeconomic Determinants in the Period 1989–2006]." *Revista Venezolana de Economia y Ciencias Sociales [Journal of Venezuelan Economics and Social Sciences]* 15(3): 37–55.

Romero, Sean. (2007). "Mass Forced Evictions and the Human Right to Adequate Housing in Zimbabwe." *Northwestern Journal of International Human Rights* 5(2): 275–97.

Romero, Simon (2007, February 17). Chavez Threatens to Jail Price Control Violators. The New York Times.

Ron, J. (2003). *Frontiers and Ghettos: State Violence in Serbia and Israel.* Berkeley, University of California Press.

Roth, K. (2004). "Defending Economic, Social and Cultural Rights: Practical Issues Faced by an International Human Rights Organization." *Human Rights Quarterly* 26(1): 63–73.

Roy, S. (2012). "Reconceptualizing the Israeli-Palestinian Conflict: Key Paradigm Shifts." *Journal of Palestine Studies* 41(3): 71–91.

Rubin, O. (2011). *Democracy and Famine.* New York, Routledge.

Rueda, J. and F. Bajak (2013, June 4). Food Rationing to Begin in Big Venezuelan State. Associated Press.

Ruggie, J. (2011). Report of the Special Representative of the Secretary-General on the Issue of Human Rights and Transnational Corporations and other Business Enterprises, United Nations Human Rights Council.

Rukini, M. (2006). The Evolution of Agricultural Policy: 1890–1990. *Zimbabwe's Agricultural Revolution Revisited.* M. Rukini, P. Tawonezvi, and C. Eicher (eds.). Harare, University of Zimbabwe Publications: 29–61.

Sabel, R. (2011). "The Campaign to Delegitimize Israel with the False Charge of Apartheid." *Jewish Political Studies Review* 23(3/4): 18–31.

SADOCC (2011, May 27). AU Credibility Questioned as Zimbabwe Set to Chair Peace Organ. Southern Africa Documentation and Cooperation Centre.

Salmeron, V. (2014, September 11). Food Inflation Climbs 210% in 24 Months in Venezuela. El Universal.

Sanchez, F. (2010, May 7). Butchers Beware: Venezuela Cracks Down on Prices. Associated Press.

(2012, January 3). Chavez's Spending Could Boost Venezuelan Inflation. Associated Press.

(2012, July 26). Venezuela to Pull out of OAS Human Rights Bodies. Associated Press.

Sandbrook, R., M. Edelman, et al. (2007). *Social Democracy in the Global Periphery: Origins, Challenges, Prospects*, New York, Cambridge University Press.

Sasley, B. E. and M. Sucharov (2011). "Resettling the West Bank Settlers." *International Journal* 66(4): 999–1017.

Satzewich, V. and T. Wotherspoon (1993). *First Nations: Race, Class, and Gender Relations*. Scarborough, ON, Nelson Canada.

Sayigh, Y. (2010). Hamas Rule in Gaza: Three Years On. Crown Center for Middle East Studies, Brandeis University: 1–8.

Schabas, W. A. (1991). "The Omission of the Right to Property in the International Covenants." *Hague Yearbook of International Law* 4: 135–70.

(2006). "The 'Odious Scourge': Evolving Interpretations of the Crime of Genocide." *Genocide Studies and Prevention* 1(2): 93–106.

Schaber, P. (2011). "Property Rights and the Resource Curse." *Global Governance* 17(2): 185–96.

Scoones, I., N. Marongwe, et al. (2010). *Zimbabwe's Land Reform: Myths and Realities*. Woodbridge, Suffolk, James Currey.

Scott, J. C. (1998). *Seeing Like a State: How Certain Schemes to Improve the Human Condition Have Failed*. New Haven, CT, Yale University Press.

Sen, A. (1981). *Poverty and Famines: An Essay on Entitlement and Deprivation*. Oxford, Clarendon Press.

(1995). "Nobody Need Starve." *Granta* 52: 213–20.

(1999). *Development as Freedom*. New York, Alfred A. Knopf.

Sengupta, K. (2012, October 8). Group of White Farmers Who Had their Land Seized in Zimbabwe Plead with William Hague not to Lift Sanctions on Robert Mugabe. The Independent.

Shachar, A. (2009). *The Birthright Lottery: Citizenship and Global Inequality*. Cambridge, MA, Harvard University Press.

Share, F. (2012, November 6). Zimbabwe: Court Bars Governor from Evicting Villagers. The Herald.

Sharp, J. M. (2008). The Egypt-Gaza Border and its Effect on Israeli-Egyptian Relations. Washington, D.C., Congressional Research Service.

Shavit, A. (2013). *My Promised Land: The Triumph and Tragedy of Israel*. New York, Spiegel and Grau.

Shaw, A. (2010, July 2). Protests at Seizure of German-owned Zimbabwe Farm. Associated Press.

Shewell, H. (2004). *"Enough to Keep Them Alive": Indian Welfare in Canada, 1873–1965*. Toronto, University of Toronto Press.

Shifter, M. (2006). "In Search of Hugo Chavez." *Foreign Affairs* 85(3): 45–59.

Shlaim, A. (2009, January 7). How Israel Brought Gaza to the Brink of Humanitarian Catastrophe. The Guardian.

Shue, H. (1980). *Basic Rights: Subsistence, Affluence, and U.S. Foreign Policy.* Princeton, NJ, Princeton University Press.

Shulman, D. (2014, May 22). "Occupation: 'The Finest Israeli Documentary.'" *New York Review of Books* 61(9): 29–32.

Sibanda, T. (2010, August 26). Zimbabwe: Nation Ranked 10th for Food Insecurity Worldwide. allAfrica.com.

Simmons, B. A. (2009). *Mobilizing for Human Rights: International Law in Domestic Politics.* New York, Cambridge University Press.

Sithole, M. (2008). Zimbabwe: History and Politics. *New Encyclopedia of Africa.* J. Middleton and J. C. Miller (eds.). New York, Thomson Gale. 5: 336–39.

Smith, D. (2012, January 9). Zimbabwe Gold Deposits 'Claimed' by Robert Mugabe's Zanu-PF. The Guardian.

(2013, September 4). Zimbabwe Facing Food Crisis, UN Warns. Irish Times.

Snyder, T. (2010). *Bloodlands: Europe between Hitler and Stalin.* New York, Basic Books.

Sohlberg, P. (2006). "Amartya Sen's Entitlement Approach: Empirical Statement or Conceptual Framework?" *International Journal of Social Welfare* 15(4): 357–62.

Soko, M. and N. Balchin (2009). "South Africa's Policy towards Zimbabwe: A Nexus between Foreign Policy and Commercial Interests?" *South African Journal of International Affairs* 16(1): 33–48.

Solidarity Peace Trust (2011, November 2). Hard Times Matabeleland: Urban Deindustrialization and Rural Hunger. kubatana.net.

Song, J. (2010). "The Right to Survival in the Democratic People's Republic of Korea." *European Journal of East Asian Studies* 9(1): 87–117.

Southern African Development Community Tribunal (2008, November 28). Mike Campbell (Pvt) Ltd and Others v. Republic of Zimbabwe. *SADCT 2, 2007*, Southern African Development Community.

Southern Rhodesia Constitutional Conference (1979). Lancaster House Agreement. Lancaster House, London.

Southwick, K. G. (2005). "Srebrenica as Genocide? The Krstic Decision and the Language of the Unspeakable." *Yale Human Rights and Development Law Journal* 8: 188–90.

Stacy, H. M. (2009). *Human Rights for the 21st Century: Sovereignty, Civil Society, Culture.* Stanford, CA, Stanford University Press.

Stanton, G. and H. Fein (2008). Letter to the Editor, The New York Times, International Association of Genocide Scholars.

Starr, B. (2011, January 18). North Korea Willing to Resume U.S. Missions to Recover Remains of MIAs. CNN.com.

Statistics Canada (2013). Household Food Insecurity, 2011–2012. Ottawa, Government of Canada.

Staub, E. (1989). *The Roots of Evil: The Origins of Genocide and Other Group Violence.* New York, Cambridge University Press.

Stefanini, A. and H. Ziv (2004). "Occupied Palestinian Territory: Linking Health to Human Rights." *Health and Human Rights* 8(1): 160–76.

Steinberg, G. M. (2011). "The Politics of NGOs, Human Rights and the Arab-Israel Conflict." *Israel Studies* 16(2): 24–54.

Sullivan, T. (2012, September 12). Is North Korea Experimenting With Change? Associated Press.

Supreme Court of Appeal of South Africa (2012). National Commission of the South African Police Service and National Director of Public Prosecutions vs. South African Human Rights Litigation Centre and Zimbabwe Exiles Forum: Case No: 485/2014.

Tafadar, S. (2003). The Legal Case against Ariel Sharon. Wembley, UK, Islamic Human Rights Commission.

Taghdisi-Rad, S. (2011). *The Political Economy of Aid to Palestine: Relief from Conflict or Development Delayed?* New York, Routledge.

Tarasuk, V., A. Mitchell, et al. (2014). Household Food Insecurity in Canada 2012.

Tauger, M. B. (1991). "The 1932 Harvest and the Famine of 1933." *Slavic Review* 50(1): 70–89.

— (2006). "Arguing from Errors: On Certain Issues in Robert Davies' and Stephen Wheatcroft's Analysis of the 1932 Soviet Grain Harvest and the Great Soviet Famine of 1931–1933." *Europe-Asia Studies* 58(6): 973–84.

Taylor, I. (2008). "Sino-African Relations and the Problem of Human Rights." *African Affairs* 107(426): 63–87.

Taylor, I. and P. Williams (2002). "The Limits of Engagement: British Foreign Policy and the Crisis in Zimbabwe." *International Affairs* 78(3): 547–65.

Tendi, B.-M. (2010, September 1). After Robert Mugabe. The Guardian.

Terry, F. (2001). Feeding the Dictator: Food Aid to North Korea Only Props up Kim Jong-il's Grotesque Regime. It Should be Stopped. The Guardian.

Tevera, D., J. Crush, et al. (2010). Migrant Remittances and Household Survival in Zimbabwe. *Zimbabwe's Exodus: Crisis, Migration, Survival*. J. Crush and D. Tevera (eds.). Kingston and Cape Town, Southern African Migration Programme and International Development Research Centre: 307–21.

Thaxton, R. A., Jr. (2008). *Catastrophe and Contention in Rural China: Mao's Great Leap Forward Famine and the Origins of Righteous Resistance in Da Fo Village*. New York, Cambridge University Press.

The Elders (2008, November). The Elders' Zimbabwe Initiative: Report on the Visit to Southern Africa.

The Herald (2011, December 27). Zimbabwe: Cartoons Depict National Question.

— (2013, July 10). Zimbabwe: President Donates to Orphans, the Elderly.

The Small Business Newswire (2013, August 12). New Market Research Report: Venezuela Food and Drink Report Q3 2013.

Thein, B. (2004). "Is Israel's Security Barrier Unique?" *The Middle East Quarterly* 11(4) 25–32.

Torpey, J. (1997). "Revolutions and Freedom of Movement: An Analysis of Passport Controls in the French, Russian and Chinese Revolutions." *Theory and Society* 26(6): 837–68.

(2000). *The Invention of the Passport: Surveillance, Citizenship and the State.* New York, Cambridge.

Totten, S., W. S. Parsons, et al. (1997). *Century of Genocide: Eyewitness Accounts and Critical Views.* New York, Garland.

Transparency International (2014). Corruption Perception Index.

Trottier, J. (2007). "A Wall, Water and Power: The Israeli 'Separation Fence.'" *Review of International Studies* 33(1): 105–27.

Truth and Reconciliation Commission of Canada (2015). The Survivors Speak: A Report of the Truth and Reconciliation Commission of Canada. Ottawa, Library and Archives Canada.

Tungwarara, O. (undated). Sanctions: In Aid of Transition or an Obstacle to Democracy, Open Society Initiative for Southern Africa.

Turner, B. S. (1993). Contemporary Problems in the Theory of Citizenship. *Citizenship and Social Theory.* B. S. Turner (ed.). London, Sage: 1–18.

Turner, M. (2006). "Building Democracy in Palestine: Liberal Peace Theory and the Election of Hamas." *Democratization* 13(5): 739–55.

UN-Habitat (2005, July 27). UN Special Envoy on Zimbabwean Evictions Briefs Security Council.

UN Sub-Commission on the Promotion and Protection of Human Rights (2003). Norms on the Responsibilities of Transnational Corporations and other Business Enterprises with Regard to Human Rights. New York, United Nations.

UNAIDS (2008). Zimbabwe.

UNHCR (2014). 2014 UNHCR Regional Operations Profile–Latin America.

UNICEF (2008). UNICEF Humanitarian Action: Zimbabwe in 2008.

United Kingdom Parliament (2004, March 2). House of Commons Hansard Written Answers: "Zimbabwe."

United Nations (1951). Convention Relating to the Status of Refugees. Geneva (1960). Convention Relating to the Status of Stateless Persons.

(1977). Standard Minimum Rules for the Treatment of Prisoners, Economic and Social Council.

(1993). World Conference on Human Rights: Vienna Declaration and Program of Action.

United Nations Development Programme (1994). Human Development Report 1994. New York, Oxford University Press.

United Nations General Assembly (1948a). Convention on the Prevention and Punishment of the Crime of Genocide: Entry into force 12 January 1951.

(1948b). Universal Declaration on Human Rights.

(1973). International Convention on the Suppression and Punishment of the Crime of Apartheid: Entry into Force 18 July 1976.

(1981). Convention on the Elimination of All Forms of Discrimination against Women.

(1984). Convention against Torture and Other Cruel, Inhuman or Degrading Treatment or Punishment.

(1986). Declaration on the Right to Development.

(1990). Res. 45/98: Respect for the Right of Everyone to Own Property Alone as well as in Association with Others and its Contribution to the Economic and Social Development of Member States.

(2010, August 3). The Human Right to Water and Sanitation. Res. 64/292.

(2012, March 29). Resolution Adopted by the General Assembly, 66/174. Situation of Human Rights in the Democratic People's Republic of Korea.

(2012, December 4). Resolution Adopted by the General Assembly, 67/19. Status of Palestine in the United Nations.

(2013, February 7). Compilation Prepared by the Office of the High Commissioner for Human Rights in Accordance with Paragraph 5 of the Annex to Human Rights Council resolution 16/21: Canada. Geneva, Human Rights Council.

(2013, February 8). National Report Submitted in Accordance with Paragraph 5 of the Annex to Human Rights Council Resolution 16/21: Canada. Geneva, Working Group on the Universal Periodic Review, Human Rights Council.

(2014, December 18). Situation of Human Rights in the Democratic People's Republic of Korea.

United Nations High Commissioner for Human Rights (2011, September 13). How Can Israel's Blockade of Gaza be Legal?-UN Independent Experts on the "Palmer Report".

United Nations News Centre (2013, March 15). External Aid Essential for Subsistence of Millions in DPR Korea-UN Official.

United Nations Security Council (1980, June 5). Resolution 471. New York, United Nations.

(2006, April 28). Resolution 1674. New York, United Nations.

(2006, October 14). Resolution 1718. New York, United Nations.

(2008, June 23). Press Release: Security Council Condemns Violent Campaign against Political Opposition in Zimbabwe: Regrets Failure to Hold Free, Fair Election, in Presidential Statement. New York, United Nations.

(2008, July 11). Press Release: Security Council Fails to Adopt Sanctions against Zimbabwe Leadership as Two Permanent Members Cast Negative Votes. New York, United Nations.

(2009, June 12). Resolution 1874. New York, United Nations.

(2013, January 22). Resolution 2087. New York, United Nations.

(2013, March 7). Resolution 2094. New York, United Nations.

UNRWA (2013a). Gaza, United Nations Relief and Works Agency for Palestine Refugees in the Near East.

(2013b). West Bank, United Nations Relief and Works Agency for Palestine Refugees in the Near East.

USAID (2009, February 13). Zimbabwe-Complex Emergency. United States Agency for International Development.

(2012). Foreign Assistance Fast Facts: FY2012. United States Agency for International Development

Usher, G. (2001). "Gaza Agonistes." *Middle East Report* 218: 2–5.

Van der Kloot, W. (2003). "Ernest Starling's Analysis of the Energy Balance of the German People during the Blockade, 1914–1919." *Notes and Records of the Royal Society of London* 57(2): 185–93.

Vanderklippe, N. (2013, December 4). North Korea Finds Itself at Economic Crossroads. Globe and Mail., A17.

Verini, J. (2012). The Tunnels of Gaza. *National Geographic*.

Verma, S. (2008, July 1). Mugabe Gets Quiet Nod from African Leaders. Globe and Mail.

Vigil (2011, October 5). World Ignores Zimbabwe: Vigil. The Zimbabwean.

Vincent, C. P. (1985). *The Politics of Hunger: The Allied Blockade of Germany, 1915–1919*. Athens, Ohio, Ohio University Press.

Vivanco, J. M. and D. Wilkinson (2008, November 6). "Hugo Chavez Versus Human Rights." *New York Review of Books* 55(17): 68.

von Burgsdorff, D. (2012, April 11). Strangling the Lifeline: An Analysis of Remittance Flows from South Africa to Zimbabwe, PASSOP (People against Suffering Oppression and Poverty).

Vyas, K. (2015, April 8). Venezuela's Maduro Takes Petition Against U.S. Sanctions to Summit. Wall Street Journal.

Wallace, R. (2012, December 19). Footage shows North Korea Famine. The Australian.

Walton, D. (2007, July 31). Were Bison One of Globalization's First Victims? Globe and Mail.

Weisbrot, M. (2008). "Poverty Reduction in Venezuela: A Reality-Based View." *ReVista: Harvard Review of Latin America* 8(1): 1–8.

Weisbrot, M. and J. Johnston (2012). Venezuela's Economic Recovery: Is It Sustainable? Washington, D.C., Center for Economic and Policy Research.

Weisbrot, M. and L. Sandoval (2007). The Venezuelan Economy in the Chavez Years. Washington, D.C., Center for Economic and Policy Research.

Weissbrodt, D. (2015). Human Rights of Non-Citizens. *The Human Right to Citizenship: A Slippery Concept*. R. E. Howard-Hassmann and M. Walton-Roberts (eds.). Philadelphia, University of Pennsylvania Press: 21–30.

Weissbrodt, D. and C. de la Vega (2007). *International Human Rights Law: An Introduction*. Philadelphia, University of Pennsylvania Press.

Weitz, E. D. (2003). *A Century of Genocide: Utopias of Race and Nation*. Princeton, N.J., Princeton University Press.

Werth, N. (1999). A State against Its People: Violence, Repression, and Terror in the Soviet Union. *The Black Book of Communism: Crimes, Terror, Repression*. S. Courtois, N. Werth, J.-L. Panne, et al. (eds.). Cambridge, MA, Harvard University Press: 33–268.

Whande, T. J. (2010, July 8). Opinion. The Zimbabwe Mail.

Wheatcroft, S. G. (2004). "Toward Explaining Soviet Famine of 1931–33: Political and Natural Factors in Perspective." *Food and Foodways* 12: 107–36.

WikiLeaks Press (2011, December 1). Cablegate in Africa–First Part: Zimbabwe.

Wilkinson, R. and K. Pickett (2009). *The Spirit Level: Why More Equal Societies Almost Always Do Better*. London, Allen Lane.

Williams, P. D. (2007). "From Non-Intervention to Non-Indifference: The Origins and Development of the African Union's Security Culture." *African Affairs* 106(423): 253–79.

Williams, S. (2006). "Has International Law Hit the Wall-An Analysis of International Law in Relation to Israel's Separation Barrier." *Berkeley Journal of International Law* 24(1): 192–217.

Willows, N. D., P. Veugelers, et al. (2008). "Prevalence and Sociodemographic Risk Factors Related to Household Food Security in Aboriginal Peoples in Canada." *Public Health Nutrition* 12(8): 1150–56.

Wilpert, G. (2006). Land for People Not for Profit in Venezuela. *Promised Land: Competing Visions of Agrarian Reform.* P. Rosset, R. Patel, and M. Courville (eds.). Oakland, California, Food First Books: 249–64.

Wilson, R. A. (2005). "Judging History: The Historical Record of the International Criminal Tribunal for the Former Yugoslavia." *Human Rights Quarterly* 27(3): 908–42.

Windfuhr, M. (2010). The World Food Crisis and the Right to Adequate Food. *Universal Human Rights and Extraterritorial Obligations.* M. Gibney and S. Skogly (eds.). Philadelphia, University of Pennsylvania Press: 130–56.

World Bank. World Bank World Data Profile.

(2009). World Development Indicators Database. Washington, D.C.

(2013a). Statistical Database.

(2013b). World Development Indicators.

(2013, September 16). West Bank and Gaza: Strengthening Public Institutions for Service Delivery.

World Food Conference (1974, December 17). Universal Declaration on the Eradication of Hunger and Malnutrition. New York, United Nations General Assembly.

World Food Programme (2009, February 24). WFP in Zimbabwe–Facts and Figures.

(2010). Korea, Democratic People's Republic (DPRK).

(2013, June 21). UN Agency Heads Raise Alarm At Rising Levels of Food Insecurity in Palestine.

(2013, October). Special Focus: Zimbabwe. Rome.

World Food Programme, Food and Agriculture Organization, et al. (2011). WFP/FAO/UNICEF Rapid Food Security Assessment Mission to the Democratic People's Republic of Korea, World Food Programme.

World Health Organization (2013). Water Sanitation and Health: What Is the Minimum Quantity of Water Needed?

Worster, W. T. (2011). "The Exercise of Jurisdiction by the International Criminal Court over Palestine." *American University International Law Review* 26(5): 1–41.

Wright, N. G. (2008). Zimbabwe: Geography and Economy. *New Encyclopedia of Africa.* J. Middleton and J. C. Miller (eds.). New York, Thomson Gale: 5, 329–33.

Wyss, J. (2014, March 31). Fingerprints for Food: Venezuela Rolls out New Plan to Keep Shelves Stocked. Miami Herald.

Yaari, E. (2013). Hamas in Crisis: Isolation and Internal Strife. Washington, D.C., Washington Institute.

Yiftachel, O. (2009). "'Creeping Apartheid' in Israel-Palestine." *Middle East Report*(253): 7–15, 37.

YNet news.com (2014, August 8). Comptroller: Nearly 900,000 Israelis Facing Malnutrition.

Yoo, A. (2013, August 26). What do North Korean Rice Prices Say about the Supreme Leader's Power? South China Morning Post.

York, G. (1989). The Dispossessed: Life and Death in Native Canada. Toronto, Lester and Orpen Dennys.

(2006, March 4). China Keeps Bad Company. Globe and Mail.

Zartal, I. and A. Eldar (2007). *Lords of the Land: The War for Israel's Settlements in the Occupied Territories.* New York, Nation Books.

Zhai, K. and S. Kim (2015, January 13). North Koreans Walk Across Frozen Border River to Murder Chinese. Bloomberg News.

Zhakata, T. (2006, January 27). ICC Prosecution of Mugabe Urged. London, Institute for War and Peace Reporting.

Ziegler, J., C. Golay, et al. (2011). *The Fight for the Right to Food: Lessons Learned.* New York, Palgrave Macmillan.

Zimbabwe Independent (2009, August 20). Cash Crunch Hits Farmers As Planting Season Nears.

Zimbabwe Reserve Bank (accessed January 26, 2015). no title. Harare.

Zimmerer, J. (2009). "From the Editors: Genocide in Zimbabwe?" *Journal of Genocide Research* 11(1): 1–3.

Zuma, J. (2009). Opening Speech of the SADC Meeting. Southern Africa Development Community. Kinshasa, 29th Summit.

Index